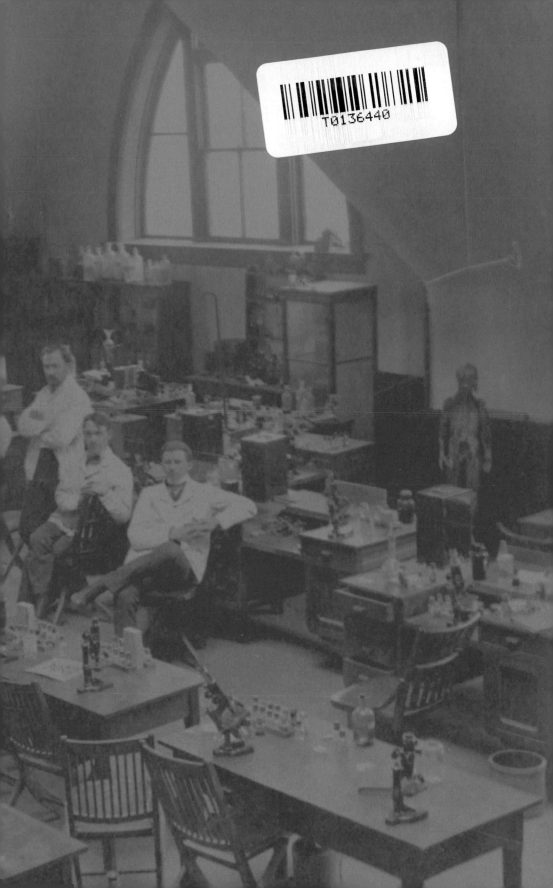

REFORMING MEDICAL EDUCATION

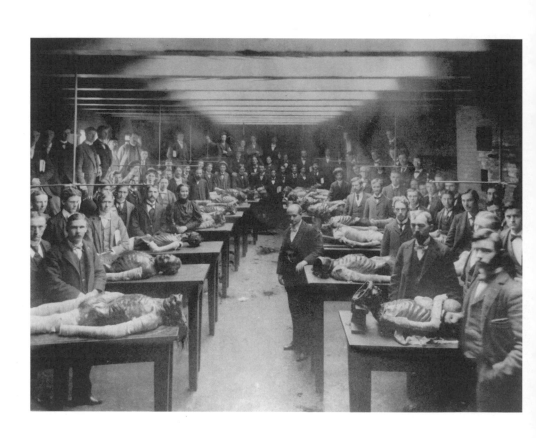

Reforming
Medical Education

The University of Illinois
College of Medicine
1880–1920

WINTON U. SOLBERG

UNIVERSITY OF ILLINOIS PRESS
URBANA AND CHICAGO

Endpapers photo: Physiology and Biophysics Laboratory, Urbana.
Courtesy of the University of Illinois at Urbana-Champaign Archives.

Frontispiece: William T. Eckley's dissecting class. Photo courtesy of
Special Collections and University Archives, the University Library,
University of Illinois at Chicago.

⊗ This book is printed on acid-free paper.

Library of Congress Cataloging-in-Publication Data

Solberg, Winton U., 1922–
Reforming medical education : the University of Illinois College of
Medicine, 1880–1920 / Winton U. Solberg.
p. cm.
Includes bibliographical references and index.
ISBN 978-0-252-03359-9 (cloth : alk. paper)
1. University of Illinois Chicago Professional Colleges. College of
Medicine—History. 2. Medical colleges—Illinois—Chicago—History.
3. Medical education—Illinois—Chicago—History.
I. Title.
[DNLM: 1. University of Illinois Chicago Professional Colleges.
College of Medicine. 2. College of Physicians and Surgeons of
Chicago. 3. Schools, Medical—history—Chicago. 4. Education,
Medical—history—Chicago. 5. History, 19th Century—Chicago.
6. History, 20th Century—Chicago. W 19 S6865r 2008]
R747.U683373S65   2008
610.71'177311—dc22   2008035617

To my grandchildren

Suzanne Beril Solberg

Alexander Tarkan Solberg

Giulia Costanza Nicita

Marta Cristina Nicita

John Winton Seyler

Matthew Kamuran Solberg

Stuart Andrew Seyler

Benjamin Tolgahan Solberg

CONTENTS

PREFACE

The history of medical education is primarily a matter of the history of education, not a matter of medicine, and I am a historian, not a medical doctor. I began work on this book intending it to be a chapter in a third volume on the history of the University of Illinois that I have under way. The topic proved far more challenging than anticipated. The present account draws heavily on primary sources in many archives. The materials in the University of Illinois Archives, Urbana-Champaign, are scattered and hard to locate and bring under control. I discovered most of the evidence that went into this book by diligent digging, but I also found important documents by serendipity. This book is laden with facts, and the citations are numerous. I have shaped the facts into an interpretive framework, and what was intended as a chapter has become a book.

This history of the University of Illinois College of Medicine is set within the context of the intellectual and scientific transformation that occurred in the Western world from 1880 to 1920. In 1880 Europe, and especially Germany, was the center of medical research and education, while the United States was regarded as a backwater in these areas. By 1920, however, America had emerged as the world center of medical research and education.

The Prologue states the theme of this book, and the first three chapters trace the historical and cultural background of the College of Physicians and Surgeons of Chicago, the forerunner of the University of Illinois College of Medicine. The chapters describe the training of doctors by the apprentice system and by proprietary medical colleges and also describe the varieties of sectarian medicine that competed for public attention. They demonstrate that Chicago, destined to become one of the great cities of the world, was home to medical colleges that taught sectarian medicine of one kind or another and turned out far more doctors than the nation needed. And they outline the history of Rush Medical College, which affiliated with the University of Chicago, and the Chicago Medical College, which became the Northwestern University Medical School. The history of the University of Illinois College of Medicine became closely intertwined with these institutions, and especially Rush.

Chapters 4–6 depict the history of the College of Physicians and Surgeons during its formative years. For a decade after the college's opening in 1882 troubles threatened its viability. However, in the early 1890s it gained stability, and in

1897 it affiliated with the University of Illinois and began anew. The discussion of the faculty, students, library, and related matters is primarily chronological but to some extent topical.

Chapters 7–9 discuss the College of Medicine from the arrival of Edmund J. James as president of the university in 1904 to 1912. James had been devoted to the reform of medical education since 1874. He believed that a medical school should be part of a university and that a medical school should be devoted to medical research as well as medical education. As president of the university he pursued two goals with respect to reforming medical education in Chicago. His main objective was to gain control of the College of Physicians and Surgeons, win a legislative appropriation for its support and maintenance, and raise academic standards in the college. He met organized opposition to his request for a legislative appropriation as well as obstacles that were inherent in the system of medical education at the time. During these years the Flexner Report depicted the city of Chicago in respect to medical education as the "plague spot" of the nation. James believed that the evaluation was not sufficiently critical. In 1912 the College of Physicians and Surgeons severed its affiliation with the university and reverted to proprietary status.

Chapters 10–12 describe events from 1913, when the University of Illinois opened its own College of Medicine, to 1920, when the University of Illinois Medical Center began to take shape on the West Side of Chicago. During these years James pursued the same twin goals as before. He finally obtained a legislative appropriation to support the college, whereupon he reorganized the institution and revitalized its academic offering. At the same time he sought to consolidate the leading university-related medical schools of Chicago in order to make Chicago a world center of medical research and education. His efforts along this line focused on a union of the University of Illinois College of Medicine with Rush Medical College. His prospects seemed favorable when they suddenly evaporated for reasons beyond his control.

James strove to strengthen the University of Illinois College of Medicine by erecting a clinical building and acquiring a hospital. He was able to realize these goals when the Illinois Department of Public Welfare and the University of Illinois agreed to cooperate in building and staffing the Illinois Educational and Research Hospitals on the West Side.

An Epilogue draws together the strands that constitute the story of reforming medical education and the University of Illinois College of Medicine from 1880 to 1920 and assesses the contribution made by Edmund J. James.

ACKNOWLEDGMENTS

Scholarship is truly a collective enterprise. In my research I have become newly convinced that if you seek the truth you must go to the archives, and I am pleased to thank the many archivists who have assisted me in working on this book.

I am heavily indebted to William J. Maher, Christopher J. Prom, and Linda Stahnke of the University of Illinois Archives, Urbana-Champaign; Ann C. Weller, Douglas Bicknese, Krystal M. Lewis, Susan R. Glover, and Kevin O'Brien at the Library of Health Sciences, University of Illinois at Chicago (Professor Weller deserves special thanks for identifying the church steeple in the illustration of the West Side Grounds in this book as that of St. Francis Assisi Church); Julia Gardner at the Special Collections Research Center of the University of Chicago; Kathleen A. Zar of the John Crerar Library of the University of Chicago; Heather J. Stecklein at the Rush University Medical Center Archives; Kevin B. Leonard of the Northwestern University Archives; Susan Rishworth of the American College of Surgeons; Kathy Young at Loyola University of Chicago; Debbie Vaughan of the Chicago History Museum (formerly the Chicago Historical Society); and members of the staff in the Manuscripts Library of the Library of Congress in Washington, D.C.

Among the librarians who helped me in various ways were Mary P. Stuart, History, Philosophy, and Newspaper Librarian, University of Illinois, Urbana-Champaign, and Victoria G. Pifalo and Mary Shultz of the Library of the Health Sciences-Urbana, University of Illinois at Chicago.

The Research Board of the University of Illinois, Urbana-Champaign, and Dean Joseph Flaherty of the University of Illinois College of Medicine offered financial assistance that enabled me to conduct research in Chicago, and Dean Flaherty provided a subvention to facilitate publication of this book. Arnim Dontes, assistant dean in the College of Medicine, cheerfully facilitated my work in countless ways.

I owe much to Dr. Willis G. Regier, director of the University of Illinois Press, for advice as to how to bring my manuscript to the highest state of readiness for publication. I appreciate the process by which Dr. Regier tries to assure the quality of the books published by the University of Illinois Press. The outside reviewers of my manuscript for the press have held me to an exacting standard. I have benefited greatly from their comments and suggestions.

I am pleased also to thank Jodi K. Kiesewetter, Jason Hamilton, Sharif Islam, and Kelvin Touchette of the Internet Technology Help Desk in the University of Illinois Library for their expertise in solving computer-related problems.

This book is based largely on primary sources, most of which are located in the University of Illinois Archives, Urbana-Champaign. Many additional primary sources relevant to this study are held in the city of Chicago. The most valuable of these are in the University Archives, University of Illinois at Chicago, and the Special Collections Research Center, University of Chicago Library. Other primary sources for this topic are found in the Rush University Medical Center Archives, the Northwestern University Archives, the Northwestern University Medical Center Archives, the American Society of Surgeons Archives, the Loyola University of Chicago Archives, and the Chicago History Museum. The Manuscript Library of the Library of Congress in Washington, D.C., holds the papers of Herman S. Pritchett and Abraham Flexner, which are vital in understanding the medical situation in Chicago in the early twentieth century.

To place the reform of American medical education in context, this study draws on a wide variety of secondary sources. The articles and books used for this purpose are cited in the notes. Since readers will easily be able to find references to points of interest in the notes, a conventional bibliography does not seem necessary.

The documentation is extensive because scholarly obligations require an author to show the source of the evidence for important facts and conclusions. The following abbreviations are keyed to published works and to frequently cited primary sources in archives.

Publications

Alumni Record	Carl Stephens, ed., *The Alumni Record of the University of Illinois: Chicago Departments. Colleges of Medicine and Dentistry. School of Pharmacy* ([Urbana]: University of Illinois, 1921).
Council	Council of the Chicago Medical Society, *History of Medicine and Surgery and Physicians and Surgeons of Chicago* (Chicago: Biographical Publishing Corp., 1922).
Cutler	H. G. Cutler, ed., *Medical and Dental Colleges of the West: Historical and Biographical: Chicago* (Chicago: Oxford Publishing, 1896).

ooth Report	University of Illinois, *ooth Report of the Board of Trustees of the University of Illinois.* Citations give the number of the report in Arabic numerals, the year of publication in parentheses, and page references: for example, *25th Report* (1911), 602.

RECORDS SERIES, UNIVERSITY OF ILLINOIS ARCHIVES, URBANA-CHAMPAIGN

The number and the name of a Record Series cited less than five times are given in the note. For Records Series cited more than five times, the number is in the note and the name is given here:

2/5/3	Edmund J. James General Correspondence
2/5/4	Edmund J. James General Letterbooks
2/5/5	Edmund J. James Subject Files
2/5/6	Edmund J. James Faculty Correspondence
2/5/7	Edmund J. James Diaries
2/5/10	Edmund J. James General Scrapbooks
2/5/11	Edmund J. James Subject Scrapbooks

RECORD GROUPS, UNIVERSITY OF ILLINOIS AT CHICAGO

027/01/01	F:1	Minutes of the College of Physicians and Surgeons of Chicago, 4 May 1881 to 20 October [1881]
027/01/01	F:2	Minutes of the Corporation of the College of Physicians and Surgeons of Chicago, 30 June 1881 to 11 July 1891
027/01/01	F:3	Minutes of the Corporation of the College of Physicians and Surgeons of Chicago, 11 August 1891 to 11 February 1915
027/01/05/01	F:1	Executive Faculty Minutes, 11 August 1899 to 14 February 1905
027/01/05/01	F:2	Executive Faculty Minutes, 11 April 1905 to 5 May 1911
027/01/05/02	F:1	Teaching Faculty Minutes, 8 June 1891 to 18 April 1902

REFORMING MEDICAL EDUCATION

Prologue

One of the momentous transformations of modern times occurred from 1880 to 1920, a period that witnessed the emergence of the United States as a world center of medical research and education. In 1880 Europe, and in particular Germany, was recognized throughout the world for its preeminence in medical research and education. The strength of the German system rested on the experimental method. German medical men relied on laboratory research as the way to the understanding of the human body and healing, and they viewed such fundamental medical sciences as anatomy, pathology, and physiology and those later known as bacteriology, biochemistry, and pharmacology as indispensable aids in understanding disease and therapeutics. In addition, the German people believed that the government had an obligation to promote public health as a means of advancing the general welfare.[1]

In the early part of this period the United States was a medical backwater. The nation harbored a multitude of medical colleges, most of which were frankly commercial enterprises dependent on tuition and fees to meet operating expenses and return a profit. Thus, entrance requirements were kept low and were often laxly enforced. Medical faculties, usually small, were made up of practitioners who were also teachers. Instruction was largely didactic and was conducted in large groups and often in an amphitheater. Students received little or no exposure to laboratories, clinics, or hospitals. The course of study, often brief and ungraded, consisted of two periods of four months each, repeating the work of the first year in the second year.

A medical career appealed to many upwardly bound people, however, and American medical colleges trained an oversupply of mediocre physicians. "The ignorance and general incompetency of the average graduate of American Medical Schools, at the time when he receives the degree which turns him loose upon the community, is something horrible to contemplate," Charles W. Eliot, president of Harvard, observed in 1871. "The mistakes of an ignorant or stupid young physician or surgeon mean poisoning, maiming, and killing, or at the best, they mean the failure to save life and health which might have been saved, and to prevent suffering which might have been prevented."[2]

In England, France, and Germany the law regulated the business of preparing men to practice medicine. General education preceded technical training; the technical training was graded, that is, the studies of each year built on the studies of the preceding year; the instruction was practical as well as theoretical; the course was four years long; and disinterested examiners judged the fitness of candidates. In the United States all but a few schools disregarded each of these principles. Medical schools proliferated easily, and a faculty position was coveted as a way of stimulating a private practice.[3]

The year 1885 may well serve as the dividing line between an older system of medical education and what followed. By 1885 Germany had established itself as the center of medical science, and many American medical graduates went there for postgraduate study. Most of them were attracted by Germany's strength in the new medical specialties that were proliferating at the time—dermatology, gynecology, laryngology, obstetrics, ophthalmology, physiology, and surgery—while some went to study the fundamental medical sciences. The Americans also witnessed an academic and professional structure that included full-time professorships, teaching departments, institutes, clinics, hospital beds, graduate education, and research. Thomas N. Bonner estimates that between 1870 and 1914 no less than fifteen thousand American medical students, young physicians, and older practitioners undertook serious study in a German university. At least a third and perhaps a half of the best-known men (and women) in American medicine in this period received part of their training in a German institution. Berlin was a great magnet, while the universities of Göttingen, Heidelberg, Strasbourg, Leipzig, Breslau, Munich, Würzburg, and Freiburg drew a few. Vienna was a prime attraction. Of the German-speaking Swiss universities, Zurich attracted the largest number from the United States. In these places Americans absorbed German attitudes toward medical knowledge and returned home with the conviction that the key to medical discovery lay in controlled experimentation. The impact of their German experience on American medical training was long and lasting. The reformation of American medical education and consequently of American medical practice was undertaken by Americans directly acquainted with the triumphs of European medical science.[4]

By 1885 many of the great scientific discoveries of the nineteenth century were becoming established in Europe and more slowly in the United States. The germ theory of disease and the emergence of the science of bacteriology were of fundamental importance. In its modern form the germ theory was advanced in the 1860s by Louis Pasteur (1822–95). Studying the relationship between microorganisms and their environment, he put an end to the age-old belief in spontaneous generation, showed that fermentation could be traced to living organisms, and demonstrated the benefit of a sterilizing procedure. Joseph Lister

(1827–1912) applied Pasteur's discovery to the healing art by introducing antiseptic methods in the treatment of surgical wounds. And in 1876 Robert Koch (1843–1910) demonstrated that anthrax, a disease of cattle, was caused by a specific bacteriological organism. Koch proved conclusively that a bacterium could be a specific infectious agent. Soon thereafter he devised a method by which single species of microorganisms could be isolated and identified, and within the next several years investigators proved that a host of infectious diseases were microbiological in origin. These discoveries helped make laboratory medicine an exact science. Initially, some of these notable achievements met resistance by medical men who ridiculed the idea that microbes caused disease and refused to believe that asepsis was essential in the operating room.[5]

In America the reform of medical education began in 1859 with the introduction of an optional five-month graded course of study occupying three winter sessions in the medical department of Lind University in Chicago (which later become the Northwestern University Medical School) as an alternative to the standard program of two four-month terms of lectures, with the second repeating the first. Lind's innovation may have inspired a few peripheral schools, but the reform gained momentum in 1871 when Charles W. Eliot, who had become president of Harvard two years earlier, initiated drastic changes in the medical school despite strong faculty resistance. Harvard announced for 1871–72 a three-year graded course of instruction with thirty-seven weeks in each term. The University of Pennsylvania Medical Department was slow in matching this reform, but in 1874 it opened a university hospital as a medical teaching facility, and in 1877 reforms similar to those at Harvard followed. In the Midwest, Victor C. Vaughan, with the aid of President James Angell, placed the University of Michigan in the vanguard of reform. Vaughan, who received a PhD (1876) and an MD (1878) from the University of Michigan, became a full professor in the medical school in 1883 and its dean in 1891. Meanwhile, in 1888 he went to Germany, where he spent a year in Koch's laboratory learning the new science of bacteriology and also visited Pasteur. Returning home, Vaughan introduced laboratory instruction in bacteriology and set out to shape the medical school into a center of research and teaching.[6]

Johns Hopkins University, which opened in 1876, was a pioneer in the history of American higher education because it emphasized research and the discovery of new truth, and the Johns Hopkins Medical School, which opened in 1893, represented a radical departure in American medical education. A new creation unhampered by traditions and commitments, it was the first medical school in America of genuine university type. It required a bachelor's degree for admission, its classes were small, it offered two years of instruction in the basic sciences, it made laboratory work mandatory, and it gave students experience at the hospital bedside. The school aimed at training investigators and teachers as well as practitioners. The Johns Hopkins Medical School boasted the finest faculty in the country, a new hospital and medical school buildings, and a huge endowment. It was an exemplary American medical school.[7]

In the medical colleges and universities where reform was at work, authorities brought the financing of medical education under the control of the central administration. In addition, they raised the requirements for admission; lengthened the curriculum to three (and later four) years of nine months each; introduced new courses in chemistry, physiology, microscopic anatomy, and pathology; and taught the courses in an ordered sequence. They also made laboratory instruction the primary vehicle of education.

The reform of medical education required an appropriate institutional structure, one in which scientific research was regarded as being as important as teaching. The transformation of American higher education met the need. The college had been the paradigmatic form of higher education in the United States from the founding of Harvard College in 1636 to the eve of World War I. Typically, the college was small, church-related, and devoted to the liberal arts. It existed to transmit the wisdom of the past, train the mind, heighten aesthetic sensitivity, and confirm students in the Christian faith. Research in the pursuit of new knowledge was not part of its agenda. Gradually, Americans became increasingly aware that the collegiate system was little related to the democratic and practical character of the nation. Thus, a demand to transform higher education began in the 1820s, gathered momentum in the 1840s, and culminated in the Morrill Act of 1862. The act gave rise to the land-grant universities, state schools that emphasized practical studies and welcomed women and men of all races.

By the late nineteenth century the frontier, which had long been instrumental in shaping the character of American culture, had closed, and the population was increasingly concentrated in urban areas. Metropolitan centers posed pressing public health problems, and the major cities of the United States were destined to become the home of the leading medical colleges and teaching hospitals. The industrial revolution had decreed the dominance of industry, industrial growth had created huge fortunes, and wealthy individuals were able to give generously to reconstruct higher education. Donors made it possible to transform existing colleges into universities, as at Harvard, Yale, and Princeton, and to establish new universities, as at Johns Hopkins, Clark, Chicago, and Stanford. The graduate college, which emphasized research as a means of discovering new truth, was a distinguishing feature of the new universities. In 1900 a few of the leading universities cooperated to establish the Association of American Universities, an act that was in effect a declaration of American educational independence. The best of the new American universities were able to offer students advanced studies of high quality. By about 1910 the university had replaced the college as the model for American higher education.[8]

At the time, the belief that science was the key to advancing human welfare was widespread. The United States had few central scientific agencies, and industry conducted little fundamental research. Thus, the universities became the institutional home of basic research. Progress in healing depended on medical research, and a medical school came to be regarded as an integral part of a university. Almost every major university acquired a medical school by affiliation or union with an older one or created one de novo.[9]

The rise of the university accelerated the demise of proprietary medical colleges because scientific medicine and research were costly, and proprietary schools could not provide adequate facilities and equipment on the proceeds from tuition income. But the doctors who owned the schools and taught in them as a sideline to medical practice did not surrender without a struggle. Moreover, with the steady advance of scientific medicine in university medical schools and the adaptation of German medical education to American conditions, American doctors no longer needed to go to Europe for postgraduate study.[10]

This book examines the role of the University of Illinois College of Medicine in the transformation that marked the emergence of the United States as a world center of medical research and education. The story begins in 1881 with the formation of the College of Physicians and Surgeons in Chicago (widely known as P&S). The college opened in 1882, and in 1897 it became affiliated with the University of Illinois. For several years thereafter the college and the university made the best they could of an often difficult relationship. Assuming office in 1904, President Edmund J. James devoted himself to bringing the College of Medicine under the control of the university and invigorating it. James was one of several university presidents who brought medical education into the orbit of the university in the early twentieth century. He was committed to the reform of medical education long before 1910, when Abraham Flexner brought the matter to public attention. In 1912 the affiliation of P&S with the university ended, and in 1913 the university reopened its College of Medicine. President James then labored to make the college and the city of Chicago a world center of medical research and education. In large measure he succeeded. The history of the University of Illinois College of Medicine up to 1920 is best understood as part of the transformation of medical research and education that occurred in the United States during these years.

CHAPTER 1

The Medical Scene at the Turn of the Century

The College of Physicians and Surgeons of Chicago (P&S) arose out of a perceived need for another center devoted to training regular physicians in the growing metropolis. Its formation stimulated the establishment of additional medical colleges, some of which taught alternative systems of medicine. By the turn of the century P&S was but one of many medical colleges in the city of Chicago, which was "the great factory for medical degrees."[1] We can fully appreciate the origins and development of P&S by viewing the college in historical context.[2]

Medical Education in America

At the turn of the twentieth century, medical education in America was badly in need of reform. During the eighteenth century and the first half of the nineteenth century the apprentice system was the prevailing way of training doctors. Most medical students apprenticed themselves to a physician (called a preceptor) for a period of time. A number of rules governed the relationship between apprentice and preceptor. The standard program was three years at a fee to the preceptor of one hundred dollars per year, modified according to the preceptor's reputation. In the first part of the course, the apprentice read basic medical texts and assisted with menial chores, gradually learning to help with office calls, apply plasters, dress wounds, and prepare medications. In the second or clinical part of the course, the apprentice accompanied the doctor on house calls and occasionally assisted in surgeries. At the end of the term of instruction the preceptor provided the apprentice with a certificate.

The quality of apprenticeship training varied. Many preceptors were themselves poorly prepared and often used their apprentices as cheap labor. Apprentices were wont to shirk their duties. The certificate of completion meant little to anyone who did not know the preceptor. Standards were nominally maintained by medical licensing laws, which were often ineffective or lacking. And as the body of medical knowledge grew, even the best preceptors were incapable of providing quality medical education. The apprentice system survived, nevertheless, because it was popular with physicians and acceptable to students, who could find a preceptor close to home and pay relatively little for medical training.[3]

Medical schools were a more efficient and economical way of educating a growing number of medical students than the apprentice system. Their number grew rapidly during the first half of the century. In 1800 the new nation had four medical schools, all located in the Northeast (New England, New York state, and Philadelphia), and by 1850 there were forty-two. Seventeen of these were in the Northeast, with others in the South and West.[4]

A few medical schools were connected with educational institutions, as at Harvard, Yale, Columbia, and the University of Pennsylvania. In some cases a medical school was added to a liberal arts college, which enabled the medical school to use the college charter to grant degrees to their graduates. But the vast majority of the new medical schools were proprietary enterprises.

Proprietary medical colleges sprang up and flourished for many reasons. Physicians and surgeons established them to make a profit and enhance their prestige. To be known as a professor in a medical college stimulated a private practice. Proprietary medical colleges were inexpensive to operate. They needed only a small faculty, a classroom and a backroom, a few teaching aids, and a charter that conferred authority to grant degrees. The operating costs were independent of the number of students, so the more students, the more profitable the enterprise. Proprietary medical colleges offered students better medical training than the apprentice system, and their founders anticipated that the income from tuition and fees would cover expenses and leave a surplus.

While these institutions lacked uniformity, they were remarkably similar in length of training and curricula. Most proprietary colleges offered two terms of four months each. The course of study was not graded, that is, the subjects did not proceed from simple to complex. The faculty taught the basic medical sciences: chemistry, anatomy, physiology, pathology, and the diagnosis and treatment of disease, including materia medica, surgery, midwifery, and medical jurisprudence. Teaching was didactic and by the lecture method except in anatomy. Because the instruction was based on the existing state of medical knowledge, it was deficient. A preceptor taught the clinical subjects.[5]

Proprietary medical colleges became a powerful part of the medical scene in the late nineteenth century. Many licensing laws made a medical college diploma equivalent to a license to practice medicine. Thus, the number of medical schools and medical graduates greatly increased. The number of graduates of medical schools in the United States rose from 343 in the decade 1800–1809 to 17,213 in the decade 1850–59.[6]

Between 1880 and 1903 the number of medical colleges in the United States increased by 71 percent. In 1880 there were 90 medical colleges, 11,826 students, and 3,214 graduates. In 1903 the nation had 154 medical colleges, 27,615 students, and 5,698 graduates. Medical colleges were turning out twice as many graduates as were required to meet the people's needs. In proportion to population, the United States had twice as many physicians as England, four times as many as France, five times as many as Germany, and six times as many as Italy.[7]

Proprietary medical colleges were often riven by internal tensions and by rivalry with each other over how to attract students. Faculties were reluctant to raise or enforce the minimum requirement for matriculation, a high school degree or its equivalent, for fear of losing students. The resulting low standard of medical education in the United States, as compared with that of other countries, caused serious concern. In 1904, the high-water mark year in the matter, the United States had 166 medical schools, 28,142 medical students, and 5,742 graduates. The nation had too many medical schools, too many physicians, and a great oversupply of poor or mediocre practitioners.[8]

The Medical Practice of Physicians

In the nineteenth century, before scientific medicine made substantial inroads on medical practice, physicians treated the symptoms of disease rather than disease itself. They drew on a bag of familiar therapies—purgatives, emetics, bloodletting, and blistering—with such vigor that their practice became known as heroic medicine.

Bloodletting was based on the symptomatic treatment of the period. If a patient had fever, for example, the physician sought to reduce it by bleeding the patient. The opening of a vein or the application of leeches often seemed effective, but any improvement was merely symptomatic, not evidence of betterment in the patient's condition. Bleeding became a panacea. Administered to excess and over a long period of time, bleeding could be and often was fatal.

The use of purgatives and emetics to cleanse the bowels and the stomach also treated symptoms. Calomel, a chloride of mercury, was the most popular purgative. Although therapeutically useless, it did purge the system and, like bloodletting, became a panacea for all ills. Most physicians recognized that calomel's side effects damaged health, but they continued to administer it in large doses. Other popular purgatives were the minerals nitre (salt-peter), a lethal poison, and jalap. Because the action of jalap was so harsh, it was often mixed with calomel to make it more palatable. One of the most popular emetics was tartrate of antimony. In small doses it produced vomiting; in large doses it reduced the force and frequency of the heartbeat and lowered the body temperature. It too was a lethal poison. After administering heroic doses to cleanse the system, practitioners prescribed tonics to build up the system. One of the most popular was arsenic, a deadly poison, in solution. Excessive use produced toxic side effects.

Blistering was also part of the doctor's stock-in-trade. A physician raised a blister on the affected part of a patient's body with a plaster that irritated the skin. The discharge that flowed from the skin when the blister broke was viewed as "laudable pus," a desirable emission of harmful matter.[9]

Regular physicians who administered the remedies described acted in good faith. They drew on the medical knowledge that prevailed before the advent of scientific medicine, but they violated the Hippocratic precept: Do no harm.

The Rebellion against Heroic Therapy

As people lost confidence in heroic therapies and regular physicians, they turned to lay healers and alternative forms of medicine. Two main challenges arose to confront orthodox practitioners. One was botanical medicine and its progeny, physio-medicine and eclectic medicine. Another was homeopathic medicine. Of the many other kinds of alternative medicine, only osteopathy became noticeable during the period covered by this book.[10] Alternative forms of medicine had largely spent their force by the time Edmund J. James became a reformer of American medical education, but they left a legacy with which he had to contend.

Botanical Medicine, Physio-Medicine, and Eclectic Medicine

Botanical medicine has an honorable lineage. People have used leaves, roots, herbs, plants, and bark for medicinal purposes since antiquity. The botanicals were usually either dried and stored in leaf form, ground into a powder, brewed into a tea, or liquified and bottled for use as needed. In the United States people turned to these natural drugs in opposition to the mineral drugs associated with heroic medicine. In the 1820s botanical medicine became a social movement of broad public appeal during a time of Jacksonian democracy and westward expansion.

Samuel Thomson (1769–1843) was the father of the movement. Born in backwoods New Hampshire, at an early age he manifested an interest in plants and their physical effects. Learning about botanical remedies, he became skeptical about the therapeutic skills of regular doctors. In the early 1790s he discovered that lobelia, an old Indian remedy, was a potent therapeutic. Its pods usually produced vomiting. Thomson promptly designated lobelia, the "Emetic Herb," Old Number One in his system of practice.

Around 1805 Thomson became an itinerant botanical doctor. He taught a system of medicine based on a course of six numbered remedies to be given in sequence. First was a botanical emetic, lobelia, to cleanse the stomach and induce perspiration. Second was cayenne pepper in sweetened hot water to warm the patient and restore lost internal heat. Third and fourth were teas and tonics made from roots, barks, and so forth to improve digestion. Fifth and sixth were brandy or wine mixed with botanicals to strengthen the body. Thomson offered little that was new. His endeavor to clean out and then strengthen the system resembled that of orthodox physicians except for the use of botanical rather than mineral drugs.

Thomson's major innovation was his marketing system. In 1811 he established his first Friendly Society, a group of families pledged to use his remedies and to help each other. A year later he wrote a pamphlet describing his system that eventually grew into a book, *New Guide to Health: Or, Botanic Family Physician Containing a Complete System of Practice* (1822). Then Thomson sold rights, which consisted of a copy of his book and the privilege of belonging to a local Friendly Society.

Thomson's book had two parts. The first part contained recipes for drugs and gave medical advice on a wide variety of topics in language that people could understand. The autobiographical part, the prototype of the Horatio Alger story, described the successful career of a farm boy and attacked regular physicians who tried to suppress his system. The *New Guide to Health* struck a responsive chord among many Americans. Thomsonism became popular, especially on the southern and western frontiers among the poor and uneducated. Thomsonian healers, many of whom used a botanical version of heroic medicine, often became important practitioners. Thomsonism gradually changed from a social movement of laymen to a movement dominated by professional healers. The professionals who assumed leadership of the societies and botanical national conventions disagreed among themselves, and in the late 1830s Thomsonism split into factions led by Thomson's agents.[11]

Alva Curtis (1797–1881), a professional botanical practitioner, headed one faction. In 1836, wanting more structure to the Thomsonian system and more educated healers, he began instructing students in his home. In 1839 he broke with Thomson and obtained a charter for the Literary and Botanico-Medical Institute of Ohio. Its medical department opened in Columbus as the College of Physicians and Surgeons. In 1841 Curtis moved his school to Cincinnati, where it became known as the American Medical Institute. Ten years later the institute divided into the Scientific and Literary Institute and the Physiopathic College of Ohio. In 1859 the college became the Physio-Medical Institute, the name it kept until closing in 1880. Thus, the Curtis faction of the botanical movement gave rise to the physio-medical sect.[12]

Wooster Beech (1794–1868), a botanical practitioner, condemned Thomson's puke and steam methods but recognized Thomson as an intellectual anteced-ent. Beech allegedly graduated from the medical department of the University of the City of New York (New York University) and received a license from a county medical society. He and others founded a Reformed Medical College in New York City (1829–30), the first sectarian medical college in the United States. Seeking a more favorable environment, they relocated to Worthington, Ohio. There in 1830 they opened the Reformed Medical College of Ohio as part of Worthington (later Kenyon) College. Beech believed that there must be first principles in medicine, and in 1833 he published *The American Practice of Medicine*, the earliest textbook of so-called reformed medical practice. Worthington

Medical College distinguished itself from both the Thomsonian system and the botanico-medical or physio-medical school of Curtis. The college declared itself in favor of an improved botanical system of practice, but because it had no specific therapeutic philosophy it used the term "eclectic" to describe its approach to medication. By 1839 Worthington Medical College had awarded more than ninety degrees, but in that year an antidissection riot ruined its prospects, and in 1840 the state revoked the school's charter.[13]

Thomas V. Morrow, who had been educated at Transylvania University and had graduated from a regular medical college in New York City, was the second president of the Worthington Medical College. After it closed he moved to Cincinnati, where he organized a faculty and announced a course of lectures for 1842–43. In 1845 Morrow and others obtained a charter for the Eclectic Medical Institute of Cincinnati, usually called the E.M. Institute. The appointment of Wooster Beech to the faculty demonstrated continuity with the Reformed Medical College of New York City. By the mid-1840s the term "eclectic" described those persons who drew from any and every source all medicines and modes of treating disease they found to be of value. Eclecticism offered itself to the American people as the common man's access to medical education.[14]

In 1862 John M. Scudder (1829–94) took control of the Eclectic Medical Institute. An 1856 graduate of the institute who had established a successful medical practice in Cincinnati, Scudder restored harmony to a divided faculty and financial stability to the college. He was also a prolific author. By 1888 he and his colleagues had written eighteen eclectic medical textbooks. These works heightened the respectability of eclectics and the reputation of the institute. Under Scudder's leadership the institute was the largest medical school in Cincinnati for some years and by far the most influential eclectic college in the nation. Its success inspired the establishment of a number of eclectic medical colleges around the country.[15]

Eclectic materia medica was a distinguishing feature of this branch of sectarian medicine. Eclectics introduced the medium system as an alternative to the allopathic and homeopathic systems of the day. Most eclectic physicians dispensed their own medicines as tinctures made into powders or lozenges, drawing on the milder plants, the weaker vegetable acids, and mild chemical preparations. John King (1813–93), a professor at the Eclectic Medical Institute, stimulated the growth of eclectic medicine by a therapeutic discovery: the concentration of the resin of plants, especially podophyllum. Concentrated medicines, marketed from 1847, were more palatable and more transportable than other botanicals. Their extraordinary success distinguished eclectics from other practitioners. In the mid-1850s, however, people discovered that most concentrated medicines had no therapeutic value, and King himself denounced them as a "stupendous fraud."[16]

Eclectic adepts replaced their fleeting commitment to concentrated medicines with a new materia medica, specific medicines. They prescribed a specific medicine for a specific disease, making each specific medicine from a certain part of a plant. By 1930 nearly two hundred specific medicines were used in eclectic practice. Over time eclecticism formulated a set of principles that represented the reform practice of medicine. According to historian John Haller, these principles included opposing all forms of heroic therapy, using vegetable medicines, a belief in sustaining the vital forces, advocating single remedies and wherever possible using simple combinations, a predilection for kindly treatment, and a preference for dispensing their own medicines.[17]

In 1873 the United States had a total of 50,000 physicians, 2,857 (5.7 percent) of whom were eclectics. In 1902 there were ten eclectic medical colleges in the country, and eclectic practitioners constituted perhaps less than 4 percent of the total number of physicians.[18]

Homeopathic Medicine

Homeopathy appeared in the United States when the public was eager for alternatives to heroic medicine. The largest unorthodox medical sect during the nineteenth century, homeopathy posed both a meaningful alternative and a serious threat to orthodox medicine.

Homeopathy developed out of the experimental pharmacology of a German practitioner, Samuel Hahnemann (1755–1843). Disillusioned by his inability to cure his patients by traditional means, Hahnemann abandoned medical practice. In translating classical texts he became aware of medical ideas found in ancient works and began to wonder about the effects of various drugs. In experimenting with cinchona, or Jesuits' bark, that was used for fever, he developed the homeopathic law of similars (*similia similibus curantur*): disease could be cured by drugs that produced, in a healthy person, the symptoms found in a sick person.

Using himself for test purposes, Hahnemann then investigated the effects of various pharmaceuticals of the day. In extensive drug provings he employed pure and simple medications so that he could determine the exact symptoms produced. This research led him to the law of infinitesimals: the smaller the dose, the stronger the effect in stimulating the body's vital force. Diluting and diluting, Hahnemann carried this idea to an extreme. Dilutions as small as one millionth of a grain (.0648 grams), he believed, could be effective. He called these dilutions high potencies. According to Hahnemann, it took more than a simple dilution to effect the cure. The medication could not aid the vital spirit unless the vial containing the drug was succussed or struck against a leather pad several times after each dilution. Succussion, said Hahnemann, excited the medicinal properties of drugs and enabled them to act spiritually (dynamically) upon the vital forces.

Homeopathy spread to the United States by the conversion of physicians and by German-speaking immigrants. Hans B. Gram (1787–1840), who was born in Boston and received his medical training in Europe, became convinced that homeopathy was superior to orthodox medicine. In 1825 he settled in New York City. His successful practice attracted other physicians to homeopathy, and he trained apprentices in the new system. In the 1820s Henry Detweiler, a Swiss physician who had arrived in the United States in 1817, became aware of Hahnemann's ideas, and by the end of the decade Detweiler practiced homeopathic medicine. In 1833 Detweiler and Constantine Hering (1800–1880) founded a medical college in Allentown, Pennsylvania. It had little national impact and closed in 1841. In 1848, however, Hering received a charter for the Homeopathic Medical College of Pennsylvania, which opened in Philadelphia and became the center of homeopathic education in the United States.[19]

The disciples of Gram carried homeopathy northeast, while the disciples of Hering carried it south and west. In 1844 homeopaths around the country established the nation's first medical society, the American Institute of Homeopathy. By 1860 out of a total of 2,399 homeopaths in the country, New York had 699, Pennsylvania had 325, Massachusetts had 207, Ohio had 188, and Illinois had 158. In 1873 the nation had 50,000 medical practitioners, 2,955 of which (5.9 percent) were homeopathic.[20]

For various reasons, homeopathy was a greater threat to orthodox or regular medicine (which Hahnemann named allopathy) than was botanical medicine. Most homeopathic physicians had been orthodox practitioners, unlike the poorly educated and often rural healers who were attracted to botanical treatment. Homeopathy was based on a scientific approach to medicine and did not use strong mineral drugs. Moreover, homeopathic practitioners and pharmacists prepared domestic kits with remedies that gave people the opportunity to heal themselves.

Orthodox physicians initially regarded homeopathy as a valuable new approach to medical practice but soon recognized the major ideological and financial threat posed by its growth. Oliver Wendell Holmes (1809–94), poet, physician, and Harvard professor of medicine, published a classic attack, *Homeopathy and Its Kindred Delusions* (1843). Granting that the law of similars had some validity, Holmes insisted that it was not the only law of cure, and he ridiculed the doctrine of infinitesimals with its requirement of numerous dilutions.

Despite criticism, homeopathy attracted physicians and patients. The American Medical Association (AMA), organized in 1847, responded to the challenge by adopting a code of ethics that prohibited orthodox physicians from consulting with homeopaths or aiding a patient who was being treated by a homeopath. Nevertheless, homeopaths strengthened their hold on the public, and by 1880 homeopathic colleges were found in most major cities.

Later, major changes in outlook occurred among both homeopaths and allopaths. Some homeopaths abandoned dogmatic adherence to Hahnemann's original ideas, while some allopaths no longer saw the AMA's code of ethics as necessary to defend orthodox medicine. By 1900 leading voices among the allopaths and the homeopaths urged that the entire medical profession should be united. This suggestion led a minority within the homeopathic medical community to insist on remaining faithful to pure Hahnemannian doctrine.[21]

Other Forms of Alternative Medicine

The rebellion against heroic medicine and orthodox practitioners bred a luxuriant crop of quacks, fringe groups, and varieties of alternative medicine. Among them were Grahamites, hydropaths (the water-cure movement), hygeio-therapists, electropaths, mechano-paths, magnetic healers, drugless healers, Christian Scientists, naturopaths, and osteopaths.[22]

Osteopathy was founded by Andrew T. Still (1828–1917) to provide an alternative to contemporary orthodox practices. He studied medicine with his father, a Methodist minister in Kansas, and gained some practical experience as a hospital steward during the Civil War but apparently did not attend a medical college. Still's medical practice was relatively orthodox for many years, but the death of three of his children despite the ministrations of an orthodox physician caused him to look at alternative systems of medicine. For a time he found guidance in the principles of magnetic healing, later concluding that the free flow of blood constituted the key to health. This required removing obstructions in some artery or vein by spinal manipulation. In the 1870s Still severed his ties with regular medicine and became interested in bonesetting. He became a lightning bonesetter, handling a variety of chronic ailments. In 1889 he made Kirksville, Missouri, his permanent base of operations. To name his new science of healing he combined the word "os" (bone) with "pathology" to create the word "osteopathy." In 1892 he opened the American School of Osteopathy in Kirksville, charging students five hundred dollars for four months of instruction, far more than most regular proprietary medical colleges. The first class had eighteen students, but within a few years the school had seven hundred. Graduates received the Doctor of Osteopathy (DO) degree.[23]

The preceding developments help explain the distribution of medical schools and students at the end of the century. During 1896–97 the United States reportedly had 150 medical schools with a total of 24,577 students. Chicago, with a total of 2,682 students (10.9 percent, excluding postgraduate students), ranked first, followed by Philadelphia with 2,139 (8.7 percent), New York with 2,096 (8.3 percent), and St. Louis with 1,531 (6.2 percent). In number of students in regular schools of medicine, Philadelphia stood first with 1,881 students (7.6 percent), New York was second with 1,843 (7.4 percent), Chicago was third with 1,783 (7.2 percent), and St. Louis was fourth with 1,385 (5.6 percent). In the number of students who attended homeopathic and other irregular schools, Chicago was first with 899 (3.6 percent), Philadelphia was second with 258 (1.04 percent), New York was third with 253 (1.02 percent), and St. Louis was fourth with 146

(0.59 percent). In sum, Chicago had more students in irregular medical schools than the other three cities combined. The homeopathic schools enabled Chicago to stand first in total attendance.[24]

These figures helped shape the struggle that erupted between the University of Illinois College of Medicine and the proprietary schools in Chicago after Edmund J. James became president of the university. With the rise of scientific medicine, medical education became vastly more expensive. Proprietary medical schools could no longer exist on tuition and fee income. Most of them fought fiercely for their lives. The best of them became affiliated with one of the leading universities in Chicago. James was in the thick of this battle.

CHAPTER 2

The Medical Situation in Chicago

The medical situation in Chicago in the late nineteenth century is best understood from two perspectives. One is afforded by an evaluation of the extent to which those who taught and practiced medicine accepted advances in medical science. The other is offered by a survey of the medical colleges in the city and the type of medicine they taught.

Bayard Holmes, a medical doctor well acquainted with the medical colleges of Chicago, portrayed the condition of medical thought, medical practice, and hospital service in Chicago from 1871 to 1893. He criticized the medical situation in Chicago during these years because he himself was alert to advances in medical science.

In the years between the Great Fire of 1871 and the World's Fair of 1893, Holmes wrote, Chicago was but dimly conscious of the remarkable advance of medical science then taking place. Listerism, which was demonstrated in 1867, was not practiced in any hospital in Chicago before 1882, and as late as 1893 the lectures on medicine in Chicago schools were "guiltless of the teachings of bacteriology."[1] Hosmer Johnson, a professor in the Chicago Medical College, never recognized the bacterial origin of disease. Almost yearly the medical colleges in Chicago received men into the medical profession from European sources of medical advancement, but few of them were Jews. When the College of Physicians and Surgeons of Chicago (P&S) was organized in 1881, there was a notable absence on its faculty of Jews and of recent European graduates. The faculties of Rush Medical College, the Chicago Medical College, and the Woman's Medical College were "almost homogeneously American bred and educated."[2]

During this period, Holmes added, medical thought in Chicago was provincial. The educated continentals who practiced medicine in Chicago rarely visited the medical societies and rarely contributed to medical literature. The only young professor who brought an up-to-date specialty to his students was W. W. Jaggard, who taught obstetrics at the Chicago Medical College from 1882. Charles W. Earle, one of the founders of P&S, was a distinctly American product. A general practitioner and an obstetrical professor, he went to Europe in 1880 and came back beaming with antiseptic obstetrics. Rush Medical College also had its home products who were guiltless of any un-American influence. The medical schools were proprietary. The number they graduated was much smaller than the number of their matriculants. The colleges had no laboratories and no small classes except in chemistry. A few inspiring teachers had a cosmopolitan horizon.

According to Holmes, the student body was deficient in English education. Few students had graduated from high school, and fewer still had a bachelor's degree from any sort of college. They were therefore unprepared to have an international and historical view of the medical sciences or to appreciate the value of a knowledge of the growing auxiliary sciences.

Chicago was home to plenty of advertising medical quacks, and they were prosperous and occasionally fell into lucrative investments. Some made money largely in real estate; some of the others did well financially with nostrums or gum. The moral character of the medical profession was undermined by greed, the neglect of public service, and the failure of the profession to read and advance.

The County Hospital, the only institution in Chicago that could be called a free hospital, moved to Wood and Harrison streets in 1876, and medical colleges began to congregate around it. The nursing of the hospital was put in charge of the Illinois Training School for Nurses around 1880. The medical staff was appointed by the county commissioners; each commissioner appointed his own family physician. The County Hospital and the other hospitals in the city were fitted up for operations about as well as the ordinary kitchen. In the late nineteenth century, the men who practiced medicine in Chicago and held the hospital positions knew little of scientific medicine.[3]

In the early 1880s, according to Holmes, "the medical colleges of Chicago atoned for their short terms and their paucity of medical education by a grand finale—a bishop and a brass band in a theatre, an afternoon distribution of Latin diplomas engrossed on real sheepskin, and a banquet at night at the best hotel for graduates and all alumni." Each faculty member patted the outgoing student on the back, shook his hand, and whispered in his ear words that meant, "Don't forget your old Professor. He'll help you out in consultation." Bad as it was, there were no rented caps and gowns, no processions or recessions. "It was honest bombast, parvenue and crass."[4]

A second perspective comes from a survey of the number of medical colleges in the city and the type of medicine they taught. In the nineteenth century Chicago was home to a superfluity of medical schools. All were proprietary ventures. Over the years the number declined as some of the schools merged or became extinct and others were reported fraudulent or not in good standing. In 1885 the city of Chicago was home to eight medical schools.[5] In 1904, when Edmund J. James became president of the university, at least fourteen and perhaps as many as eighteen medical colleges were located in Chicago.[6]

The medical colleges in Chicago taught one or another of the systems of medicine that competed for public favor at the turn of the century. Most of them adhered to regular or allopathic medicine and did not consider themselves sectarian. In 1904, according to the *Journal of the American Medical Association*, the United States had a total of 166 medical colleges, of which 133 were regular, 19 were homeopathic, 10 were eclectic, 3 were physio-medical, and 1 offered various forms of instruction.[7] In that year Chicago had more medical students than any other American city. Chicago had a total of 2,912 students, including 2,265 undergraduates and 647 postgraduate medical students. New York was a close second with a total of 2,827 students, including 1,888 undergraduates and 939 postgraduates. Philadelphia followed with a total of 2,552 students, of which 2,075 were undergraduates and 477 postgraduates. Baltimore was fourth with a total of 1,708 students, including 918 undergraduates and 790 postgraduates. Boston followed with a total of 889 students, of which 779 were undergraduates and 110 were postgraduates.[8]

Certain subjects were basic to medical education. In the first two years sectarian medical colleges taught the fundamental branches—anatomy, bacteriology, chemistry, pathology, and physiology—and imposed their special principles on students in the clinical years. Over time the difference in practice between a regular physician and one who came out of an alternative medicine background became less significant than the quality of the instruction.

The regular medical schools in Chicago, though few in number, were the most prominent ones in the city. The three regular university-related medical schools—Rush Medical College that was affiliated with the University of Chicago, the Chicago Medical College that became the Northwestern University School of Medicine, and P&S that was for a time affiliated with the University of Illinois and later became its College of Medicine—are discussed in later chapters.

The Post-Graduate Medical School was also devoted to orthodox medicine. In 1886 it commenced instruction as the Chicago Policlinic and was a pioneer of its kind west of the Alleghenies. Two years later a group of physicians and surgeons from the leading regular medical colleges in the city withdrew from the Policlinic and organized the Post-Graduate Medical School of Chicago as a stock company. The original location was on Washington Street in the business district. By 1891 the college had moved into its own quarters at 59 Plymouth Place, and two years later it relocated to a new building it erected at 819-23 West Harrison Street, directly opposite Cook County Hospital. The college, which was only for graduates in medicine, offered superior clinical advantages to general practitioners. It had nine departments and treated only charity patients. In the mid-1890s some faculty members moved the Post-Graduate Medical School to 2400 Dearborn Street, near the Northwestern University Medical School and within a few blocks of Wesley, Mercy, St. Luke's, and Michael Reese hospitals. Other members of the faculty remained on the first two floors of the building on Harrison Street. In 1896 they incorporated the West Chicago Post Graduate and Policlinic. Another regular school with a special focus was the Chicago Eye, Ear, Nose, and Throat College. It was incorporated in 1897.[9]

Some of the colleges extant in 1904 are difficult to classify according to the system of medicine they taught. The Dearborn Medical College, incorporated in 1903, became extinct in 1907. Jenner Medical College, chartered in 1893, was a commercial enterprise and a night school. Illinois Medical College, a day school, shared its physical facilities with Reliance Medical College, which was organized in 1907 and was a night school.

The American Medical Missionary College, launched by John H. Kellogg, is also hard to classify. After receiving an MD at Bellevue Hospital Medical College in New York City in 1875, Kellogg became superintendent of the Western Health Reform Institute (later the Battle Creek Sanitarium) in Battle Creek, Michigan. He was a health reformer with affinities to botanical remedies. In 1895, with Seventh-day Adventist support, Kellogg incorporated the American Medical Missionary College under the laws of Illinois. The college was registered under the laws of Michigan as an Illinois corporation with all the rights and privileges of Michigan medical schools. Its purpose was to educate physicians for Christian missionary service. The college gave preclinical instruction in regular medicine in Battle Creek, after which the students transferred to P&S for their clinical study.[10]

The Chicago College of Medicine and Surgery, Physio-Medical, represented the physio-medical sect. It evolved out of the Chicago Physio-Medical Institute, which began offering instruction in the city of Chicago in 1885 when William H. Cook and three colleagues broke away from the Physio-Medical Institute in Cincinnati and secured recognition from the Illinois State Board of Health. In 1891, having acquired larger hospital and clinical facilities, the institute obtained a new charter and changed its name to the Chicago Physio-Medical College. From 1891 to 1895 it was located at 605 West Van Buren Street in the vicinity of Cook County Hospital and other medical colleges. In 1897 Cook and two colleagues withdrew from the school and organized a rival, with twenty-two part-time faculty. In 1899 the schism ended, and the two schools merged and became the College of Medicine and Surgery, Physio-Medical, located at 245-247 Ashland Boulevard. In 1904 the college listed a faculty of forty-four, seventy students, and eleven graduates. In 1907 the physio-medical sect had three schools in the United States, but in 1910 only the one in Chicago remained.[11]

Eclectic medicine had a strong presence in the Midwest. In 1902 the nation had ten eclectic medical colleges, two of which were in Chicago.[12] Bennett College of Eclectic Medicine and Surgery, chartered in 1868, was the pillar of reform medicine in Chicago. The college had burned to the ground in the Chicago fire of 1871, but the trustees erected a new building at the corner of Ada and Fulton streets on the West Side and established a hospital. The official organ of the college, the *Chicago Medical Times*, the second-oldest eclectic journal in existence, had the largest circulation of any medical journal in the state.[13]

John Dill Robertson became the dominant figure in the college. Born in 1871 in Indiana County, Pennsylvania, Robertson attended local schools for a few years, became a railway telegrapher, and qualified as a bookkeeper. In 1893, having read medicine for six months under a preceptor, he went to Chicago and enrolled in the Bennett College of Eclectic Medicine and Surgery, and in 1896 he graduated with an MD. A year later he completed an internship at Cook County Hospital. In his early days, Robertson said, he went to Kansas to practice medicine. In 1905 he became professor of surgery at Bennett. Robertson was active politically.[14]

In 1908 Robertson was elected president of Bennett's board of trustees. A year later Bennett College of Eclectic Medicine and Surgery was renamed Bennett Medical College and became a regular medical school.[15] Robertson's position in the college is hard to determine with certitude because evidence on the matter is fragmentary. Bennett Medical College, Abraham Flexner wrote, was "practically owned by the dean of the school: 'there are enough others to legalize the thing.'"[16] This cryptic remark leaves much unsaid. John Dill Robertson was the dean to whom Flexner refers.

In addition to Bennett, the city of Chicago was home to the Chicago Eclectic Medical College. Its history is complicated, and written accounts of it are not always based on adequate or reliable sources. The school was organized in 1901. When the Woman's Medical College of Northwestern University closed, the Chicago Eclectic Medical College bought its property from Northwestern. The property consisted of two large four-story brick and basement buildings at 333-339 South Lincoln (later Wolcott) Street, facing Cook County Hospital. The Board of Trustees of Valparaiso College (later Valparaiso University) in Valparaiso, Indiana, apparently purchased the property. In 1902 the college, known as the American College of Medicine and Surgery, became the medical department of Valparaiso University.

The college provided instruction in both Chicago and Valparaiso. Robertson was professor of general and clinical surgery in the college and was on the Board of Directors of the American College of Medicine and Surgery. His location was in Chicago. J. Newton Roe, professor of chemistry, toxicology, and pharmacy and secretary of the corporation, was based in Valparaiso, though he spent much of his time in Chicago. The new school opened on 1 October 1902 with 135 students. Its course was arranged so that students could complete two years of work in Valparaiso and two in Chicago or all four years in Chicago. In 1907–8 the total registration was 325, and 70 students graduated. In 1907 the school, now regular, was renamed the Chicago College of Medicine and Surgery.[17]

In 1909, when Robertson was president of Bennett Medical College's board, the college purchased the equipment of both the Illinois and Reliance medical

colleges, both of which then closed. By this time Loyola University, a Jesuit institution that developed out of St. Ignatius College, had obtained a charter and had
grown to the point where it wished to add new departments. Bennett Medical
College became the medical department of Loyola University by an agreement
that was to remain in force for five years.[18]

Robertson was instrumental in securing the affiliation between Bennett and
Loyola. The Reverend Henry S. Spalding, director of affiliated work for Loyola,
said that when Bennett Medical College purchased the equipment of the Illinois
and Reliance medical colleges, Robertson assumed all financial obligations of
both institutions and turned over Bennett Medical College, said to be worth
$125,000, to Loyola University. Spalding admired Robertson, especially for his
business ability. "The gift of Dr. Robertson," Spalding wrote, "was the real beginning of Loyola University."[19]

In addition to regular, physio-medical, and eclectic medical colleges in Chicago
were homeopathic medical colleges.[20] Harvey Medical College, incorporated in
1891, became extinct in 1905. The National Medical University, incorporated
in 1891 as the National Homeopathic Medical College, was a night school that
dropped the word "homeopathic" from its name in 1895. Hering Medical College, incorporated in 1897, taught homeopathic doctrine in its original purity. In
1902 it united with Dunham Medical College; a year later it dropped the name
"Dunham."[21] The most prominent homeopathic institution was the Hahnemann
Medical College and Hospital. The college was incorporated in 1855, and the
hospital was incorporated in 1872. In 1892 Hahnemann Medical College erected
new and commodious buildings.

Almost lost on the landscape of medical colleges in Chicago in 1904 was
one osteopathic school. The Littlejohn College and Hospital, an undisguised
commercial enterprise according to Flexner, boasted that it was the leading
osteopathic college of medicine in the world. It conferred the degree "M.D.
Osteopathic."[22]

In 1904, the year in which James assumed the presidency of the University
of Illinois, Chicago had a large proportion of all the medical schools in the
United States and a greater number than some European countries. The city
had too many medical colleges in relation to the needs of the public it served but
few good ones. Most of these colleges perished as university-affiliated medical
schools arose to meet the need for scientific rather than sectarian medicine. We
turn now to these harbingers of a new day.

CHAPTER 3

The University-Related Medical Colleges in Chicago

In the 1890s three university-related medical colleges dominated the medical scene in Chicago: Rush Medical College, the Chicago Medical College, and the College of Physicians and Surgeons of Chicago (P&S). Their histories are closely interwoven, and as a result each of the schools must be viewed in relation to the others. At one point President Edmund J. James came seemingly close to success in his plan for the University of Illinois to absorb Rush Medical College.

Rush Medical College, the oldest medical school in Chicago, prided itself on its seniority. Chartered in 1837, the school was named after Benjamin Rush, a medical doctor who signed the Declaration of Independence. The charter provided for a board of directors (the governor of Illinois was an ex officio member) and a faculty organization. The school opened in 1843 with a faculty of four and twenty-two students. The admissions requirement was practically nonexistent. The college mandated attendance on two annual terms of ungraded instruction of sixteen weeks each and three years of medical study for graduation (one year of credit could be by transfer). Rush met a strong demand for medical education and prospered.[1]

In the late 1850s, however, some Rush faculty members were dissatisfied with traditional medical training and the Rush curriculum. When they proposed reform, Daniel Brainard, the founder and president of Rush, resisted. So the restless spirits resigned and organized under the auspices of Lind University in Lake Forest, Illinois. In March 1859 the seceders invited Nathan S. Davis of Rush to join them, whereupon they organized and elected officers. The following October they opened the medical department of Lind University on two upper floors of a new brick building at the corner of Market (later Wacker Drive) and Randolph streets. The faculty included thirteen professors. Their revolutionary program called for attendance on at least two courses of five months each, a graded curriculum in each of several branches of medical science, full examinations at the end of each annual course, and clinical instruction by arrangement with Mercy Hospital, located on Wabash Avenue near Van Buren Street.

In 1863, with a steadily increasing student body, the faculty put up a new build-ing at 1015 State Street near Twenty-Second Street. During the summer Mercy Hospital moved into new quarters at Calumet Avenue and Rio Grande (now Twenty-Sixth) Street, facilitating continued association between the two. In that same year the trustees of Lind University changed the name of the institution to Lake Forest University, whereupon the medical department reorganized and assumed the name of Chicago Medical College. The faculty became both the incorporators and the trustees of the school.[2]

Northwestern University, which opened in 1855, was favorably disposed to medical education as an academic activity. For years the Northwestern trustees discussed union with Chicago Medical College, and in 1870 an arrangement was made by which Chicago Medical College, while retaining its name, became the medical department of Northwestern University. The college controlled its professorships and curriculum, while the university conferred the MD. In Sep-tember the college moved into a new and spacious building on the northeast corner of Twenty-Sixth Street and Prairie Avenue, adjoining Mercy Hospital that, with St. Luke's Hospital, furnished material for clinical instruction. In 1891 the Chicago Medical College became an integral part of Northwestern Univer-sity and took the name Northwestern University Medical School. The university purchased new lots, a generous benefactor provided funds, and the university erected a building to house the medical, pharmaceutical, and dental schools and Wesley Hospital at the corner of Dearborn and Twenty-fourth streets.[3]

Woman's Hospital Medical College was founded in 1870. During the late 1860s Chicago Medical College had admitted female medical students on the same terms as male students. The male students unanimously requested the faculty to discontinue the admission of women, so during the summer of 1870 Mary Thompson, in collaboration with sympathetic male doctors, organized the Woman's Hospital Medical College with a faculty of sixteen. (In 1865 Thompson, who had established herself in practice, had opened a hospital for the treatment of diseases of women and children. In 1870 she received an MD from Chicago Medical College.) The plan of organization at Woman's Hospital Medical Col-lege, also known as Woman's Medical College, was similar to that of Chicago Medical College, including the requirements of three years of medical study and attendance on three annual graded courses of instruction of six months each. In 1891 the college became the Woman's Medical School of Northwestern University.[4] Northwestern University had two medical schools until 1902, when Woman's Medical College became extinct.

For many years after the withdrawal of leading faculty members from Rush Medical College, the standard of the school was not so high, although good work was done, large classes were graduated, and the college flourished.[5] In October 1871 the Chicago fire destroyed the college building north of the Chicago River at Dearborn and Indiana (later Grand Avenue) streets, but four days later the college reopened on the top floor of the Cook County Hospital at the southwest corner of Eighteenth and Arnold (later Wentworth) streets on the South Side.

Cook County Hospital played a significant role in the life of Chicago, and it does in this history. It was the first institution in the city to be devoted exclusively to the care of poor sick people, and it provided physicians and medical students with clinical material. In 1876 both Rush Medical College and Cook County Hospital erected new physical facilities on the West Side, which still had a reputation as a fashionable neighborhood. Rush put up its building on the northeast corner of Harrison and Wood streets. The Cook County Board of Commissioners located the County Hospital nearby on Harrison Street, facing north. The hospital was bounded by Polk on the south, Wood Street on the east, and Lincoln (later, Wolcott) Street to the west. Over the years many structures were added, and in 1916 a magnificent new Cook County Hospital opened on the site. The Board of Commissioners of Cook County appointed the chief administrator, the warden, and for years politics dominated the hospital management. In the 1880s the hospital authorized a separate staff of homeopathic and eclectic physicians and surgeons along with the regular staff. Patients had no choice as to their type of treatment. With the adoption of civil service in the selection of staff members, sectarian medicine was no longer recognized.[6]

Despite its faults, County Hospital was a major force in providing health care for the sick, the poor, and the ailing. The attending staff at various times included such medical luminaries as Moses Gunn, Nicholas Senn, William T. Byford, Norman Bridge, Christian Fenger, William T. Belfield, Ludvig Hektoen, and James B. Herrick. Internships at County Hospital were highly coveted because of their educational value. The best medical students in Chicago eagerly sought them. Before civil service was adopted, an internship was obtained only by a rigid competitive examination. Students in the medical colleges organized quiz classes and drilled with quiz masters before every annual examination.

Owing to the limitations of the County Hospital, Joseph P. Ross, an eminent physician, along with other Rush faculty members and staunch Presbyterians decided to build a hospital that would afford opportunities for clinical training. Rush College donated a lot directly adjoining the college on the condition that the Presbyterian Hospital Association erect a building and maintain it perpetually as a hospital. With liberal donations of money, in September 1884 the Presbyterian Hospital of Chicago, with a bed capacity of forty-five (later more than four hundred), opened on the southeast corner of Congress and Wood streets and Hermitage Avenue just north of the Rush Medical College building.[7]

Rush Medical College, whose income from student tuition was precarious, eagerly sought affiliation with a university. On 21 June 1887 Rush struck an agreement with Lake Forest University whereby Rush became the medical department of this small school near Chicago. Lake Forest apparently hoped to gain control of a larger enterprise by providing funds to help retire Rush's debts, after

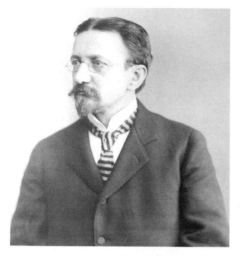

E. Fletcher Ingals. Courtesy of Special
Collections and University Archives, the
University Library, University of Illinois
at Chicago.

which ownership of Rush would re-
vert to Lake Forest without loss of academic autonomy to Rush. The hope
that Lake Forest would add a medical
school while Rush gained financial
independence never materialized.

The prospect of a more beneficial
arrangement was therefore attractive, and since Lake Forest University
decided to become a college rather
than a university, Rush began to look
· elsewhere. Ephraim Fletcher Ingals
led this effort. Born in Lee County,
Illinois, in 1848, of old New England
stock, Ingals attended local public
schools, the state normal school, and
the Rock River Seminary, a Methodist
preparatory school in Mount Morris,
Illinois, before moving to Chicago.
He studied there with his uncle, Ephraim Ingals, a member of the Rush faculty;
graduated from Rush Medical College in 1871; and then joined the Rush faculty as
assistant to the professor of materia medica. In 1874 he became a lecturer, rising in
1883 to full professor. The younger Ingals served at Rush for forty-five years, lecturing primarily on laryngology. He was a professor at Woman's Medical College
from 1879 to 1898 and at Chicago Policlinic after 1890. Ingals took a great interest in medical education. In addition to a large private practice, he was active in
various medical societies. As a member of the governing board of the American
Medical Association (AMA), he participated in the management of its affairs.[8]

Ingals, a Baptist, no doubt knew that John D. Rockefeller Sr., also a Baptist
and who, as head of the Standard Oil Company, was well on his way to amassing
the largest fortune in America, gave liberally to charities. Rockefeller needed
someone to manage his charitable gifts, and for this purpose he chose Frederick T. Gates, a former Baptist minister who had demonstrated business acumen. Rockefeller and Gates first worked together in dealing with the affairs of
the University of Chicago. Baptist leaders were interested in creating a great
university under Baptist auspices in either the eastern or the western United
States. Some suggested building it on the site of Morgan Park Theological Seminary and the remnants of the old University of Chicago on the South Side. But
Gates, as head of the American Baptist Education Society, advised that they create in Chicago a new university to provide Baptists with intellectual leadership.
In May 1889 Rockefeller announced to Gates his decision to make a gift of six
hundred thousand dollars to the University of Chicago.[9]

In the early 1890s Ingals explored the possibility of forming a bond between Rush and the University of Chicago. Before the university opened in 1892, he inquired of President William Rainey Harper, also a Baptist, about the possibility of merging their two institutions. Ingals hoped that Rockefeller would approve of such a connection.[10]

Harper wished to advance the interests of medical education by developing a medical school of the highest order in connection with the University of Chicago. He envisioned a school devoted not merely to the education of the ordinary physician but one "whose aim it shall be to push forward the boundaries of medical science." No other work, he thought, would lift the city of Chicago more quickly to "a place of honor and esteem among the cities of the world."[11]

Harper first considered a tie with Rush in 1894 but decided against it. Returning to the matter some three years later, he and others realized that a union posed legal complications. Two boards of trustees, with different terms of office, would have to deal with such questions as how to transfer property. Martin A. Ryerson, president of the Board of Trustees of the University of Chicago, did not recognize the value of an alliance with Rush. The property of Rush would never be turned over to the university, he feared, and therefore would be of no value in securing a part of the two million dollars anticipated from Rockefeller. Some of the younger Rush faculty did not see the value of the proposed affiliation, Ingals admitted, and he pleaded with Harper to keep their discussions confidential to avoid prompting two hundred or three hundred people to do everything they could to circumvent his and Harper's desires. Some of Harper's correspondents urged him to avoid the fatal mistake of making the proposed affiliation in order to get his medical department operational at once. Gates cautioned Harper, who was known to be impetuous, to take no action until he saw Rockefeller.[12]

Gates had a generally dim view of American medical practice and was skeptical about sectarian medicine, not only homeopathic medicine but also allopathic medicine as currently practiced. In 1897 he read William Osler's *Principles and Practice of Medicine*, first published in 1892, that dealt with the whole field of internal disease in light of the newest information and with a critical scientific outlook. The book convinced Gates that medicine had very few cures and that the great need was for the scientific study of medicine, which required medical research. In July 1897 he wrote a memorandum for Rockefeller in which he advocated the establishment of an institute of medical research. The memorandum was passed on to John D. Rockefeller Jr., who advised his father on philanthropic matters. Gates and the younger Rockefeller discussed the proposal.[13]

In 1897 the outlines of the proposed Institute of Research were vaguely drawn, Gates later recalled, but he associated the proposed institute with some great institution of learning and with some great medical school. Rockefeller Sr. was interested in the University of Chicago, and both he and Gates anticipated that the research institution would be associated with this young and flourishing school. In 1894, when an attempt was made to link Rush Medical College with the new university, Rockefeller Sr. discouraged the matter. He later supposed that no further attempt would ever be made to associate Rush with the University of Chicago.[14]

Gates intimated to officials at the University of Chicago that Rockefeller was beginning to think of a medical college, magnificently endowed and devoted primarily to research, conducted by the University of Chicago. Gates thought it was a mistake for the University of Chicago to connect itself with any existing institution of medicine, believing that it should delay entering the medical field until measures could be developed for realizing Rockefeller's vision. Rockefeller's plans had not yet matured, and Harper had no knowledge of them. On 1 April 1897 Harper declared that medical education was "the greatest single piece of work which still remains to be done for the cause of education in the city of Chicago," and he was eager to make some sort of beginning in medicine.[15]

Later that year the University of Chicago agreed to enter into an affiliation with Rush Medical College on certain conditions. One was that the Rush board be reorganized so as to consist of men satisfactory to the university's governing board and to have no pecuniary interest in the earnings of the school. Another was that the reorganized board pledge to increase the entrance requirements so that in 1902 they included the freshman and sophomore years of college. Affiliation was not to take place until the debts of Rush had been paid in full.[16]

The first two conditions of affiliation were speedily met, but payment of the debt of seventy-one thousand dollars remained a barrier to the alliance. Determined to wipe out the debt and to affiliate, Ephraim Ingals and Nicholas Senn of the Rush faculty each gave twenty-five thousand dollars, and about twenty-five other faculty members put up the remaining twenty-one thousand dollars.[17]

In January 1898, to their great surprise, Rockefeller Sr. and Gates were informed that official action had just been taken affiliating Rush Medical College with the University of Chicago. On 12 January Gates sent the authorities at Chicago a letter stating that "the history and the ideal of Rush College at that time rendered it an unsuitable basis on which to rear an institute of research." Gates alluded to the fact that Rush taught allopathic medicine. Rockefeller's family physician was a homeopath, and he tended to favor homeopathic medicine. Gates opposed all sectarian medicine, convinced that preconceived theories might limit the freedom of the investigator's mind. Gates probably did not know that at this very time Ingals assured Harper that Rush would be willing to teach homeopathy as well as regular medicine, but to introduce it in 1898 would greatly reduce the number of students. According to Gates, Rockefeller would favor an institution that was neither allopathic nor homeopathic but instead was simply scientific in its investigations into medical science. For that ideal the University of Chicago should wait instead of bestowing its influence, authority, and prestige gratuitously on Rush Medical College. "Such an institution," wrote Gates, "would have to be endowed and would run on a far higher principle than the principle of Rush College or any other of the ordinary institutions." The point of the letter, Gates added, was to intimate to Thomas W. Goodspeed, the official secretary of the university, that if he would quietly wait, the founder (Rockefeller Sr.) would probably endow an institute of research in connection with the University of Chicago.[18]

Goodspeed tried to justify and excuse the university's action, so Gates sent a second, more insistent letter. "The whole effect and tendency of this movement will be to make Rush ultimately the medical department of the University of Chicago," he wrote, "as against that far higher and better conception, which has been one of the dreams of my own mind at least of a medical college in this country, conducted by the University of Chicago, magnificently endowed, devoted *primarily to investigation, making practice itself an incident of investigation* and taking as its students only the choicest spirits quite irrespective of the question of funds. Against that ideal and possibility, a tremendous if not fatal current has been turned. I believed the ideal to be practical and I hoped to live to see it realized." From this time forward, Rockefeller Sr., who understood the implications of the letter, never associated the proposed institute of research with the University of Chicago.[19]

On 11 April 1898 the Rush trustees informed the University of Chicago trustees that all the conditions had been fulfilled, and on 19 April Harper arranged the proposed articles of affiliation in conference with Rockefeller Jr. and Gates. They agreed that nothing in the affiliation should be understood to give encouragement to the idea that Rush was ever to become the medical school of the university and that it was the distinct purpose of the university to establish such a medical school when funds had been provided.[20]

The Lake Forest University board agreed to waive all conditions concerning dissolution of the connection between Lake Forest University and Rush Medical College. This news freed up matters, and on 1 June 1898 the trustees of both Rush and the University of Chicago agreed that Rush should become affiliated with the University of Chicago as its medical department.[21] The agreement was for affiliation, not union.

The new entity was known as Rush Medical College in Affiliation with the University of Chicago. President Harper presided over Rush Medical College faculty meetings. In 1901 Rush transferred instruction in the first two years of medicine to the University of Chicago campus on the South Side. Instruction in the third and fourth years, the clinical years, was given on the West Side in the Rush Medical College building, at Cook County Hospital, and at Presbyterian Hospital. Thus, the Rush medical program was geographically divided.

On 14 June 1901 the Rockefeller Institute for Medical Research was incorporated, and in 1904 ground was broken on the upper East Side of New York City for the first building of the first institution in the United States devoted solely to understanding the underlying causes of disease.[22]

Officials at both Rush and the University of Chicago continued to believe that the cause of medical education would be promoted by union, so in 1902 Harper and Martin A. Ryerson conferred with Rockefeller Jr. and Gates on the matter. They understood that university authorities thought they could not do better than to make the Rush faculty the basis of the faculty of the proposed college were the university to establish de novo a medical school at the present time. They also understood that no funds would be requested from Rockefeller Sr. on account of or as a result of this union for at least five years. They thus approved the proposed union, provided the name of Rush Medical College be changed to the Medical School of the University of Chicago or to some equally suitable name. Rush, not the University of Chicago, awarded the MD to graduates of the program.[23]

In July 1903 the University of Chicago board sent Rockefeller Jr. and Gates a statement relating to a proposed union of Rush and the university. The two men did not find the statement satisfactory, so the whole matter was postponed until the fall. Before that time Rockefeller Jr. indicated considerable reluctance to accept the proposition made by the trustees, so in October Harper asked the board to consider the case anew. The original proposal had called for Rush to raise $1 million to be used in connection with the medical work already being done at Rush and the university. But only $250,000 had been raised, largely by the efforts of Frank Billings. The union, if realized, would add much prestige to medical teaching at Rush and the university and would stimulate additional contributions. Failure to effect union would probably hold back medical education for at least ten years, it was feared, and would lead Frank Billings to resign from Rush Medical College. If the $250,000 raised were used as an endowment, it would give the college about $9,000 income a year. Ingals, the comptroller, reported that with this income, tuition income, and the money in the treasury from faculty subscriptions, the college could maintain its present standard.

Harper therefore recommended that the proposed union with Rush be consummated notwithstanding the failure of the Rush trustees to complete the effort they undertook and that the university would have no further obligation to assume the conduct of Rush Medical College. Should the union be effected, the trustees would undertake the work of the college without calling on Rockefeller during the next four years for any additional help "except perhaps in the case of an unexpected emergency."[24]

Thus the union was not consummated, and Rush and the University of Chicago continued to have only an affiliation. As Abraham Flexner later wrote, the University of Chicago possessed a medical school that was neither "fish nor flesh nor good red herring." Rush was situated in a distant section of the city and had nothing to offer the University of Chicago except clinical teachers. "Mr. Rockefeller and Mr. Gates were both properly indignant," Flexner declared, "and in consequence took no interest in medicine in Chicago." This situation lasted for about twenty years. By 1924 the medical school of the University of Chicago was in the making. In May 1925 ground was broken for the buildings of the School of Medicine, and in the autumn of 1927 the hospital at the medical center was formally dedicated.[25]

While affiliated with the University of Chicago, Rush had a large faculty with many distinguished members. Frank Billings, one of the most prominent, was born on a farm near Highland, Wisconsin, in 1854, the fourth of seven children. His father died when Frank was eight years old. Working on the farm and for neighbors, he learned the discipline and determination that characterized his later career. He attended country school and for a time the Platteville Normal School and taught in a district school and a high school. A physician-preceptor kindled an interest in medicine, and at the age of twenty-four Billings entered the Chicago Medical College. He graduated in 1881 and gained an internship in Cook County Hospital by winning first place in the competitive oral examination. From 1882 to 1885 he practiced medicine and was a demonstrator of anatomy at Northwestern. Christian Fenger persuaded Billings to study in Europe, so Billings spent some eighteen months abroad, chiefly in the clinics of Vienna but also in Paris and London. He engaged in bacteriological experimentation in Europe and brought home equipment for this purpose. Some Chicago doctors viewed his stained slides and cultures of bacteria as a medical fad.

In 1886, on resuming medical practice, Billings was made lecturer of physical diagnosis in the Chicago Medical College. A year later he rose to full professor, and in 1888 he became a member of the attending staff of Mercy Hospital. Billings, in his lucrative private practice, treated many of the prominent and wealthy families of Chicago. In the late 1890s he was the spokesman for a group of younger faculty men in appealing to the president of Northwestern for financial aid to the medical school. In 1898, when the request was not encouraged, Billings resigned. In that same year Rush became affiliated with the University of Chicago, and Billings accepted an offer from Rush to become professor of medicine. In 1899 he was made dean and head of the medical department. He also held appointments in the University of Chicago, first as professorial lecturer (1901) and later as professor of medicine (1905). At the university Billings came in contact with President Harper and was inspired by Harper's vision and idealism. Billings was a builder of medical institutions and organizations. He assumed important roles in many of them, and in 1903–4 he served as president of the AMA.[26]

Arthur D. Bevan was born in 1861 in Chicago and was the son of a physician. In 1878–79 he attended the Sheffield Scientific School at Yale, and in 1883 he graduated from Rush Medical College. He served with the United States Marine Hospital Service for a few years and in 1886–87 was professor of anatomy at Oregon State University. In 1887 Bevan joined the Rush Medical College faculty as professor of anatomy. He became associate professor of surgery in 1889 and professor of surgery in 1902. Bevan was one of a group of eminent surgeons of his generation who played an important part in making Chicago a medical center. As chairman of the Council on Medical Education of the AMA, he contributed to elevating the standards of medical education throughout the country.[27]

In 1898 E. Fletcher Ingals, who eagerly promoted affiliation or union of Rush with the University of Chicago, became the comptroller of Rush. The position strengthened his authority in college affairs. Ingals viewed Rush as an exemplary medical college, one whose past gave promise as to its future. He jealously viewed P&S as a competitor and was reluctant to grant any concession to it or to the University of Illinois.[28]

CHAPTER 4

The Early Years of the College of Physicians and Surgeons

The College of Physicians and Surgeons (P&S), the youngest of the three leading medical colleges in the city of Chicago, began with bright hopes. The founders viewed themselves as reformers of medical education. They opened the door to ambitious youths who aspired to become physicians or surgeons, and they believed that a faculty appointment would enhance their prestige while also yielding a profit. After opening, however, the enterprise fell on hard times. Later it regained its footing and became affiliated with the University of Illinois. President Edmund J. James, who preceded Abraham Flexner as a reformer of American medical education, labored hard to elevate the standards of the school and to obtain public funds to support it. In 1912 when a legislative appropriation was not forthcoming and the medical school could not meet James's demands to improve its quality, it cut its ties with the university and reverted to proprietary status. A year later the university gained control, and the school became the University of Illinois College of Medicine.

Beginnings, 1881–82

The story of the beginnings of P&S has often been told but not always well. The historiography of the subject is complicated, and why this is so requires explanation. Two of the founders, Daniel A. K. Steele and Charles W. Earle, wrote about the early years, as did William E. Quine, who joined the faculty a year after the school opened.

In October 1893 Earle published "The College of Physicians and Surgeons" in the *Chicago Clinical Review*.[1] His brief essay, which historians have overlooked, devoted one paragraph to the organization of the college in 1881 and the remainder to a description of the college building and its laboratories. Earle does not mention any individual by name.

In June 1911 Quine gave an address to the Society of Medical History in Chicago that was published that year as "History of the College of Physicians and

Surgeons of Chicago."[2] Quine traced the early years of the college. Having been on its faculty since 1883, he was familiar with the events he treated.

For a decade thereafter the challenge of writing the history of the college was ignored. In 1920, however, John M. Krasa, president of the Alumni Association of the College of Medicine, took it up again. Carl Stephens, secretary of the General Alumni Association, joined him. Their original plan was to ask Steele to cover the period from the beginning to 1897; Quine to cover the period 1897–1912; Charles Davison, a surgeon who had joined the faculty in 1897, to cover the period 1912–14; and Albert C. Eyclesheimer, then the dean of the college, to cover the recent years. Since Quine had already published a history of the college, he declined to join in the venture. The others prepared their contributions, which were published in the *Alumni Record* in 1921.[3]

Since Quine did not contribute, Steele was asked to carry his account to 1912. His essay provided valuable details about the founders, the origins of the college, and its development to 1913, when P&S became the College of Medicine of the University of Illinois. Steele mentions Quine only briefly, in reference to Quine's role in seeking affiliation with the University of Illinois.[4] The essays of Davison and Eyclesheimer followed the original plan.[5]

Much of what has been written about the early history of P&S has been based on the articles by Steele and Quine.[6] However, we need to get behind these secondary accounts. One important primary source is the minutes kept by the founders of P&S from 4 May to 20 October 1881. Another is a letter dated 26 August 1882 "To the future Historian of Medical Colleges" that was found in a lead box in the cornerstone of the original P&S building when it was razed in 1938. The authors attested that the letter was "correct."[7] In addition are two large volumes of the minutes of the corporation of P&S from 30 June 1881 to 11 February 1915, some loose items, two bound volumes of the minutes of the Executive Faculty from 11 August 1899 to 5 May 1911, and a volume of the minutes of the Teaching Faculty from 8 June 1891 to 18 April 1902.[8]

According to the traditional account, A. Reeves Jackson, Charles W. Earle, Samuel A. McWilliams, Daniel A. K. Steele, and Leonard St. John founded P&S. They were all doctors who had settled in the Midwestern metropolis and were ambitious for success. In the 1870s the city of Chicago was home to six medical schools: three regular ones (Rush Medical College, Chicago Medical College, and Woman's Hospital Medical College) and three irregular ones (two homeopathic and one eclectic). Earle, in 1876, allegedly first broached the question of establishing a new medical college on the West Side near the Cook County Hospital. Notwithstanding his enthusiasm, Earle did not arouse sufficient interest to make a start, so the project was dropped. Early in 1881 Earle spoke to Jackson about the advisability of proceeding with the enterprise. Jackson, then a lecturer in Rush Medical College, readily assented to Earle's proposition, and on 4 May 1881 a preliminary meeting was held to consider establishing a new school.[9]

The 26 August letter sheds further light on these events. "For the last few years," it relates, "several gentlemen M.D.s at various times and places in Chicago have met and tried to start another Regular Medical College. They failed, because they wanted someone else to build it, to equip it, and to pay them a salary for lecturing in it." These enthusiasts made no progress, the letter adds, until Jackson, Steele, and McWilliams, the men who wrote the letter, took hold and associated with them St. John. They appointed McWilliams chairman of a committee to select and purchase a suitable site for a college building, and on 8 August 1881 they paid $5,541.78 out of their own pockets for grounds and taxes for a lot ninety-seven by one hundred feet.[10] Actually, four founders and their wives purchased the lot. According to the corporation records, in May 1882 Jackson, Steele, McWilliams, St. John, and their wives, jointly owners, transferred lots number 15, 16, 17, and 18 in the Ashland second addition to Chicago (the northwest corner of Harrison and Honore streets) to the corporation for $5,806.96, the cost of the lots.[11]

Abraham Reeves Jackson, the oldest of the five founders, was born in 1827 in Philadelphia, where he graduated from Central High School. After a brief stint as a machine-shop apprentice, he began the study of medicine under a preceptor and then attended the medical department of Pennsylvania College, a Lutheran institution at Gettysburg whose medical department was in Philadelphia, from which he obtained an MD in 1848.[12] For several years he was a general practitioner in Pennsylvania and New Jersey. In 1862 he volunteered for medical service in the U.S. Army and rose to become the assistant medical director of the Army of Virginia. He was discharged in 1864. In 1867 he was appointed surgeon to the ship *Quaker City* and in that capacity was Mark Twain's companion on the trip made famous by Twain's *Innocents Abroad* (1869). In May 1870 Jackson moved to Chicago with a view to limiting his practice to gynecology. He was among the founders of Woman's Hospital Medical College and was its surgeon-in-chief. In 1872 Jackson was appointed a lecturer in gynecology at Rush Medical College. He published a number of important papers on medical topics.[13]

Charles W. Earle was born in Vermont in 1845 and migrated with his family to Lake County, Illinois, at the age of nine, after which he divided his time between farmwork and attendance at the country school. In 1861, though underage, he enlisted in the 15th Regiment, Illinois Volunteers. In the fall he was discharged on account of an injury, but the following spring he enlisted again. Wounded in the Battle of Chickamauga and taken captive, he escaped from Libby Prison, made a harrowing flight to the Union lines, and returned to battle. In June 1865 he was mustered out, and that fall he entered Beloit College, receiving a BA in 1868. Earle next entered a doctor's office in Chicago as a medical student and matriculated at the Chicago Medical College, from which he received an MD in 1870. He had a private practice on the West Side specializing in gynecology, obstetrics, and diseases of children. Earle was among the founders of Woman's

Hospital Medical College. On its first faculty he was dean and professor of diseases of children and clinical medicine. At age twenty-five he may have been the youngest member of the faculty.[14]

Samuel A. McWilliams was born at Newtownards, County Down, near Belfast, Ireland, on 7 February 1836. He prepared for college at Pictou, a small town in northern Nova Scotia, and graduated from the University of Michigan with a BA in 1861. He attended the medical department there in 1863, taught high school in Wisconsin, and received an MA from the University of Michigan in 1864. In 1866 he graduated from the Chicago Medical College, taking first prize for his medical thesis, and was then on the faculty of the college, first as an assistant and lecturer on anatomy, next an assistant in operative surgery, and later as a lecturer on physical diagnosis. He was professor of anatomy in Woman's Medical College from 1870 to 1875, and for a decade from 1876 he was attending physician at Cook County Hospital. He had a practice in medicine and surgery in Chicago.[15]

Daniel A. K. Steele was born in Eden, Ohio, on 29 March 1852 and was the son of a Presbyterian clergyman. He grew up near Pinckneyville in Perry County, Illinois, dividing his time between the farm and country school until the age of fifteen. In 1866 he went to Oakdale Academy in the town of Oakdale and then moved with his father to Rantoul, Illinois, where he taught school for a time, clerked in a drugstore, and began to study medicine with a local doctor. In 1870 Steele entered the Chicago Medical College, from which he graduated in 1873. During his last year as a student he was prosector of anatomy in the college, and after graduating he was demonstrator in the Chicago School of Anatomy. Eager to learn operative surgery, he took a competitive examination for appointment as an intern in the Cook County Hospital and received an appointment as house physician and surgeon. He held the position for two years, demonstrating skill for surgery, and then engaged in general practice. In 1876 he became a lecturer on surgery in the Chicago Medical College.[16]

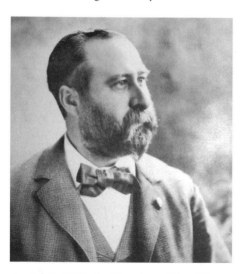

Daniel A. K. Steele. Courtesy of Special Collections and University Archives, the University Library, University of Illinois at Chicago.

Leonard St. John was born on 28 September 1852 in St. Catharines, Ontario. He was educated in private schools, in an academy at St. Catharines, and at McGill University. He graduated from the medical department of McGill in 1872 at the age of twenty and from the College of Physicians and Surgeons of Ontario in that same year. He began practice in New York in 1874–75 and moved to Chicago in December 1875, where he was a surgeon at St. Anthony's Hospital and on the staff of Cook County Hospital.[17]

As the minutes of the organizers reveal, the beginnings of P&S are more complicated than Quine, Steele, and secondary accounts suggest. The minutes show that thirteen men interested in organizing a new medical college attended one or more of eight meetings held for the purpose between 4 May and 20 October 1881. Six of the eight meetings were held in the Grand Pacific Hotel at the corner of Clark Street and Jackson Boulevard, and two were held in a doctor's office at 207 Clark Street. Jackson presided at all eight meetings. Steele and McWilliams attended all eight, Earle attended seven, and St. John attended four. In 1881 Jackson was fifty-four years old, McWilliams was forty-five, Earle was thirty-six, Steele was twenty-nine, and St. John was not yet twenty-nine.

The other eight of the thirteen interested parties attended the meetings in varying degree. Daniel R. Brower attended four. Born in Philadelphia in 1839, he graduated from the medical department of Georgetown University in 1864. He served for two years as an assistant surgeon during the Civil War and later as superintendent of the Eastern State Hospital for the Insane in Williamsburg, Virginia. In 1875 he settled in Chicago and became an important figure in the medical life of the city. At various times he was on the faculties of P&S, Rush Medical College, Woman's Medical College, and the Post-Graduate Medical School.[18]

Ezekiel P. Murdock also attended four meetings. Born in 1845 in Indiana, he earned a BA, an MA, and allegedly a PhD from Mt. Union College in Ohio. He served with the 47th Illinois Infantry during the Civil War and was superintendent of schools in various places before studying medicine. He graduated from Rush Medical College with an MD in 1876 and then engaged in a general practice in Chicago.[19] William J. Maynard, an allopathic physician, attended four meetings. His office at 207 Clark Street was the site of the second and third meetings.[20]

William T. Montgomery was present for three meetings. Born in Indiana in 1843, he served with Indiana volunteers during the Civil War and graduated from Rush Medical College in 1871 with first prize for the best anatomical preparation. He was an intern at Cook County Hospital from 1871 to 1873 and then engaged in general practice in Chicago. As professor of ophthalmology and otology, he was a member of the first faculty at Woman's Medical College.[21]

Ferdinand C. Hotz attended two meetings. Born in Germany in 1843, he received his medical training at Heidelberg and Berlin, receiving an MD at Heidelberg in 1865 after which he studied medicine in Vienna, Paris, London, Glasgow, and Dublin. In 1869 he migrated to America, settling in Chicago. From 1876 to his death in 1908 he was an ophthalmic surgeon at the Illinois Charitable Eye and Ear Infirmary.[22]

Three men attended only one meeting. Abram M. Carpenter, a Kentuckian born in 1834, graduated from Jefferson Medical College in Philadelphia in 1854 and then established himself in practice in Keokuk, Iowa. In 1865 he was elected to the faculty of the College of Physicians and Surgeons in Keokuk.[23] W. C. Maull was said to be of Middleton (a place name used at the time by several Illinois communities). We know no more about him. Alexander J. Stone (b. 1845) received his early education in the public schools of his native Maine. In 1867 he graduated from the Berkshire Medical Institute in Pittsfield, Massachusetts, and then received special training in the rapidly developing field of gynecology in Boston. In 1868 he settled in Minnesota, first in general practice in Stillwater and then in his specialty in St. Paul. At various times he was the editor and proprietor of the *Northwest Medical and Surgical Journal* and the *Northwestern Lancet.* Called the pioneer of medical teaching in the Northwest, in 1871 Stone organized a preparatory medical school, the success of which led to the establishment in 1879 of the St. Paul Medical College. He was closely identified with practically every venture in medical education in Minnesota until the University of Minnesota established its College of Medicine in 1888.[24]

In sum, thirteen relatively young men explored the possibility of casting their lot with a fledgling enterprise.[25] They were eager to improve their professional and pecuniary prospects by becoming part of a new medical college. For reasons to be noted, only five of the thirteen became founders of P&S.

The eight meetings began with general considerations and gradually became more specific. At first those present discussed the aims and objects of the proposed organization and agreed to name it "The College of Physicians and Surgeons of Chicago."[26] They appointed committees to procure a license to incorporate, to find a suitable location and ascertain the price of property for a site, and to report on chairs, lectureships, and similar matters. At the third meeting (23 June), having learned that the lot at the corner of Harrison and Honore streets was available, they appointed a committee to purchase it at the lowest possible price. They also learned that a number of doctors expressed a willingness to accept a chair in the new venture.

The avowed purpose of the fourth meeting (14 July) was to settle the plan of organization and teaching, the method of raising the necessary funds, the size and style of the building, and selection of a board of trustees. McWilliams reported that a contract had been made to purchase the lot at the corner of Harrison and Honore streets for five hundred dollars down in cash, and Earle reported that a license to incorporate had been obtained. The subject of minimum requirements for admission provoked a lively controversy. Brower and Stone proposed that a BA or BS be required to matriculate. Earle suggested that matriculants merely show evidence of a good English education or in lieu thereof pass an examination before a faculty committee. The result was a compromise, which the minutes do not describe. We know, however, that the proposed high standard would have meant low attendance and that the lower standard was common in the 1880s. Those present agreed that the college should have a four-year graded course, one in which each subject offered built upon previous courses, and that all examinations for a degree should be conducted by outside examiners.

The organizers established twenty-five named chairs and recommended fourteen men to "the Unknown Power" to occupy them. The thirteen men who had attended one or more organizational meetings each indicated a "preference of title" for one of the posts. Nicholas Senn, a highly reputed surgeon who had not attended any of the meetings, was the fourteenth person. The records do not reveal whether the entrepreneurs hoped to enlist him or he expressed an interest. Senn's preference was listed as "Operative Surgery."[27]

Two schemes for raising the necessary funds were considered. One was for a corporation of fifty thousand dollars' worth capital stock, with thirty thousand dollars subscribed by the faculty and the other twenty thousand dollars by capitalists. Another was for each faculty member to give one thousand dollars to the college (for a total of twenty thousand dollars) and then solicit contributions from the public to raise a sum sufficient for the purpose. Jackson presented a subscription agreement. After hours of fruitless discussion his proposal was withdrawn, and a finance committee was appointed. Brower urged it to present some feasible scheme, not such extravagant ones as had been offered. At this point Stone submitted his resignation, saying that it would be impossible for him to assume any financial burdens in connection with the new college. The matter was left unresolved.

The fifth meeting (19 July) dealt first with the composition of a board of trustees. Brower proposed selecting four eminent physicians who were ineligible for college positions and let them add a merchant, a minister, and a lawyer. The board was to select, retain, and dismiss the faculty, which was to consist of twenty-four men, each of whom was to donate five hundred dollars the first year, three hundred dollars the second year, and two hundred dollars the third year, with the board of trustees furnishing an additional eight thousand dollars. After receipts exceeded expenses, the surplus would be divided equally among the faculty. Any faculty member dismissed would leave his money behind as a donation. McWilliams declared the proposal inadequate and impracticable.

Those present discussed Jackson's subscription plan. It called for each faculty member to subscribe not less than two thousand dollars, paying 25 percent on subscribing and the balance in three equal installments at intervals of not less than three months. In return, subscribers would receive bonds of the college secured by a second mortgage on the property of the college and bearing interest at 7 percent a year, not payable until five years after date of issue. Brower objected to any modification of his plan. St. John saw benefits in the stock plan. Hotz objected to subscribing to any amount. Steele and St. John were appointed a committee on stock subscription.

The sixth meeting (30 August) was for the purpose of subscribing the capital stock of the corporation. Jackson, McWilliams, Earle, St. John, and Steele subscribed the entire capital stock of thirty thousand dollars. Each man subscribed sixty shares at one hundred dollars a share, a total of six thousand dollars each, in consideration of having the faculty positions that the minutes attached to their names. Jackson was professor of gynecology and clinical professor of gynecology; McWilliams was professor of clinical medicine, diseases of chest, and physical diagnosis; Steele was professor of orthopedic surgery; St. John was professor of minor surgery, surgical anatomy, and bandaging; and Earle was professor of diseases of children and clinical obstetrics. These five men subscribed to the capital stock of the corporation, thereby purchasing their chairs. They became known as the founders of P&S.

The stockholders then met on 11 October and elected themselves to the board of directors for terms of two years each. The seventh meeting of what was now called the faculty immediately followed the stockholders' meeting. McWilliams and St. John proposed that no person be allowed to occupy a chair in the college who held a position in any other medical college, but Earle and Jackson opposed the idea, and it was dropped. Multiple faculty appointments brought financial gain, but later they led to problems with accrediting agencies. Nicholas Senn wrote declining a college position "on account of business and financial engagements."[28] Steele was authorized to spend up to one hundred dollars in advertising for medical teachers in the leading medical journals.

At the eighth meeting (20 October) the four founders present (St. John was absent) named Steele and Jackson to a committee on preliminary announcements and advertising, and as members of the board of directors they elected Jackson as president, McWilliams as vice president, Steele as secretary, and St. John as treasurer. Earle was the only founder with no office on the board.

In late 1881 the founders began to implement their proposals. After considering several architects, they chose George Edbrooke, agreeing to pay him one thousand dollars for drawing the plans and supervising construction plus two hundred dollars when done if everything was satisfactory. On 29 December they adopted bylaws, and early in 1882 the board of directors began to assemble a faculty. They received many letters of application. Board members themselves had to apply, after which they received letters of acceptance. Candidates were often asked to demonstrate their fitness by presenting a twenty-five-minute lecture. Some of those appointed had attended organizational meetings. For example, Abram M. Carpenter of Keokuk was elected to the chair of the practice of medicine, and Ezekiel P. Murdock was named assistant to the chair of surgical diseases of women and clinical gynecology. Professors were to pay two thousand dollars for their chairs, lecturers were to pay one thousand dollars for their positions, and demonstrators were to pay five hundred dollars for their appointments. Professors held their chairs as one held title to property, and each adjunct lecturer or demonstrator was nominated by and subject to the direction of the person occupying the corresponding chair. Those elected had to sign an application for the number of shares of capital stock assigned to the chair, such chairs to be paid for immediately either with cash or its equivalent. By 12 April twelve chairs had been filled; six remained to be filled. The income from the appointments came to thirty-eight thousand dollars. However, expenses were heavy, so in June the directors authorized the finance committee to secure a loan of thirty thousand dollars for five years. Shortly thereafter the stockholders voted to increase the capital stock to sixty thousand dollars. A faculty organization consisting of all full professors was created. Its duty was to transact all college business not properly belonging to the board of directors. In July a proposal to make attendance at three years of lectures a requisite of graduation was rejected on the grounds that the faculty was not quite ready for so advanced a standard. Often the name of a person elected to the faculty was stricken from the list for "failure to meet the requirements," meaning that the person had not subscribed to the proper amount of stock. Frank Billings, for example, then a young doctor, withdrew from election as a demonstrator of anatomy because he could not obtain the money to pay up.[29]

In a preliminary announcement the founders boasted that they had organized the college "in the interest of a more thorough and practical education" than the nation's medical schools usually furnished, and in deference to the demand of the profession they had adopted a system of instruction extending over three years and including two or more graded winter sessions of six months each and a brief summer session.[30] Credit was given for one year in another medical school.

These goals identify the founders as reformers of medical education. The reminiscence of Hugh T. Patrick, sometime member of the Northwestern University Medical School faculty, illustrates the point. In 1884, he recalled, he "graduated from one of the best colleges in the country [Bellevue Hospital Medical College], after attending two classes of lectures, each the exact duplicate of the other, without having looked through a microscope; without having seen a case of labor; and being utterly devoid of practical training in physical diagnosis, never having taken a medical history, and having received no vestige of bedside instruction."[31]

According to Charles W. Earle, in addition to the reform of medical education the founders agreed that the college "should absorb as many teachers as possible who had been connected with other schools, but who at that time had no college connection."[32] Here Earle portrays the enterprise as an opportunity for ambitious medical men to find employment. William E. Quine wrote that "the avowed object of the corporation was to improve standards of medical education but the real object was to provide teaching positions for ambitious members of the profession who could not find accommodations in the colleges then

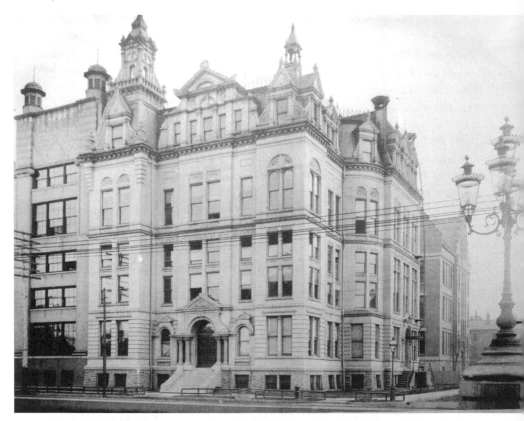

College of Physicians and Surgeons building. Courtesy of Special Collections and University Archives, the University Library, University of Illinois at Chicago.

existing. At that time the policy of nearly every medical college in the United States was frankly commercial," Quine added, "and the College of Physicians and Surgeons took a position among them a little above mediocrity."[33] Although not a founder, Quine was close to the situation. But his evaluation may have been a bit harsh. The two objectives—reforming medical education and providing positions for enterprising doctors—were not incompatible.

P&S opened on Tuesday evening, 26 September 1882. We can fix this occasion in time by recalling some notable aspects of the year 1882. In Britain, Queen Victoria was on the throne; in the German Empire the chancellor, Otto von Bismarck, was introducing state socialism to wean workers away from other variants of socialism; in Berlin, Robert Koch discovered the germ of tuberculosis; at the Vatican, Leo XIII was the pope; in Russia, Czar Alexander III was repressing revolutionary activity; and at the Bayreuth Festspielhaus in Bavaria, Richard Wagner's music drama *Parsifal* had its premier. In the United States, Chester A. Arthur was president; the Edison system of central station power production gave the commercial impetus to electric power production; the Chicago Academy of Fine Arts was renamed the Art Institute of Chicago; the reorganized Marshall Field and Co. was one year old; Mrs. Potter Palmer (née Bertha Honore) was the undisputed leader of elite society in Chicago; and in Illinois, Edmund J. James, the reformer of medical education, was the twenty-seven-year-old publisher of a crusading educational journal.

The college opened in its partially completed building in the heart of the West Side medical district. The building, which cost nearly sixty thousand dollars, faced south and was directly opposite Cook County Hospital. Edbrooke, the architect, had visited the principal medical colleges in the East to obtain ideas for use in Chicago. The brick and stone structure in the Queen Anne style covered a lot that measured seventy by one hundred feet.[34] Its four stories and basement were surmounted by a Gothic tower one hundred feet in height. The fronts on both Harrison and Honore streets were of Lemont limestone. The building was heated by steam, lighted by electricity, and ventilated. The basement included a janitor's apartment, a dining room and kitchen, and a refrigerated dead house (mortuary) with a capacity of 100. The first floor contained the college office, a large waiting room and storerooms, and the clinic rooms of the West Side Free Dispensary, with its door on Honore Street. The second floor had a lecture room that seated 226, three professors' rooms, a large clinical operating room, three rooms for clinical patients, and a microscopical laboratory. On the third floor were the chemical and physiological laboratories, the library, five professors' rooms, and prosectors' rooms. The fourth floor contained an amphitheater with a seating capacity of 450, dissecting rooms, and a room for vivisection. The building, which compared favorably with that of Rush Medical College nearby at the corner of Wood and Harrison streets, visually proclaimed that P&S was an enterprise to be taken seriously.[35]

Six hundred people attended the opening exercises in the amphitheater. After a musical overture and a prayer, Edbrooke presented the keys to the building to McWilliams, chair of the building committee. After several musical interludes, President Jackson delivered an introductory address, and Mayor Carter H. Harrison spoke in a rather humorous vein.[36]

The college opened with a total faculty of twenty-seven, including twenty professors plus seven in lower academic ranks. The founders must have been optimistic about their prospects, because in 1882–83 Rush Medical College, with a total faculty of thirty-three, had only twelve professors, with twenty-one in lower ranks.[37]

The original P&S faculty covered a variety of medical subjects. Among the founders, Jackson held the chair of surgical diseases of women and clinical gynecology, Earle held the chair of obstetrics, Steele held the chair of orthopedic surgery, McWilliams held the chair of clinical medicine and diseases of the chest and physical diagnosis, and St. John held the chair of demonstrations of surgery, surgical appliances, and minor surgery.

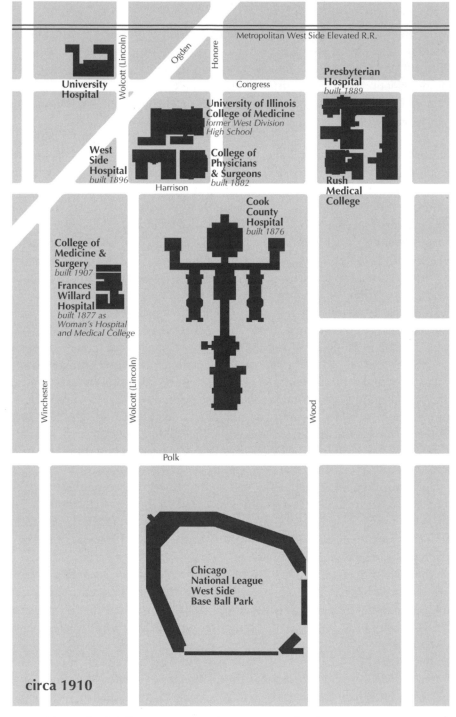

Map of the Medical College area. Drawn by Dennis McClendon, Chicago CartoGraphic.

The other fifteen professors covered as many subjects. Henry Palmer of Janesville, Wisconsin, was to teach surgery and clinical surgery; R. L. Rea was to teach the principles and practice of surgery and clinical surgery; Frank E. Waxham was to teach diseases of children; John E. Harper was to teach opthalmology and clinical diseases of the eye; Abram M. Carpenter of Keokuk, Iowa, was to teach the practice of medicine; J. J. M. Angear was to teach principles of medicine; A. W. Harlan was to teach dental surgery; W. A. Yohn of Valparaiso, Indiana, was to teach inorganic chemistry; Albert E. Hoadley was to teach descriptive anatomy; Pinckney French was to teach surgical anatomy; F. B. Eisen-Bockius was to teach medical jurisprudence; Theodore A. Keaton was to teach genito-urinary diseases; C. C. P. Silva was to teach therapeutics; Oscar A. King was to teach diseases of the mind and the nervous system; and Romaine J. Curtiss of Joliet, Illinois, was to teach state medicine and hygiene. The chair in physiology was vacant.

In addition to one demonstrator of anatomy there were six lecturers, five of whom were MDs. They assisted in gynecology, surgical anatomy, obstetrics, ophthalmology and otology, and genito-urinary diseases. The sixth lecturer, a PhG (graduate in pharmacy), was to assist in chemistry.[38]

Several members of the initial faculty served at P&S for many years. John E. Harper, who was born in Kentucky in 1851, graduated with an MD from New York University in 1878 with a prize for the best examination on diseases of the eye and ear. He then went to Europe to pursue his specialty in London, Paris, and Vienna. Harper served on the faculty until 1913.[39]

Albert E. Hoadley, who was born in Chenango County, New York, in 1847, grew up in Illinois. A former bricklayer, he graduated from the Chicago Medical College in 1872 and engaged in private practice before joining the P&S faculty. In 1893 Hoadley, who became professor of orthopedic surgery at P&S, was elected vice president of the college.[40]

John James M. Angear, who was born near Plymouth, England, in 1829, came to the United States in 1845 and settled in Racine County, Wisconsin. In 1860 he graduated from Rush Medical College. Angear had considerable experience in private practice, as an army surgeon, and on the faculty of the College of Physicians and Surgeons in Keokuk, Iowa, before joining P&S.[41]

Oscar A. King was born on a farm near Peru, Indiana, in 1851. He studied medicine under preceptors before graduating from Bellevue Hospital Medical College in New York City in 1878. After a short time in private practice he became an assistant in the Wisconsin State Hospital for the Insane in Madison. He spent the greater part of 1880 and 1881 at the University of Vienna and in the hospitals of that city devoting himself to the study of neurology and psychiatry. Returning home, he resumed work in Madison before joining the faculty of P&S as professor of diseases of the mind and nervous system. In 1883 King founded the Oakwood Springs Sanitarium in Lake Geneva, Wisconsin, that opened in

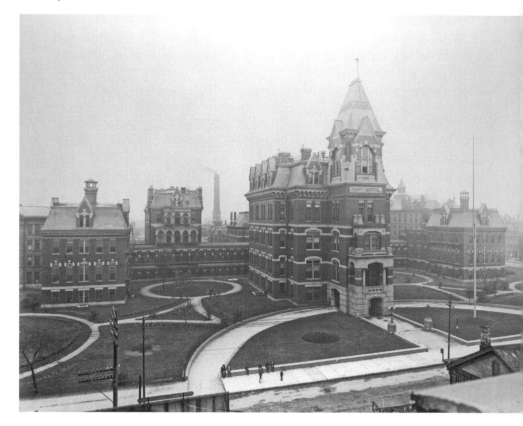

Cook County Hospital (1876). Courtesy of the Chicago History Museum.

1885. King was one of the founders and the first president of the Post-Graduate Medical School and also physician-in-chief of the Department for Nervous Diseases in the West Side Free Dispensary.[42]

In 1882 Henry P. Newman began at P&S as a lecturer in obstetrics. Born in New Hampshire in 1853, he read medicine under a preceptor, and after one year (1875) in the medical department of Dartmouth College he matriculated at Detroit Medical College, graduating in 1878. He pursued further study in the universities of Strasbourg, Leipzig, and Bonn. Returning to the United States, he settled in Chicago where he gained a reputation as a progressive member of the medical profession. Newman, later a full professor of clinical gynecology, was an influential faculty member.[43]

G. Frank Lydston also joined the first faculty of P&S as a lecturer. Born in California in 1857, he graduated from the Bellevue Hospital Medical College in New York City in 1879. In 1881, after serving in two hospitals in New York, he moved to Chicago to practice his profession. In 1891 he became a full professor. Lydston published frequently on medical topics.[44]

Boerne Bettman began at P&S as a lecturer on ophthalmology and otology. Born in Cincinnati, Ohio, in 1856, he studied in Miami Medical College before going to Europe in 1878 to study his specialty in clinics in Vienna, Heidelberg, and Paris. In 1880 he opened an office in Chicago and soon thereafter became a surgeon at the Illinois Charitable Eye and Ear Infirmary. At P&S he rose to become a full professor of diseases of the eye and ear and of clinical ophthalmology.[45]

Frank E. Waxham was born on a farm near La Porte, Indiana, in 1852. He had a rather meager literary education before graduating in medicine from the Chicago Medical College in 1878. A nose and throat specialist, for a time he maintained a general private practice on the southwest side, where his attention was called to the terrible deaths from laryngeal stenosis in diphtheria. His practice was almost exclusively with the poor. At P&S he was professor of laryngology and rhinology. Learning about a technique for intubation of the larynx for stenosis from diphtheria, Waxham rushed off to New York, took a course under the originator of the method, and made a conspicuous reputation with the technique. After successfully treating the son of a retired millionaire for a "putrid sore throat," using as an analogy a real estate agent's fee Waxham submitted his bill for twenty-five hundred dollars. The father questioned the fee. Arbitrators were appointed to deal with the matter, and the bill was paid. Waxham served on the faculty for ten years and later became a professor at the University of Colorado in Boulder.[46]

Perhaps some early faculty members were the best that could be recruited, but the eight just discussed possessed solid credentials, and four of them had pursued postgraduate study in Europe. They would have raised the level of the faculty a "little above mediocrity." King, Newman, and Lydston all gave long and distinguished service to P&S.

With the faculty assembled, the college was ready for students. For admission a student had to be at least eighteen years of age and of good moral character and had to pass an examination showing preliminary education and training sufficient to study medicine. Exempt from the examination were graduates of a high school or the equivalent. In effect, the entrance door was wide open. The costs included an annual matriculation fee of five dollars, a general lecture ticket of forty dollars, a dissection ticket of ten dollars, and a final examination fee of thirty dollars. A ticket to the Cook County Hospital was five dollars. Seats in the amphitheater were numbered and, except for seniors who got preferential treatment, assigned in the order in which students paid the fees. Rooms in the neighborhood of the college cost from two dollars to three dollars a week; with board, rooms cost from four dollars to six dollars per week. Students who formed a club and employed a cook could lessen their expenses. Rush Medical College was more expensive. The Rush matriculation fee was the same, but the ticket to lectures was seventy-five dollars, and room and board were said to be from three dollars to five dollars a week.[47]

According to the first college announcement most medical colleges largely ignored graded instruction, but at P&S instruction was to extend over three years and to include two or more graded winter sessions of six months each. The first regular session was to begin on 26 September 1882 and continue for twenty-four weeks.

The elementary studies of the first year included descriptive and practical anatomy, physiology, histology, general chemistry, materia medica, and therapeutics. In the second year, along with review of the fundamental branches of the first year, advanced courses in the medical and surgical specialties were added. The third year consisted entirely of practical subjects. Students were permitted to pursue their studies in all forms of laboratory work, for which facilities were provided. All important subjects were presented at least a second time, and students could attend lectures in some branches even more often. The faculty advised students to attend not less than three full winter courses of lectures. As of 1882, those who had studied medicine for two years and who had attended one course in a recognized medical school would be admitted as students of the third year by undergoing satisfactory examinations in anatomy, physiology, chemistry, materia medica, and therapeutics. For clinical instruction students could witness the examination and treatment of patients in the college amphitheater, the West Side Free Dispensary, the Cook County Hospital, and the Illinois Charitable Eye and Ear Infirmary.

Instruction was by didactic and clinical lectures, practical work in the dissecting room, chemical and physiological laboratories, daily quizzes on the subject of the preceding lectures, and, when possible, illustration by means of diagrams, charts, models, and instruments. These methods were adapted as necessary for different courses. Surgery in all of its branches was presented by means of systematic lectures and operations in the presence of the class on the living subject and the cadaver. Advanced students were required to perform the various operations in minor surgery and to become familiar with the use of instruments and the performance of surgical manipulations. Orthopedic surgery gave instruction by way of lectures, quizzes, exhibition, and demonstrations in the use of the most approved apparatus for the treatment of deformities. Clinical cases illustrating the different varieties of clubfoot, spinal curvatures, and hip-joint diseases were presented to the class.[48] College announcements listed two or three textbooks for each subject in the course of study.

In addition to the winter term of six months, the college offered practitioners' and spring courses, each of which followed the winter course and lasted four weeks. The lectures in the practitioners' course were adapted to the needs of practitioners and conducted by the regular faculty. The spring course, for students, was also instructed by members of the regular faculty. Attendance was optional, but students were encouraged to take advantage of this offering, in which about one-third of the work of each year could be done and the final examinations passed.[49]

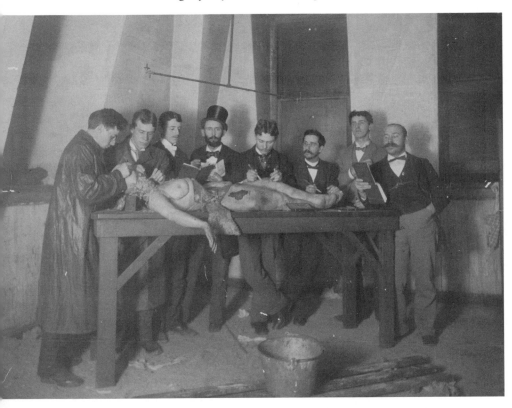

Dissecting, College of Physicians and Surgeons, circa 1890. Courtesy of Special Collections and University Archives, the University Library, University of Illinois at Chicago.

The requirements for graduation were good moral character; having reached the age of twenty-one; three full years of medical study under the direction of a physician in regular standing; attendance at two or more courses of lectures, the last of which must have been in P&S; dissection of each part of the cadaver; two years of attendance in some recognized hospital; satisfactory examination in all branches of medicine taught in P&S; and deposit of the final examination fee.

P&S was a new creation. As such, the founders might well have been bold innovators in medical education. They announced their intention to be more thorough and practical than the other medical colleges of the day, but in fact they were thoroughly traditional. They were not rigorously devoted to graded instruction, they relied on didactic teaching, and they permitted rather than encouraged students to pursue laboratory work. But P&S was in good company. In 1882–83 Rush Medical College, older and more prestigious, offered the same kind of medical education.

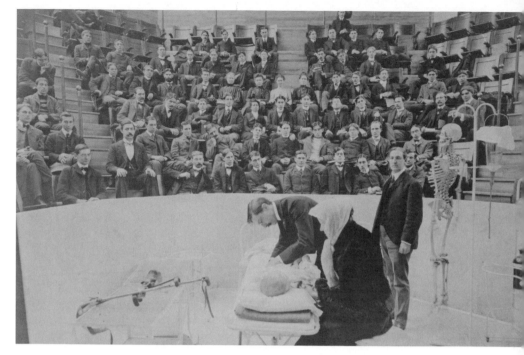

Surgical Clinic, College of Physicians and Surgeons, 1890s. Courtesy of Special Collections and University Archives, the University Library, University of Illinois at Chicago.

The college opened with a class of 100, gradually increasing during the year to 165. At the close of the year 52 men who had been admitted to the senior class graduated. They ranged in age from eighteen to fifty-two. Three were born in the 1830s, 3 in the 1840s, 27 in the 1850s, and 4 in the 1860s. We know the birth place of 15 of the 52: Iowa, 4; Illinois, Ohio, New York state, and Pennsylvania, 2 each; and Kentucky, Missouri, and England, 1 each. As the available evidence indicates, most of the graduates came from the Midwest but not from the city of Chicago.

Some of the group came with far more than the minimum required preparation. John Jay Crittenden, for example, had an MA from Evansville College in Indiana. Two men had MDs from the College of Physicians and Surgeons in Keokuk, Iowa (1870 and 1878). Presumably they wished to improve their skills or to earn a more valuable degree or both. Two men had studied at Rush Medical College in 1881–82, one of whom had also studied in 1877–78 at Kalamazoo College and in 1879–81 at the University of Michigan. Three men had a prior affiliation with the University of Michigan. William H. Weaver studied there before earning a BS at Carthage College, Clifford B. Wood had prepared in Chicago's South Division High School and at the School of Pharmacy of the University of Michigan in 1877–78, and Henry C. Darby had attended the University of

Michigan from 1880 to 1882. The older, well-prepared graduates no doubt imparted gravity to both the class and the college.[50]

A Time of Troubles, 1882–92

For a decade after it opened, P&S experienced much faculty turnover and considerable turmoil.[51] Some new professors joined the faculty, while others departed for one reason or another. The faculty remained about the same size as before (twenty-three or twenty-four). In 1883–84 E. E. Holyroyd was added in physiology, Wallace K. Harrison in medical chemistry, William E. Quine in practice of medicine, and James T. Jelks of Hot Springs, Arkansas, in surgical diseases of the genito-urinary system. New assistants also joined the staff. These additions, a college announcement boasted, greatly augmented the efficiency of the faculty. A year later the new appointees included Frank O. Stockton in laryngology and Henry J. Reynolds in dermatology. The chairs of histology and microscopy, materia medica, and surgical anatomy were vacant.[52] The college was still embryonic.

Describing this period, Quine wrote that "the policy which limited the right to teach in a particular field to the person who had bought the stock covering that field was responsible for some of the discord; intriguing for official prominence on the part of one or two was responsible for a little more; vehement and persistent opposition on the part of others to some of the policies of the governing board, and to some of the official acts of one or two of its members, caused a great deal; while overshadowing all was the general uneasiness and disaffection resulting from the known financial insecurity of the enterprise." Year after year deficits piled up. Earle, Steele, and Quine pledged their private funds for the debts of the college, Quine recalled, and if any one of them had failed during this trying period the college would have gone under.[53]

Contemporary records supplement Quine's account. In March 1883 the directors met to elect a permanent faculty. Presumably all faculty members had been on probation the first year. Discussions on the retention or rejection of faculty members for other than the inability to purchase their chair were rancorous. Earle was the only founder not present at many meetings, but when present he often objected to the proceedings. The board reelected a majority of the provisional faculty by ballot, but some of them "withdrew." Abram M. Carpenter of Keokuk, professor of practice of medicine, was among those not reelected. Records do not reveal the reason for his departure, but if it was not because he didn't pay his subscription the reason must have been lack of qualifications. Earle protested against any such action being taken without consultation with members of the temporary faculty and against the refusal to reelect Carpenter.[54] The most important addition to the faculty was that of Quine, who had been on the faculty of the Chicago Medical College for thirteen years. On 1 April

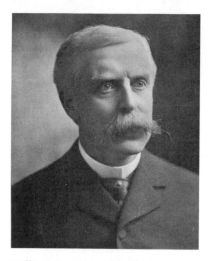

William E. Quine. This photo was published in the *Illio 1907*. Courtesy of the University of Illinois at Urbana-Champaign Archives.

1883 the trustees of that college accepted his resignation from the chair of materia medica, and on 12 June Quine attended his first faculty meeting at P&S.[55]

How do we account for the fact that Earle, Steele, and Quine supported the college as they did? Earle had a personal as well as a pecuniary interest in the college. He had proposed its establishment and had stock in the enterprise. Steele was a founder as well as a successful practitioner with a heavy investment in P&S and such medical enterprises as the West Side Hospital and University Hospital. Quine had resigned from a long tenure at the Chicago Medical College and taken a position at P&S. His career at P&S demonstrated his complete confidence in the school.

In the session of 1885–86 S. K. Crawford was appointed in surgical anatomy, Nicholas Senn in principles and practice of surgery and clinical surgery, and Christian Fenger in clinical surgery. Ludvig Hektoen became an assistant in the clinical laboratory. At the time the clinical work in the college was conducted in twelve departments.[56] A year later Charles A. Kelsey joined the faculty in pathology; Edward F. Wells joined in materia medica and pharmacology; and Charles B. Gibson, PhG, an assistant in chemistry since 1882, was named professor of inorganic chemistry and director of the chemical laboratories.

The appointments of Senn, Fenger, and Hektoen greatly strengthened the faculty. Senn, who was born in Switzerland in 1844, immigrated to Wisconsin with his family in 1852. He graduated from the Chicago Medical College in 1866, served as resident physician at Cook County Hospital for eighteen months, and then commenced private practice in Wisconsin, settling in Milwaukee in 1874. Gaining fame as a surgeon, in 1878 he went to Europe to complete his education at the University of Munich. In 1890 he left P&S to become a professor at Rush Medical College.[57] (At the time medical faculty often moved from college to college for reasons the available evidence does not explain.)

Christian Fenger, born in Copenhagen, Denmark, in 1840, graduated in medicine from Copenhagen University in 1867. He was in hospital practice in Copenhagen until the Franco-German War, in which he was a surgeon in an international ambulance unit. After the war he was a prosector for three years in Copenhagen Hospital and later in Egypt, where he was a medical officer in both Alexandria and Cairo. In 1877 he came to America, settled in Chicago, and established himself in the front ranks of the surgeons and pathologists of the nation. Fenger served on the P&S faculty until 1891 and then went to Rush.[58]

Ludvig Hektoen was born to Norwegian parents in Westby, Wisconsin, in 1863. His early years were those of a farm boy in a Norwegian community in which English was spoken only in school. He received a general education with no training in science in six academic years at Luther College in Decorah, Iowa, graduating with a BA in 1883. During vacation periods Hektoen had become acquainted with a young Norwegian physician practicing in Westby whose encouragement may have helped him decide on medicine as a career. Following graduation Hektoen spent a year at the University of Wisconsin taking premedical courses. He began his medical studies at the relatively new P&S in the autumn of 1885, selecting the college mainly because two or three physicians from Wisconsin who were favorably known in the state were on the faculty there. He earned high grades and was elected valedictorian of his class when he graduated in the spring of 1887. Hektoen won first place in the competition for an internship in Cook County Hospital, and in the autumn of 1887 he took up this position, in which he came more closely under the instruction of Christian Fenger and other prominent Chicago pathologists. In 1889 Hektoen was appointed pathologist to the Cook County Hospital, a position he held until 1903. In 1891 Hektoen became professor of pathology and pathologic anatomy at P&S. In 1894 Rush offered him a professorship of morbid anatomy on the understanding that he study abroad for a year. By 1895 Hektoen had studied new developments in Upsala, Prague, and Berlin. In 1901 he became professor and head of the Department of Pathology at the University of Chicago, and for years he served at both Rush and the University of Chicago. In 1902 he became head of the John McCormick Institute of Infectious Diseases in Chicago. Hektoen was a pioneer in the field of immunology.[59]

In the session of 1887–88, while the chairs of both medical jurisprudence and materia medica and pharmacy stood vacant, John A. Benson joined the faculty as professor of physiology. Born in Hoboken, New Jersey, in 1859, Benson graduated in 1880 from the College of Physicians and Surgeons of New York, during which time he was assistant in physiology to John C. Dalton, a famous physiologist. After serving in the U.S. Marine Service, Benson came to Chicago. "A handsome man of fine physique, with a polish that comes from generations of good breeding, he was a gentleman of the old school," according to *Plexus*. "Gracious and affable and genial, he had that charm of manner that puts one at his ease at once."[60]

In 1888 Henry P. Newman, an assistant since 1882, become professor of diseases of children; Clarendon Rutherford was appointed in descriptive anatomy; Charles E. Caldwell was appointed in surgical anatomy; and John S. Simonds was appointed in medical jurisprudence. Thomas A. Davis joined the faculty as a lecturer.[61] In the session of 1889–90 William C. Caldwell, an 1885 graduate of P&S, joined the faculty as professor of materia medica, and both Wallace K. Harrison and Thomas Kelly were appointed professors of medical chemistry.

During the 1880s the college provided opportunities for clinical instruction. Students could witness the examination and treatment of patients in several places. One was in the clinics conducted by faculty members in the hospital established in the college building by 1888. Two wards, one for men and one for women, in addition to single rooms were fitted up for hospital purposes. The hospital made possible the performance before students of all the major operations in surgery and gynecology. Another was the West Side Free Dispensary, which was under the control of the faculty. It occupied the first floor of the college building with its entrance on Honore Street. There students could learn the details of actual practice as the faculty members in charge of the work treated poor patients for diseases of every kind. From the time it was organized in 1882 to 1 June 1887 the dispensary treated 66,625 cases. Still another place was the Cook County Hospital, to which students had access through P&S faculty members on the staff. The large number of patients treated at County Hospital made the clinical advantages unsurpassed.

Faculty turnover remained a problem, however, and so too was Charles W. Earle. "No one could paint Earle in somber colors," testified Quine, who added that "his mirthfulness, cheerfulness, ready wit, and effusive friendliness" contributed to his success in life. Earle had "pushing audacity and a self-assurance before which frowning dignity warmed and melted."[62] He was one of the strongest men in the college and was generally well liked, according to his friend Quine, but he was also "one of the stormiest and most persistent of the insurgents." Quine explained how others treated Earle. "The directors decided every detail of administration of the college," Quine wrote, "and [Jackson, McWilliams, Steele, and St. John] entered into a secret alliance whereby they intended to maintain permanency of control."[63] So colleagues ousted the obstreperous Earle. Quine does not explain when or why this occurred, but corporation records reveal what happened.

On 24 September 1888 at a directors' meeting, Jackson reported that he had told Earle, who was not present, "that in the opinion of his colleagues the best-interests of the College demanded his resignation from all the positions he now held in the institution." McWilliams, on behalf of the other three directors, then offered several resolutions. They began by declaring that the four directors believed that "any and all further connection" between the college and Earle would be "prejudicial to the best interests of the College, and likely to be in the future as it has been in the past, destructive of such peaceful and harmonious spirit as should prevail among and characterize the actions of persons engaged in a common work." The four directors justified their belief by citing details. First, Earle had frequently betrayed the interests of the college by divulging the proceedings of both the board of directors and of the faculty to persons unauthorized to receive such knowledge in violation of the bylaws of the board and the faculty. Second, Earle had often arrayed himself against the college in issues between the college and adverse interests. Third, Earle had maligned and injured the character and reputation of colleagues by spreading reports about them, and when the victims were vindicated by a unanimous vote of faculty members to whom the facts in the case were presented, he declined to retract his injurious statements on the "absurd ground that 'he would like to have more time.'" Fourth, in conversations with stockholders he had charged fellow directors with improperly purchasing and selling the stock of the college, even though it was at his own instigation that the stock in question was purchased. Fifth, he had denounced his colleagues for purchasing the stock of a stockholder, though he admitted that he had received his share on the sale of the stock; this had set him to thinking, the result of which was that he kept the money in his pocket. Sixth, Earle had "cruelly, wickedly and falsely accused his colleagues of dishonest practices, and endeavored to injure their reputations, and lessen their influence." The four directors therefore requested that Earle "resign his membership in the Board of Directors, and his Professorship in the College at once." Jackson, McWilliams, Steele, and St. John all voted to adopt the resolutions.[64]

Since Earle declined to resign any of his college positions, St. John declared that it was the opinion of the board that the further connection of Earle with the college as a teacher would be prejudicial to the best interests of the institution, and since the board's bylaws gave the board the power to remove any teacher by a four-fifths vote, the four directors voted to remove Earle at once from his position as professor of obstetrics at P&S. In order to allay the upheaval in the faculty caused by this act, the dominant four elected Quine, Earle's close friend, to the governing board, and the administration proceeded with its duties.

In January 1889 the secretary of the board of directors sought legal advice on the question of a director who was not a stockholder retaining his position. On 17 April at the annual meeting of the stockholders, Earle was not present. Quine, who was present, objected to the treatment of Earle's stockholdings on the grounds of illegality. John A. Benson offered a resolution asking for Earle's resignation as a director. It carried by 330 yeas to 160 nays. Quine then tendered Earle's resignation, which was accepted by 375 to 90. Quine and Romaine J. Curtiss were nominated to fill the vacancy on the board caused by Earle's resignation. Quine got 370 votes (Curtiss got 120) and was declared a director. Quine then offered a resolution saying that all candidates for director be required to state before balloting that if elected they would be guided by the wish of the faculty as expressed by a majority vote in deciding all questions pertaining to making and filling vacancies on the faculty. The proposal lost by 330 nays to 160 yeas. The stockholders were unwilling to surrender control.[65]

Reconstituting the faculty proceeded from year to year. In 1889 William A. Evans was appointed. Born in Alabama in 1865, he earned a BS at the Mississippi

Agricultural and Mechanical College in 1883 and an MD from Tulane University two years later. He then went abroad for postgraduate study after which he settled in Chicago. A stranger in a great city, he began to practice medicine. He was well qualified to become an ideal practitioner, but his ambition was on the scientific side of the art, and in 1889 he secured the chair in pathology at P&S. A distinguished member of the faculty, he remained at P&S until 1908, when he went to the Northwestern University Medical School as professor of preventive medicine. In 1907 Evans became health commissioner of the city of Chicago, a position he held until 1911 when he became health editor at the *Chicago Tribune*.[66]

In the session of 1890–91 Robert W. Jones, an 1884 graduate of the college, joined the faculty as professor of therapeutics, and Charles M. Burrows was added as professor of medical jurisprudence. New material on hygiene and germ theory was added to the course of study, which was overdue but surely a sign of progress.

We do not know how faculty turnover and internal conflicts affected the student body, but we do know that the number of matriculants as well as the number of graduates remained fairly steady during the 1880s. During these years the number of new students ranged from 148 to 228, while the number of graduates ranged from 42 to 71, as shown in Table 1.[67] In 1891–92 there were 17 nonresident students. In addition, the practitioners' course had several graduates over the years. In 1884–85, for example, there were 10, in 1885–86 there were 14, and in 1886–87 there were 10. During these years P&S admitted and graduated far fewer students than Rush Medical College. In 1891–92, for example, Rush Medical College counted 641 matriculants and 142 graduates.[68]

Annual college announcements listed the name of matriculants, their state of residence, and the name of their preceptor, and we have information on the age and educational preparation of students from other sources. In 1882–83, the opening year, 5 of 152 students came from Canada (Ontario, 3; Nova Scotia, 2), a sprinkling came from widely scattered states (Pennsylvania, 3; Massachusetts,

Table 1. Matriculants and graduates, 1882 to 1892

	Matriculants	Graduates
1882–83	152	52
1883–84	167	52
1884–85	168	60
1885–86	159	71
1886–87	150	54
1887–88	162	46
1888–89	175	50
1889–90	148	57
1890–91	153	43
1891–92	228	42

New York, South Carolina, Colorado, and California, 1 each), and the great majority came from the Midwest (Illinois, 65; Iowa, 28; Wisconsin, 19; Indiana, 8; Missouri, 7; Minnesota, 3; Kansas, 3; Ohio, 2; Michigan, Kentucky, Nebraska, and Dakota Territory, 1 each). Illinois was the residence of 42.8 percent of the matriculants. We do not know how many of these were from Chicago.[69]

The composition of the classes was similar throughout the decade. Analysis of the students who matriculated in the 1885–86 session demonstrates the point. Three of the 159 matriculants came from outside the country (Ontario, 2; England, 1), and another 15 came from widely dispersed states (New York, 6; Pennsylvania, 3; Washington Territory, 2; Connecticut, Tennessee, Arkansas, and Arizona, 1 each). The overwhelming majority came from midwestern states: Illinois, 67; Wisconsin, 23; Minnesota, 12; Michigan, 10; Iowa, 9; Missouri, 5; Indiana, 4; Ohio, 4; Dakota Territory, 3; Kentucky, 2; and Kansas, 2. Illinois was the residence of 42.1 percent of the class, the same as three years earlier.[70]

For the academic year 1890–91 the list of matriculants was broken down by class. In the third-year class, Illinois was the state of residence of 27 of 51 members (52.9 percent). One student was from Russia, while most of the others were from the Midwest. In the second-year class Illinois was the state of residence of 26 of 48 matriculants (54 percent). In the first-year class Illinois was the state of residence of 30 of 54 (55.5 percent) members of the class, while 1 or more students came from each of the following places: Winnipeg, Ontario, Massachusetts, New York, Virginia, and California.[71] As these figures demonstrate, over time the matriculants were coming in larger proportion from the state of Illinois.

The available data on the age and educational background of members of graduating classes enable us to describe the composition of the student body. In 1884, for example, the graduating class numbered fifty-two. The birth dates of thirty-four of them ranged from 1835 to 1865 (the record lists the birth date of one graduate as 1874, surely an error). The oldest graduate was forty-nine years old, and the youngest was twenty years old. Six others were born in the 1840s, eighteen in the 1850s, and eight in the 1860s. Many graduates were not raw youths. We know the birth place of ten members of the class. One was born in Ireland, two in New York state, one in Connecticut, and six in the Midwest (Illinois, two; Indiana, Michigan, Ohio, and Wisconsin, one each). We can infer that most of the graduates were born in the Midwest. Four (one of whom had been dentist to the czar of Russia) can be identified as living in Chicago when they entered P&S.

Several men had far more than a high school education. One had attended Becton College in London, England; one had attended Carthage College in Illinois; another had attended Illinois State Normal School at Macomb; another had attended Upper Iowa University in Fayette, Iowa; and still another had attended Albion College in Michigan for two years and the University of Michigan for one year. William H. Wilson had prepared in Keokuk, Iowa, in 1880–81, in Chicago in 1881–82, and in New York in 1882–83. Samuel L. Brick had an MD from the College of Physicians and Surgeons in Keokuk (1875). Wallace K. Harrison had a Yale BA and an 1877 MD from Bennett Medical College of Chicago, while Frank M. Sawyer also had an MD from Bennett (1878). For graduates of Keokuk and Bennett, P&S was a step up. R. H. Chittenden had an MD from the Long Island College Hospital (1866).[72]

The class that graduated three years later (1887) was also richly diverse. The birth dates of twenty-nine of the fifty-four members (53.7 percent) show that the oldest one was born in 1839, making him forty-six years old when he graduated. Eleven others were born in the 1850s and seventeen in the 1860s. Most graduates were not beardless boys. We know the birth place of ten members of the class. One was born in Toronto, Canada; one was born in Pennsylvania; and the other eight were born in the Midwest (Iowa, Illinois, and Minnesota, two each; Indiana and Ohio, one each). We can infer that most members of the class were born in the Midwest, but not in Chicago. Several members recorded that they had prepared through high school, but many had advanced preparation. One had prepared in the Amsterdam schools and at the University of Amsterdam in 1881. One reportedly had studied at Valparaiso, Indiana. One had studied in the Hospital for the Insane in Mendota, Wisconsin, in the summer of 1885 and in Oakwood Sanitarium in the summer of 1886. One had studied in a normal school in Dixon, Illinois, and another at Mt. Morris College in Mt. Morris, Illinois. Two had prepared at Illinois Wesleyan University in Bloomington, Illinois (another earned a PhB there in 1900). One had prepared in Harris Institute in Mt. Sterling, Kentucky, and at the University of Missouri in 1882–84. One had prepared in the medical school of the University of Michigan. One had attended the College of Physicians and Surgeons of New York. One (Ludvig Hektoen) had earned a BA at Luther College in Decorah, Iowa, and had attended the University of Wisconsin in 1883–84.[73]

In 1890 a total of fifty-seven men graduated from P&S. The birth dates of forty-nine (86 percent of the total) ranged from the 1840s (two) to 1870 (one), with seventeen in the 1850s and twenty-nine in the 1860s. The oldest graduate was forty-four years old, and the youngest was twenty years old. Five of the twenty-three graduates whose birth places are known were foreign-born. Denmark was the birthplace of two, and Canada, Germany, and Scotland of one each. Among the native born were one each from Vermont, Connecticut, New York state, and Pennsylvania. The remaining fourteen were sons of the Midwest. Illinois was the birthplace of five, including three born in Chicago. Four were born in Wisconsin, three in Indiana, and one each in Kentucky and Ohio. Chicago was a magnet that drew aspiring physicians and surgeons from the immediate hinterland and beyond.

While many members of the class reported having been prepared through high school, others went beyond that level. One man had gone from an American high school to the Vienna Allgemeine Krankenhaus. Another had a BA

(1886) and a PhB (1887) from Copenhagen University. One man had prepared in Koensberg and Berlin in 1882–87. Among different places, others had prepared at Northwestern University; Lawrence University in Appleton, Wisconsin; Western Reserve University in Cleveland; and Eureka College in Eureka, Illinois. One man had attended the University of Michigan (1885) and Chicago Medical College (1887) and had experience in three Chicago hospitals. One man had attended Indianapolis Medical College (1878). Another had an MD from Bennett Medical College (1886). In sum, the graduates ranged widely in age, place of origin, and degree of preparation. P&S attracted a large number of well-prepared medical students.[74]

"During the first ten years of its existence," a medical doctor close to the scene later wrote, P&S "was a two-ring circus of the conventional sort, and then it suddenly added a multitude of side shows in the form of laboratories, seminars, and dispensary clinics. During the following ten years this aggregation became scholasticized." This evaluation strives for effect, but it helps put developments in perspective.[75]

A Period of Stability, 1892–97

The time of troubles gradually but unmistakably gave way to a period of stability. The faculty was now reconstructed. Quine, who had won the respect of his colleagues by his "disinterested strong personality" and fairness, was named president of the faculty. He led in strengthening and enlarging the instructional force. In 1891 two of the founders, St. John and McWilliams, retired, and members of the faculty submitted their resignations en masse. The resignations were referred to the board of directors, which accepted some and rejected others, reappointing only those who were highly valued. On Quine's motion Earle, who had landed on his feet when ousted from P&S,[76] was brought back to fill the chair of obstetrics. The collective faculty read the flood of applications for an appointment and referred them to the board for action. Quine exerted great influence in selecting those who were appointed. They included John H. Curtis in therapeutics; James A. Lydston in inorganic and medical chemistry; Elmer E. Babcock in surgical anatomy; Robert H. Babcock in clinical medicine, diseases of the chest, and physical diagnosis; and James Madison Gore Carter of Waukegan, Illinois, in pathology and hygiene. The titles of some professors were changed in the interest of accuracy, and G. Frank Lydston and Boerne Bettman, lecturers since 1882, were promoted to full professor.

As will become clear later, five new appointees were of special importance. They were Bayard Holmes in surgical anatomy and pathology, Ludvig Hektoen in pathology, Weller van Hook in surgical pathology and bacteriology, Thomas M. Hardie in miscroscopy and histology, and Albert P. Ohlmacher in comparative anatomy and embryology.[77]

In addition to the faculty, the college organization was reconstructed. In July 1892, at the urging of Steele and Jackson, Quine remodeled the structure of the college so as to end the board of directors' complete control over the institution. Quine established two interrelated bodies. The teaching faculty, made up of all members of the instructional corps, was charged with educational operations, subject to financial restraints imposed by the executive faculty or the board of directors. The executive faculty, which included members of the teaching faculty who held stock in the corporation, had final say in finances and appointments. When Jackson died in November 1892, Earle became president of the board of directors, and Quine remained president of the faculty.[78]

When Earle died on 19 November 1893, Steele succeeded him as president of the board with the title of actuary, and Quine's title was changed to dean of the faculty. For more than twenty years Steele and Quine were dominant in the affairs of the college. In 1893 Steele was forty-one years old, and Quine was forty-six years old. Born in 1847 on the Isle of Man, Quine came to the United States in 1853. His family settled in Chicago, where the boy attended public schools and graduated from high school in 1863. He served an apprenticeship in pharmacy for a total of four years in Chicago and Memphis, and in 1869 he graduated from the three-year course in the Chicago Medical College at the head of his class. Before graduating he won an internship at Cook County Hospital by competitive examination. He served in that capacity from October 1868 to March 1870 and was then elected a member of the medical board of the Cook County Hospital (an appointment he held for ten years) and professor of materia medica and therapeutics in the Chicago Medical College.[79]

Steele and Quine were instrumental in setting the college on a new course. They worked through the faculty and the board of directors. In August 1892 the board was enlarged to include nine members. Earle, King, Fenger, and Hoadley were added to the governing body.[80]

In the early 1890s the faculty, including all ranks, averaged thirty-eight members.[81] When Romaine J. Curtiss resigned in September 1891 the directors paid him cash for his stock. The following April the directors asked Charles M. Burrows, professor of medical jurisprudence, to resign because of unsatisfactory performance.[82]

Among other new appointments in the early 1890s were Samuel B. Buckmaster in medical surgical electricity, Adolph Gehrmann in bacteriology, John B. Murphy in surgery, Henry T. Byford in gynecology and clinical gynecology, Charles S. Bacon in obstetrics, William A. Pusey in dermatology, Walter S. Christopher in diseases of children, William T. Eckley in anatomy, and Henry T. Tolman in medical jurisprudence.[83]

Observance of the first public Class Day on 12 April 1893 marked the close of the tenth year of the college. About five hundred people gathered in the large assembly room of the college for the occasion. The main event was the presentation of a bronze bust of A. Reeves Jackson, a founder, a president of P&S, and a conscientious advocate of higher medical education. Since Jackson had been instrumental in the founding of Woman's Hospital Medical College in Chicago, it was appropriate that the bust was modeled by a woman, Ella Rankin Copp.[84]

On 13 April 1893 eighty-seven graduates of the college received their diplomas from President Charles W. Earle in commencement exercises at the Grand Opera House. A large faculty contingent was seated on the stage, members of the class occupied the orchestra chairs, and friends of the students crowded the theater. The Reverend J. M. Caldwell opened and closed the exercises with prayer. Professor James Madison Gore Carter gave the doctorate address, after which prizes were awarded and hospital appointments were announced.[85]

No evidence suggests that either the Panic of 1893 or the World's Columbian Exposition of that year significantly impacted the operations of the college or the student body. Fees had risen over the years. In the session of 1893–94 the general lecture ticket cost one hundred dollars, the laboratory ticket cost twenty-five dollars, and textbooks cost from twenty-five dollars to fifty dollars a year. But the World's Fair, ten miles from the college on the South Side, had no perceptible influence on expenses in the neighborhood of the college.[86]

While reconstructing the faculty and the organizational structure, college officials dealt with other pressing problems. One was institutional expansion. In the 1890s many proprietary medical colleges sought some sort of tie with a university. Rush Medical College, as we saw earlier, affiliated first with Lake Forest College and then with the University of Chicago. In October 1891 Earle, having interviewed William Rainey Harper, president of the University of Chicago, and Thomas W. Goodspeed, secretary of the university, reported that "everything looked favorable for the union of the College of Physicians and Surgeons with the University." Earle and others had also discussed affiliation with a hospital. Earle preferred a connection with the Baptist Hospital rather than with Temperance Hospital, which Quine had suggested. Quine thought that a connection of P&S, the University of Chicago, and both of the hospitals might be established. This is the first evidence we have of efforts made by P&S to affiliate or unite with a university.[87]

Another pressing problem was physical expansion. The P&S building was becoming crowded, and the need for more laboratory space was urgent. In October 1891 the faculty agreed that the college should purchase the lot to the west of the P&S building for twenty-one thousand dollars. They named Holmes and Hoadley as a committee to purchase the property for new laboratories. The following April, when stockholders dealt with the financial aspects of the transaction, only twenty-six stockholders attended the meeting in person, but 420 of 495 shares of stock were represented. Steele, Quine, and John B. Murphy, each of whom owned 25 shares, were among the largest stockholders. After the stockholders authorized the board of directors to borrow sixty thousand dollars to make improvements in the old building and erect a new building, the board issued bonds in that amount.[88] The directors used the proceeds to build a well-equipped laboratory adjoining the college building. Finished in 1892, it was the first laboratory building in Chicago and the first one erected by a private medical college in the United States. The first floor contained a reading room, quiz rooms, a coat room, and a hall. The second floor housed the histology laboratory, which was connected with the microscopical laboratory of the main building. The third floor housed the pathological laboratory. The fourth floor contained the chemical laboratory, and the fifth floor housed the biological laboratory. The sixth floor was occupied by the anatomical departments.[89]

The P&S faculty of the early 1890s included many strong and some outstanding members. Bayard Holmes, one of the most interesting, helped invigorate the enterprise. Born in Vermont in 1852, he grew up in northern New York and in Minnesota, attended Carleton College, and in 1871 went to Chicago, where he briefly attended the old University of Chicago. He taught in the public schools in Waterman and Ottawa, Illinois, and in 1882, having decided to study medicine, visited Rush, Chicago Medical College, and P&S but was not impressed with any of them. The Chicago Medical College had "horribly dirty and inadequate equipment[;] . . . dusty, dirty and deserted amphitheaters[;] . . . [a] foul smelling and gruesome anatomy laboratory;" and a few "almost ludicrously antiquated" microscopes. Rush also failed to make a favorable impression. P&S was "destitute of pedagogic armamentarium, but alarmingly clean and new." Impressed by the microscopes, clean rooms, and friendly instructors at the Homeopathic Medical College, Holmes matriculated there and received his MD in 1884.

Holmes won an internship in the Cook County Hospital by examination. Having never doubted the bacterial origin of disease, he set up at once a bacteriological laboratory in a bathroom of the new administration building. During his eighteen months at the County Hospital, the happiest time in his life, he discovered that regulars had strong feelings about homeopaths, so in 1885 he matriculated at P&S. But college officials did not honor arrangements that the secretary had made with him, so Holmes withdrew. His first research paper, on antisepsis in abdominal operations, with the eminent Christian Fenger as coauthor, was published in 1887. In demonstrating "some bacteriology" at a meeting of the Chicago Gynecological Society he met W. W. Jaggard, a Chicago Medical College faculty member who was the permanent secretary and later president of the Chicago Gynecological Society. Jaggard made it possible for Holmes to enroll at the Chicago Medical College. Finally, in 1888, at the age of thirty-six, Holmes obtained a regular medical degree.[90]

Bayard Holmes thus had rich experience with various styles of medical education, and he had thought about the subject. After joining the faculty in 1891, he pushed for change in P&S. He disparaged didactic teaching, emphasized laboratory instruction, and urged the introduction of a course in bacteriology.

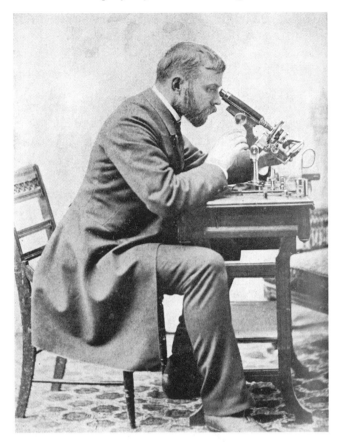

Bayard Holmes. This photo was published in *Medical Life* 34 (June 1917): 316.

Leslie B. Arey, the historian of the Northwestern University Medical School, wrote that during the early 1890s P&S "for a time, became a leader in emphasizing demonstrations and laboratory teaching."[91] Holmes prodded his colleagues to rearrange the college work according to the university plan (which resulted in a tie vote), to amplify and lengthen the course of study, to admit ladies to the laboratories (which lost by a tie vote, with Quine voting nay),[92] and to set aside one floor of the college building for hospital purposes. Holmes was appointed to a committee on a new hospital for the college. He moved to abolish final examinations and grade students on the basis of class records and attendance (his motion passed).

As corresponding secretary of the college, a position to which he was elected in June 1891, Holmes revolutionized the method of recruiting students. To discover the name and address of every young man in the six-state tributary to Chicago who proposed to study medicine, he sent a letter of inquiry to every physician, druggist, school superintendent, high school principal, and college secretary, enclosing a postal card with a return address. These cards came back, at the rate of seventy-five a day, for months. Each card had two to six names and addresses of young men who were good material for medical education. Holmes then sent each a questionnaire designed to discover their preparation for and interest in medical education. By this method, in seven weeks he came into correspondence with more than 1,000 prospective medical students. Before the college opened in September 1891, said Holmes, 314 had matriculated, and others followed.[93]

Holmes, a man of lively intellect, was an innovator in medical education. His influence on the college was beneficial but not always welcome. Holmes, Hektoen, Weller Van Hook, Ohlmacher, and Hardie, all of whom joined the faculty in 1891, collaborated in an effort to revivify medical education at P&S. Holmes was an enthusiast for bacteriology and for laboratory methods. Hektoen had been a brilliant student at P&S before joining its faculty. Weller Van Hook, who was born in Greenville, Indiana, in 1862, had a BA from the University of Michigan (1884) before receiving an MD at P&S in 1885. Albert P. Ohlmacher was born in Sandusky, Ohio, in 1865. His parents were of North German stock—German was the language used in the home—and the family moved to Sycamore, Illinois, a New England community in DeKalb County. The activating event in Ohlmacher's education was a teachers' institute in which he was introduced to the new science of biology. Ohlmacher graduated from the Chicago Medical College in 1890. He and Holmes had met when Holmes was an intern at Cook County Hospital. Thomas M. Hardie was born in New Castle, Maryland, in 1862. He earned both a BA (1884) and an MD (1888) from the University of Toronto, Canada, then pursued postgraduate work in Berlin, Vienna, and London, and in 1888 he established a general medical practice in Chicago.

Holmes, Hektoen, Van Hook, Ohlmacher, and Hardie were the products of a pedagogy that emphasized didactic instruction. Revolting against it, they initiated the laboratory method of instruction. Joining forces in the spring of 1891, each man prepared for the opening of the college year in September by making out a synopsis of his 120 hours of laboratory work, sixty sessions of 2 hours each, and a list of material required for the course. Holmes took bacteriology and surgical pathology, Hektoen took pathology, Van Hook took surgical pathology, Ohlmacher took embryology, and Hardie took histology. David H. Galloway, PhG, a student at Harvard in 1887–89 and a former professor in the Chicago College of Pharmacy who matriculated at P&S and graduated from there in 1893, systematized the plans, ordered the laboratory supplies, and put things in order.

When the laboratories opened in September, each student received his equipment and the key to his desk. "The early laboratory exercises," Holmes reported, "were difficult for the teachers and trying to the students. The classes were large, the rooms crowded, the work unprecedented. We had talked much together of educational rather than disciplinary methods, of the cultivation of curiosity, and of the development of mental continuity and integrity." But medical students did not appreciate the new approach. "The problem was radically pedagogic, against which method the high schools and colleges had almost completely immunized our students by their didactic system. . . . Our laboratory men tried to give as little instruction as possible to the student, but to arouse as much action as possible. . . . This strenuous novelty in medical education was not only unappreciated by many of the students . . . but it appeared ridiculous to some of the clinical teachers and to the older members of the faculty who had been for years bottle-feeding an amphitheatre full of narcotized worshippers at the shrine of Aesculapius."[94]

A year later, in September 1892, the innovative five had a new laboratory building, and they continued the fight by putting in a library of cataloged medical books and serials and adding to some of the lecture courses the seminar method with the production of theses instead of an examination. They struggled to work the students into intellectual and professional self-reliance and to cultivate an intellectual professional modesty by making them acquainted with the world's medical literature.

"Probably few of the clinical faculty of the College of Physicians and Surgeons ever knew what Ohlmacher, Hardie, Hektoen, Van Hook and I had in mind in the early years of medical laboratory teaching," Holmes surmised. "They did know, however, that it was a sort of education, strange in its paradoxical methods of withholding as far as possible all instruction and dictation, of avoiding as far as possible all catechising and of preventing as far as possible the use of catch words and reiteration. Obviously it was an education inimical to the vested interests of the stockholding professorship, and it must be choked into apnea. This was done."[95]

According to Holmes, the introduction of the laboratory method was a failure. "When the opposition to this educational method made the position of the laboratory enthusiast increasingly uncomfortable and when the demand of competing colleges called for experienced and tried out teachers, one after another of this first laboratory faculty went away. Hektoen was the first, and he went over to Rush. . . . Ohlmacher went to Cleveland. . . . Van Hook went to Northwestern where his enthusiasm was slowly drowned out by the economic and pedantic exploitation of the splendid foundation laid so patiently, ideally and devotedly by N. S. Davis, H. A. Johnson, Edmund Andrews and James J. Jewell."[96]

Holmes remained at P&S for many more years. His efforts at invigorating the college won him a reputation. "Three years of his life was spent in building up the College of Physicians and Surgeons," a local newspaper reported. "He entered the institution when it was badly run down. Within three years it had been so stimulated that it was in a prosperous condition." But Holmes lost some of his enthusiasm for pedagogic reform. His proposals to the faculty were often rebuffed, he was not elected to the board of directors, and he rarely attended meetings of the teaching faculty. He continued to write on medical topics, and he gradually became active in politics. In 1895 the People's Party nominated Holmes as their candidate for mayor of Chicago.[97]

Along with the experiment in medical education went continued revitalization of the faculty. Henry T. Byford joined the college in 1892. Born in Evansville, Indiana, in 1853, he was the son of a famous Chicago gynecologist, William H. Byford, a Rush Medical College faculty member and an ardent champion of medical education for women. When Henry was eleven years old his parents sent him abroad to take the classical course in a Berlin gymnasium. He spent one term at the old University of Chicago and then went to Williston Seminary, an all-male private school in Easthampton, Massachusetts, with both classical and scientific faculties. In 1870 Byford graduated from the scientific department. In 1873 at the age of nineteen he graduated from the Chicago Medical College. Beginning in 1890 he was for eighteen years president of the staff of Woman's Hospital of Chicago. At various times he was professor of clinical gynecology at Woman's Medical College (Northwestern University) and at the Post-Graduate Medical School, of which he was a founder. With his father he was coauthor of *The Practice of Medicine and Surgery, Applied to the Diseases and Accidents Incident to Women* (4th ed., 1888), and with John M. Baldy and others he co-authored *An American Text-Book of Gynecology, Medical and Surgical, for Practitioners and Students* (1896 and later editions). He published many papers on gynecology as well as the *Manual of Gynecology* (1895).[98]

Adolph Gehrmann also joined the faculty in 1892. Born in 1868 of German parents in Decatur, Illinois, Gehrmann moved to Chicago at the age of sixteen and in 1887 graduated from the South Division High School. As a student at the Chicago Medical College, from which he graduated in 1890, he rapidly mastered the details of the most modern scientific investigation and developed individual methods and original results under the guidance of Bayard Holmes. For the next two years he served as an intern in Cook County Hospital. Early in his career he established a laboratory in his home for personal research and also established the Columbus Medical Laboratories to assist physicians in the work of accurate diagnosis. Gehrmann was professor of bacteriology and hygiene. His original research led to the publication of highly regarded articles and monographs on bacteriological subjects.[99]

A year later John B. Murphy joined the faculty as professor of clinical surgery. Born in 1857 near Appleton, Wisconsin, Murphy was the fifth of six children of Irish Roman Catholic parents. He attended the district school and the high school in Appleton, graduating in 1876, and after briefly teaching in a district school he began to study medicine with a local preceptor. On graduating from Rush Medical College in 1879 he won an internship in Cook County Hospital by competitive examination. There he gained clinical experience under the guid-

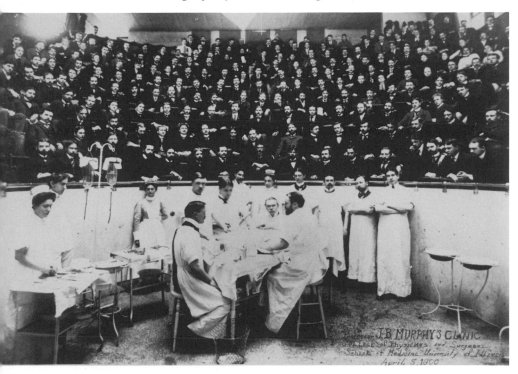

John B. Murphy's clinic. Courtesy of Special Collections and University Archives, the University Library, University of Illinois at Chicago.

ance of Christian Fenger. Murphy practiced medicine with a well-established Chicago doctor until 1882, when he pursued postgraduate study in clinics in Vienna, Munich, Berlin, and Heidelberg. Returning to his medical partnership in April 1884, he also became a lecturer in surgery at Rush Medical College. In the late 1880s he established his own office in the Loop (the business center of the city), limiting his practice to surgery. Ambitious and abrupt, Murphy was both envied and disliked. As did others, he held many academic posts. Listed as a lecturer of surgery at Rush from 1891 to 1893, Murphy then joined P&S as a clinical professor of surgery. He served on its board of directors for several years but did not always attend board meetings.

On 15 October 1892 in a paper read to the Mississippi Valley Medical Association, Murphy announced to the medical world the original research that revolutionized intestinal surgery, and in 1896, at the request of the senior class at P&S, he demonstrated the use of his world-renowned procedure, the Murphy button. He first showed how bad results often followed old methods of suturing in operations on the intestines because of the great amount of cicatrical tissue that was formed in healing, due to the fact that there was not good coaptation of the parts. The button obviated this difficulty by allowing like parts to heal together. With the assistance of two colleagues Murphy then demonstrated to the class the technique of the button operation both end-to-end and lateral. In an extended analysis Adolpho Luria described this surgical procedure as "a new cornerstone in the . . . advancement of American surgery." Murphy was in demand for appendectomies and intestinal surgery, which made him both famous and rich.[100]

Murphy was a pioneer in surgery of the appendix, gallbladder, and intestine. He maintained an experimental surgical laboratory in his home. The Murphy button for a time provided the safest technique for intestinal anastomosis throughout the world. The Murphy drip for rectal feeding was a standard for postoperative care for two generations. He introduced artificial pneumothorax treatment of tuberculosis and espoused it vigorously.[101]

Speaking to the P&S graduating class in 1896, Murphy celebrated the tremendous progress made during the nineteenth century in medicine and surgery, with emphasis on the genius "of American surgeons, yes, *of Western American surgeons.*" In 1900 Murphy became professor of clinical surgery at Northwestern. In 1905 he returned to Rush, but his colleagues did not fully accept him, so in 1908 he went back to Northwestern. Murphy, regarded by many as the foremost surgeon and teacher of his time, received many honors, including the presidency of the American Medical Association (AMA) in 1911.[102]

Murphy's brilliance, flamboyance, and independence led a biographer to call him the "stormy petrel of American surgery." He was initially proposed for election as a fellow of the American Surgical Association in 1895 but was blackballed then and on three other occasions up to 1901. In 1902 he was finally elected a fellow. Murphy, a prime adviser in the formation of the American College of Surgeons, was sufficiently aware of his own reputation to refuse a position on the founding committee.[103]

Another outstanding appointment was that of William A. Pusey. Born of Quaker parents in Elizabethtown, Kentucky, in 1865, he attended local schools and made an excellent record at Vanderbilt University, graduating with a BA. He spent another year at Vanderbilt in medical studies and literary pursuits and earned an MA. In 1886 he entered the medical college of New York University. Disillusioned by the course work, he stopped attending lectures by the end of his first year and studied alone. He graduated in 1888, among the first ten students in a class of two hundred. In 1891 he wrote an article criticizing the system of didactic lectures.[104]

To prepare himself for his specialty, dermatology, Pusey spent two years at the Skin and Cancer Hospital in New York and then went to Europe for postgraduate studies. But within a few months his father, an old-time country doctor, died, and Pusey hurried home to take over his father's practice.[105] A year later he returned to Europe and spent nearly two years continuing his studies in clinics in Vienna, Berlin, Paris, and London. Concluding that he was now sufficiently prepared to practice dermatology, in 1893 he settled in Chicago. To supplement his income he was an examiner for the New York Life Insurance Company.

In 1894 at the age of twenty-nine, Pusey joined a number of medical celebrities on the faculty of P&S as professor of dermatology. He was scheduled to give a one-hour lecture and to conduct clinics each week throughout the year for the third-year medical students. In 1896 he became secretary of the faculty.

Pusey won recognition in 1895 with two addresses that attracted attention. In "The Social Position of the Medical Profession" he offered facts to show the ways in which physicians drank cream rather than skim milk. In a speech to medical students titled "The Capacity of Medicine," he insisted that medicine had kept abreast with the advancement of other arts and sciences.

Pusey's achievements in medicine won him a reputation. He was one of the first in the United States to use roentgen rays in the treatment of cutaneous diseases. Roentgen's discovery was made in 1896, and in 1899 Pusey went to Vienna to discuss with two men their work with the therapeutic application of roentgen rays. A year later he reported on his experiments in an article titled "Lupus Treated with Roentgen Rays." In February 1902 at a meeting of the Chicago Medical Society he presented a paper titled "Cases Treated by X-rays" that was "one of the two most dramatic and exciting in the annals of the society." The medical men present acclaimed his success, and the news spread to the profession. A year later, with Eugene W. Caldwell, Pusey published *Practical Application of the Roentgen Rays in Therapeutics and Diagnosis*.[106] This book, called one of the foundations of American roentgenology, long remained standard. Pusey's pioneer work in the field of roentgen therapy was perhaps the decisive factor in establishing him as a national figure in medicine.

In 1905 Pusey suggested the use of solid carbon dioxide (carbon dioxide snow) for the treatment of certain lesions of the skin by freezing. Carbon dioxide snow was readily available and inexpensive, and it produced speedy results. Pusey pointed a way that other dermatologists followed.

For fifteen years starting in 1895 Pusey was attending dermatologist at the Cook County Hospital. He regarded his work there as his most valuable in clinical dermatology outside of his office. Pusey also saw cases at the West Side Free Dispensary of P&S. In 1907 Pusey published *The Principles and Practice of Dermatology*. Described as an indispensable volume, it went through several editions.

In addition to his expertise in radiation therapy, Pusey was an outstanding syphilologist. Early in his practice he had treated venereal diseases, but he never liked the work and gave it up as soon as he could. A few years later the organism of syphilis was discovered, and the Wasserman test was announced. In 1910 Paul Ehrlich (1854–1915) introduced a synthetic arsenical compound called salvarsan that was used for the treatment of syphilis. Confusion followed: clinical acumen gave way to the Wasserman test, and arsenic was injected indiscriminately.

Pusey, sensing the dangers, called attention to the fallacy of such practices. One of the articles he wrote on the subject, "The Present Situation in Syphilis" (1913), occasioned a great deal of discussion, much of which was severely critical. In 1915 at a congress of the AMA in San Francisco, Pusey's paper "Syphilis As a Modern Problem" considered syphilis not primarily as a disease that medicine was called on to treat but a disease that must be treated because of its impact on society. Herbert Ratner, who describes the paper as "undoubtedly the best exposition of the subject that had been made up to that time," adds that it gave Pusey "the authoritative position in syphilology and public health matters that his textbook had given him in dermatology."[107]

Pusey richly contributed to the advancement of medicine, especially dermatology. In 1912 he published *The Care of the Skin and Hair*. In 1915 he retired from P&S and became professor emeritus, but he continued his professional activities. For sixteen years he edited the *Archives of Dermatology and Syphilology*, described as one of the great journals of medicine. He published more than one hundred articles on medical subjects in addition to *The History of Dermatology* (1933), the first work on the subject in the English language; *The History and Epidemiology of Syphilis* (1933); and *High Lights in the History of Chicago Medicine* (1940).[108] Pusey held leadership positions in many medical societies and was president of both the American Dermatological Association and the AMA.

Thomas A. Davis, who was born in Ontario, Canada, in 1858, graduated from P&S with honors in 1885. He gained experience as an intern at Cook County Hospital and as an assistant to Christian Fenger. In 1887 Davis entered private practice and became a lecturer in surgery at P&S. In 1896 he became a full professor of surgery.[109]

College officials had long acknowledged a need for a hospital under their control, and in January 1896 several physician entrepreneurs formed the West Side Hospital Corporation with a capital stock of fifty thousand dollars. Two-thirds of the incorporators—including D. A. K. Steele, president; John B. Murphy, vice president; Thomas A. Davis, secretary; and Charles Davison, treasurer—were members of the P&S faculty, while some others were not directly connected with the college. In February the incorporators purchased the Post-Graduate Medical School building next to the college laboratory building at 819-823 West Harrison Street. The new owners obtained immediate possession of the two upper floors, which were furnished to receive patients by the following May. Work began on an enclosed passageway connecting P&S and the new hospital building. Members of the Post-Graduate Medical School then divided. One part relocated on the South Side of the city, while the other part occupied the lower floors of the building and took a new name, the West Chicago Post-Graduate School and Policlinic, also known as the Chicago Clinical School.[110]

Those involved in the planning thought that the hospital would be under the auspices of the Young Men's Christian Association, but after discussion of how

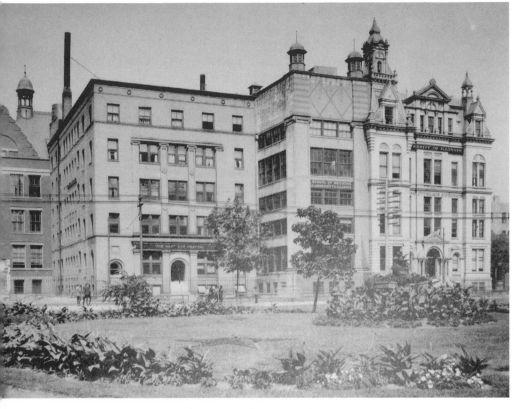

West Side Hospital. Courtesy of Special Collections and University Archives, the University Library, University of Illinois at Chicago.

best to proceed the planners decided that West Side Hospital was to be run in connection with P&S but as a private corporation separate from the college. The authorities converted the upper floors into a hospital with two operating rooms and eventually 150 beds. The hospital was intended to provide clinical instruction to P&S students and medical assistance to the poor of the vicinity. The staff included five surgeons, four gynecologists, two oculists and aurists, an orthopedic surgeon, and a doctor of internal medicine. Physicians in the city could bring their cases to the hospital and have full charge of their treatment. The founders intended to use profits from paying patients to maintain free beds for the large number of needy people on the West Side. West Side Hospital was the first hospital in Chicago owned and conducted by physicians and surgeons.[111]

A strong faculty and a teaching hospital deserved a worthy student body. We gain some idea of its quality by examining the eighty-seven members of the 1893 graduating class. The oldest one, born in 1850, was forty-three years old when he graduated, and four others were born in the 1850s. Fifty-three had been born in the 1860s and twelve in the 1870s. The average age cannot be calculated, but callow youths were not a majority. We know the birth place of thirty-nine (45 percent) of the graduates. Seven were foreign born: two each in Canada and Germany and one each in Ireland, Scotland, and Norway. One student each was born in Vermont, New Jersey, and Maryland. Twenty-nine (33 percent) were midwestern in origin. Ten listed their birth place as Illinois and another three as Chicago. Iowa was the birth place of six, Ohio of four, Minnesota of two, and Indiana, Kentucky, Missouri, and Wisconsin of one each. P&S, a magnet, drew students from widely scattered places.

Many members of this graduating class were formally well prepared. Thirty-four of the eighty-seven (39 percent) had more, sometimes considerably more, than a high school education. At least twenty had prepared in college for varying lengths of time. Three men had attended foreign colleges, among them Heriot-Watt College in Edinburgh, Scotland; the University of Aberdeen, Scotland; and Aars and Voss College in Christiana (later Oslo), Norway. The Norwegian student took a BA in Oslo and then attended the University of Minnesota for a year. Three graduates had prepared in the eastern United States: one had trained in the medical department of the University of Buffalo; one had a BA from Alfred University in Alfred, New York; and one had studied at Harvard for two years (1887–89) and became a lecturer on chemistry at P&S (1892–93). Others had prepared in colleges scattered around the Midwest: Iowa, Illinois, Indiana, Kansas, Minnesota, Missouri, Nebraska, Ohio, and Wisconsin. In addition, several graduates had either attended or graduated from a medical college. One man had attended Chicago Medical College (he previously had a DDS from the University of Michigan), while another had an MD from Chicago Medical College. One man had attended the Homeopathic Medical College in Chicago, three others had attended Rush Medical College for one or two years, and another had a certificate from Rush. Even more impressive, five graduates already had MDs: one from the University of Michigan (1892); one from the University of Virginia (1892); one from Bennett Medical College (1877); one from the College of Physicians and Surgeons of Keokuk, Iowa (1873); and one from the Homeopathic Medical College in Chicago (1886). P&S attracted a variety of students who were at least formally well prepared. They deserved able teachers.[112]

Carl Beck, a notable addition to the faculty, exemplified the transformation in medicine that is the theme of this book. For years American medical graduates had found it necessary to go to Europe for advanced study in their specialties, but in time the United States itself became a center of medical research and education. Carl Beck, a European-trained surgeon, immigrated to the United States and made an impact on American medicine.[113] Beck was born in 1864 in Milin, Bohemia (later Czechoslovakia). His parents died when Beck was sixteen, leaving him to care for three younger brothers and a sister in conditions of stringent poverty. He attended a gymnasium where he became proficient in

Greek and Latin. In 1889 after working his way through school by tutoring other students, he graduated summa cum laude with a medical degree from the Royal German Carlo-Ferdinandia University in Prague. Beck subsequently served as an assistant in the Pathological Institute under Hans Chiari, a noted pathologist, and at the Schauta clinic in Prague under Professor Carl I. Gussenbauer. Beck was also an assistant in the surgical clinic of Theodor Billroth in Vienna. A traveling fellowship enabled Beck to visit European surgical clinics and pathologic institutes.

Owing to an attack of hemoptysis ascribed to tuberculosis, Beck went to sea as a surgeon on a ship of the Red Star Line plying between Antwerp and New York. On his second voyage he met Henry P. Newman, a P&S faculty member, who invited him to teach in Chicago. In 1891 Beck accepted a position as instructor of surgery at the Post-Graduate Medical School on the West Side with which Newman was connected. Surprised to learn that the position paid no salary, Beck practiced medicine to support himself. His facility in European languages enabled him to build a large surgical practice in the polyglot Chicago of the day. He brought two of his brothers to join him and saw them through P&S. Joseph C. Beck (b. 1870) graduated in 1895, and Emil G. Beck (b. 1866) graduated in 1896.

Carl Beck joined the P&S faculty in 1898 as an instructor in surgical pathology. A year later he became a full professor. He was probably the first Jew on the faculty. Beck served as attending surgeon at Cook County Hospital along with the surgical greats Fenger, Senn, and Murphy and was part of a group that conducted experimental operations in the animal laboratory. He was one of the first to use bismuth subnitrate in petrolatum jelly to visualize sinus tracts and fistulas with roentgenograms, to develop a repair of hypospadias, and to transplant the ureters into the appendix and colon. A successful orthopedic surgeon, Beck contributed to the scientific literature, notably *Principles of Surgical Pathology* (1905) and *The Crippled Hand and the Arm* (1925). He was a founding member of the American College of Surgeons.

In July 1904 Carl Beck and his brother Joseph, who joined the P&S faculty that year as associate professor of surgery in otology, rhinology, and laryngology, went to Montreal for a prearranged meeting with Alexis Carrel, a young French scientist who was there to attend a medical congress. Carrel presented a paper on vascular operations that stirred great interest in the subject. Carl Beck invited Carrel to come to Chicago to work with him. Carrel arrived in Chicago the following September. He was a guest in the home of Carl Beck for over a year. The arrangement was for Carrel to work with Beck not only in the small animal laboratory but also in the operating room and in practice. Photographs have been published showing Carrel giving an anesthetic while Beck operated. Beck and Carrel experimented on dogs in an effort to form a new esophagus from the greater curvature of the stomach. Beck was determined to find a way to replace the esophagus of a patient who, as a child, had swallowed lye and whom Beck had operated on at the Gussenbauer Clinic in Prague. By the time they had perfected the operation, the patient, an adult who was running the elevator at the West Side Hospital, had disappeared. Although Beck and Carrel published reports of their procedure in 1905, Amza Jianu, a Romanian surgeon who had visited the Beck laboratory, reported it as his own in 1910. The gastrosotomy is now called the Beck-Jianu operation.

Beck gave Carrel his start in Chicago, but as an assistant Carrel left much to be desired. He read English well, but his lack of command of spoken English was a drawback in patient care. Beck introduced Carrel to George N. Steward of the Hull Laboratory of Physiology at the University of Chicago. There Carrel and Charles C. Guthrie worked together for about six months during which time they jointly wrote several papers, and then Carrel left for a position at the Rockefeller Institute. In 1908 Carl Beck was asked to propose a candidate for the Nobel Prize in Physiology and Medicine. Beck recommended Carrel. While at Chicago, Carrel had perfected his triangulation technique for vessel anastomosis that, together with his work in transfusion and organ transplantation, won him the Nobel Prize for Physiology and Medicine in 1912. Carrel was the first scientist working in an American laboratory to win this prize.[114]

Joseph C. Beck was professor of otology and rhino-laryngology at P&S. His contributions to medical literature included numerous publications on neoplasms, plastic surgery, and pathology. A tonsillectomy known as the Beck tonsil snare or ring was his invention. Emil G. Beck, a specialist in roentgenology, introduced new methods of treating tuberculous sinuses and abscessed cavities by the injection of bismuth paste (Beck's method). The three brothers together founded and operated North Chicago Hospital.[115]

Carl Beck retained his roots in European culture. "A magnetic personality," his son recalled, "he demanded unquestioning obedience and recognition of his authority and that of a few respected friends. His dogma demanded rational thought, logic, and self control. . . . He knew no doubt. Strictly observing Sundays, he wore a Prince Albert coat with grey-striped trousers and attended . . . the Rationalist services in Chicago's Orchestra Hall." Beck believed only what could be proved, his son wrote, and doubted everything else. The senior Beck typified the philosophical system known as positivism, which attracted certain kinds of educated people in the late nineteenth century. Beck and his wife frequently entertained at small formal dinner parties in their home where those present spoke French or Italian. Among his memorable guests were the sculptor Lorado Taft; Jan Masaryk, later president of Czechoslovakia; and Albert Einstein.[116]

Beck was friendly with the Mayo brothers, who established a private group practice of medicine that brought fame to Rochester, Minnesota. Beck first met Charles H. Mayo after a postgraduate clinic that Beck presented in Chicago. Dr. Mayo stayed to discuss what had been described. Amazed by the younger

Mayo's knowledge of surgical procedures, Beck told Nicholas Senn, his former teacher, about his encounter with Charles Mayo. Senn, who knew that William J. Mayo had a broad knowledge of surgery, suggested that Beck accept Dr. Charles Mayo's invitation to visit Rochester and observe the brothers' work, which Beck did. He was favorably impressed with the Mayo brothers' work and their friendliness and formed a long-lasting friendship with the Mayo family. He visited them in Rochester periodically. In a birthday greeting to Beck in March 1939, they paid tribute to the position Beck had occupied "in guiding the advancement of medical and surgical science in our country." Beck responded by saying, "Next to my brothers, I have always regarded you as the most valuable friends I have had in my lifetime."[117]

In 1908 after seven weeks visiting medical schools in France, Germany, and Austria, Beck returned to the United States firm in his conviction that American medical schools were far in advance of their transatlantic rivals. "There is no doubt," Beck averred, "that we are ahead of them not only in methods of teaching but in scientific achievement as well."[118]

In the late 1890s shortly after Carl Beck joined the faculty, P&S responded to the changes taking place in medical education by increasing the admissions requirements. In addition to a certificate of good moral character from a reputable physician and a diploma or certificate from a recognized college or high school or the equivalent, matriculants were asked to pass a satisfactory examination in English, physics, mathematics, and Latin. In Latin, students were to be examined on the rudiments of Latin grammar and to translate Caesar's Commentaries from Latin into English. The entrance examination was open to the public. These requirements were probably not taken seriously.

Each academic year consisted of a winter term of twenty-eight weeks and a spring term of eleven weeks. The plan of instruction included four annual courses. The studies of the first year were biology, embryology, human anatomy, histology, materia medica, general chemistry, and physiology, a total of twelve and one-fourth credits. The studies of the second year were human anatomy, general pathology, pathological anatomy, bacteriology, surgical pathology, general therapeutics, organic chemistry, and toxology, a total of eleven and one-half credits. In the third year the courses were orthopedic surgery, physical diagnosis, practice of medicine, practice of surgery, surgical anatomy, dental surgery, medical jurisprudence, gynecology, obstetrics, dermatology, and hospital and dispensary clinics, a total of twelve and one-half credits. The fourth-year studies were practice of medicine, practice of surgery, operative surgery, obstetrics, diseases of the chest, gynecology, genito-urinary surgery and venereal diseases, ophthalmology, otology, laryngology and rhinology, diseases of children, diseases of the mind and nervous system, hospital and dispensary clinics, medical clinic, surgical clinic (in the college, with Steele), surgical clinic (in Cook County Hospital), surgical clinic (in the college, with Holmes), surgical clinic (in Cook

Table 2. Matriculants and graduates, 1892 to 1897

	Matriculants	Graduates
1892–93	186	87
1893–94	285	93
1894–95	244	80
1895–96	233	54
1896–97	309	83

County Hospital, with Davis), gynecological clinic, eye clinic, and nerve clinic, a total of seventeen and three-fourths credits. The work of four years came to fifty-four credits, each credit consisting of sixty recitation or lecture hours or of twice that number of laboratory or clinic hours.[119]

Despite internal tensions, the number of matriculants and the number of graduates had remained fairly steady during the 1880s, as we saw earlier. In the 1890s with the reinvigoration of the college, the number of matriculants gradually increased, and the number of graduates, with one exception, varied within a narrow range. These trends are illustrated in Table 2.[120] In addition, thirteen people graduated from the practitioners' course in 1894–95, and ten graduated the following year.

The college gained considerable strength during the years of stability, and its future prospects appeared to be favorable. In fact, however, the sun was setting on proprietary medical colleges. Medicine was being established on a foundation of basic sciences, and universities were becoming the institutional home of medical research and education. Perceptive observers at P&S read the signs of the times.

CHAPTER 5

Affiliation

The College and the University

Bayard Holmes discerned the shape of the future, and in 1891 he took the initiative in seeking a connection between the College of Physicians and Surgeons (P&S) and the University of Illinois. On 8 December he pleaded his case in a meeting with the board of trustees but failed to arouse any interest. Holmes was not alone in perceiving that proprietary medical colleges and universities needed each other. In 1892 the Democrat John P. Altgeld was elected governor of Illinois. He wanted to make the state university, the capstone of the state's public school system, "a complete University in the highest meaning of the term." Apparently believing that a true university should have a medical school, Altgeld was eager to affiliate P&S with the University of Illinois since P&S was the only one of the leading medical colleges in the city that was not already connected to a university. Thus Altgeld opened negotiations with Quine (the dean) and Holmes, and they made a proposition to the university.[1]

The University of Illinois, a land-grant college, had opened in 1868. It developed slowly for a quarter century and was primarily a school for engineers. In the early 1890s the board of trustees decided to expand the course offerings, attract more women students, and gain institutional visibility. To lead in a new direction the board searched for a new president for three years. Meanwhile, in December 1892 Acting Regent Thomas J. Burrill informed the board that a movement was afoot to consolidate the two leading colleges of medicine in Chicago (Rush and Northwestern) and to make the combined institution a department of the University of Chicago. This movement, Burrill added, might have a bearing on the question of establishing a medical department in connection with the University of Illinois.[2]

In 1894 Andrew S. Draper, who had made a reputation as a school administrator in New York state and in Cleveland, Ohio, became the new president. Draper had no college or university experience before taking office. During his ten-year tenure the university acquired the structure of a university by adding professional schools, but it lacked the spirit of a university in that both the trust-ees and the president refused to encourage or support research.

In 1894 the board appointed James E. Armstrong, its president, and Draper to consider the matter of bringing a medical college in Chicago, or elsewhere, into relations with the university. They reported that "the interests of the University, of higher professional education in Illinois, and of medical practice, would be promoted by such a step." After investigating various medical institutions in Chicago, Armstrong and Draper advised that the school best suited for such an arrangement was P&S, the only one of the three prominent medical colleges in Chicago not already affiliated with universities. The board adopted the report. It then heard from Quine. In late December, Quine observed, the board of direc-tors of P&S had agreed to sell the property and goodwill of the college to the Board of Trustees of the University of Illinois for a price not to exceed $160,000, and the stockholders had approved the decision. The university's board favored the absorption of P&S by the university for its fair market value and agreed to apply to the legislature for an appropriation to pay for the same. The board of directors of P&S then agreed to sell the property and goodwill of the college at the stipulated price and not to engage in negotiations with any other univer-sity pending the action of the legislature. On 12 February 1895 the university's board approved the text of a bill for the purpose to be introduced in the General Assembly.[3]

On 7 March 1895 David Revell, a Chicago Republican, introduced in the House a bill for an act to enable the University of Illinois to acquire the prop-erty and goodwill of P&S and to establish a professional medical department in connection with the university. The bill was referred to the Committee on Ap-propriations, where it died.[4] The people of Illinois were not yet ready to move in this direction. Time passed before Illinois legislators recognized that medical education was an integral part of a university and that the state had an obliga-tion to support it.

Noting the failure of the bill, E. Fletcher Ingals, the comptroller of Rush, who feared competition and kept himself well informed about P&S, informed Presi-dent Harper of the University of Chicago about it. "From very reliable sources," Ingals wrote, "I have to report that there seems to be no prospect whatever that the Chicago College of Physicians & Surgeons will succeed in its effort to attach itself to the State University. I may be over confident, but think I have good reason for my belief."[5]

Renewed efforts were made to unite the two schools. The P&S board em-powered Quine to negotiate a lease on behalf of the college. He informed his colleagues that the lease required the resignation of all faculty members with no guarantee of reemployment, although no change in the faculty was contem-plated. In late March the P&S stockholders approved the terms of the lease, and on 1 April 1897 the two parties signed an understanding in which the university agreed to lease the property of the college for a period of four years beginning on 21 April 1897 in order to establish a medical department in Chicago. The lease gave the university and the college the use of each other's name.[6]

On 11 March Ingals sent President Harper a newspaper clipping describing the lease, in which Harper had expressed interest. "This on its face," said Ingals, "appears a bad thing for other medical schools, but it seems to me the advantages are more than the disadvantages. The State of Ill. cannot be allowed to maintain a poor school or even to endow one, therefore, this school must hereafter hold up the grade. If it receives no financial aid it will not be an objectionable competitor."[7]

When the lease was signed, conditions in the college seemed favorable. To be sure, internal problems intruded. In 1896, for example, John A. Benson, professor of physiology, was fired for being absent eighteen out of twenty-five hours during the term. In elections for the board of directors in May 1898 John B. Murphy led in the vote, while Bayard Holmes trailed three others. Perhaps his continuing call for internal reforms irritated colleagues. In 1898, with earnings exceeding expenses, the corporation declared a 3 percent dividend on stock, followed in 1900 with a 10 percent dividend. Murphy, who had been accumulating stock, now owned seventy shares. And yet, for whatever reason, in 1899 Steele advanced the college $25,800.[8]

The progress of the times and an increased number of students required changes in the medical school. In 1899 both the faculty and the curriculum were reorganized. The new measures included establishment of a physiological laboratory, dropping four men from the faculty list (they had not been active teachers for years, and their names had been carried in recognition of their property interests in the corporation), accepting the resignations of five professors, and transferring seven faculty members to other departments. The chairs of hygiene, otology, dental surgery, and general diagnosis were abolished as separate departments; hygiene was united with bacteriology, otology was united with rhinology and laryngology, dental surgery was included in junior surgery, and general diagnosis became microscopical and chemical diagnosis.

The school year was to be divided into three terms of sixteen weeks each, credit was to be given for not more than two terms of attendance in any year, and attendance for at least eight terms was to be required. This change would require attendance of eight months a year for four years instead of seven months as hitherto. The amphitheater was to give way to the classroom and the lecture to personal instruction.

The reorganization led to discord in the faculty, owing in large measure to intolerance on the part of some faculty members to the new methods of administration, Quine observed, but he believed that the troubles had been cured and the faculty organization had emerged stronger than ever in respect to "unity of purpose" and "professional standing and efficiency."[9]

Along with reorganization, P&S sought to define its relations with the university.[10] In April 1899 William A. Pusey raised the question of the locus of ultimate authority within the university. Basically, Draper replied, the board of trustees had authority over appointments to the instructional staff, setting salaries, and determining educational policy. And yet Draper and the university wanted to give the medical college as much freedom to make policy as possible.[11]

On 5 May 1899 D. A. K. Steele and Walter S. Christopher, who had joined the faculty in 1892 as professor of diseases of children, spoke to the board of trustees in relation to what was described as "certain matters concerning the School of Medicine." The board referred their concern to its Committee on the School of Medicine, asking it to investigate and report and to consider at the same time "the entire question of sustaining a medical school."[12] Also in May, a committee of the medical faculty devised a set of rules on relations with the university, and the faculty adopted them.[13]

Quine had labored under the strain of reorganizing the medical school and its relations with the university, and on 12 May he submitted his resignation as dean of the School of Medicine and professor of the practice of medicine to take effect on or before the forthcoming meeting of the board of trustees. Apparently Quine's health was not good, and he felt overworked; he had gone to Finch House in Kilbourn, Wisconsin. Draper, the faculty and students of the medical college, and the board of trustees all requested that Quine withdraw his resignation.[14]

Meanwhile, on 13 June Steele and Oscar King of the School of Medicine presented to the board of trustees the rules proposed by the medical faculty regarding relations between the medical school and the university, and the chairman of the board's Committee on the School of Medicine submitted sundry papers regarding the reorganization then going on in the medical school.[15]

The earnings of P&S had largely increased owing to its affiliation with the university, and board members thought that the university should share in the increase. At its meeting on 13 June the trustees instructed their Committee on the School of Medicine to confer with the stockholders of P&S to determine the sum for which said stockholders would dispose of their stock to the university and indicated that if a satisfactory sum could be agreed on, such a portion of the surplus earnings as might be agreed on be set aside each year as the property of the university to be used as a sinking fund with which the university might in time purchase said stock and become the owner of the property and the school.[16]

These developments alarmed the medical faculty. "The prosperity of the school," a resolution adopted by the medical faculty on 19 June declared, "the devotion of the individual members of the faculty and the safety of their property interests require that the wishes of the faculty should be consulted in all matters pertaining to the filling of vacancies in and dismissal from the corps of instruction, and in the expenditures of all monies from the treasury of the School of Medicine so long as the school remains affiliated with the University through the instrumentality of a lease."[17]

On 27 June Quine withdrew his resignation as dean and asked for a leave of absence from official duties for a year. The board granted his request.[18] On that same day the board adopted "Rules to Govern Relations between the School of Medicine and the University" based on those drafted by the medical faculty. The rules stipulated that the general statutes of the university applied to the School of Medicine with some exceptions during the continuance of any lease between the college and the university. The rules divided the faculty of the school into a teaching faculty and an executive faculty. The former, consisting of the president of the university and the entire instructional corps, was given legislative functions pertaining exclusively to the internal work of the school. The latter, which included the president of the university and members of the teaching faculty who held stock in P&S, was to have an advisory relation to university officials and the board of trustees with respect to all matters pertaining to the School of Medicine. The executive faculty was empowered to nominate from among its members an actuary, a dean, and a secretary for the school; the nominations were made through the president of the university to the board of trustees. The executive faculty also had the right to nominate candidates for faculty positions and to cooperate through official channels in determining the school's educational policy. The dean, with the advice and consent of the executive faculty, was to deal with resignations or dismissals from the faculty and to recommend the discontinuance or establishment of chairs of instruction or the change of title of any chair. The actuary, with the advice and consent of the executive faculty, was to recommend the salary for faculty members and employees of the school. Finally, a sum not exceeding one thousand dollars from the net earnings of the School of Medicine of the previous year, not otherwise appropriated, could be spent on athletics if authorized by the executive faculty. The rules spelled out the limited extent to which the university controlled the School of Medicine.[19]

In September 1899 with time on the lease running out and optimism about affiliation high, a university committee conferred with the officers and stockholders of P&S about a permanent union with a view to the university acquiring title to the property without assuming financial responsibility and without spending the state's money. The negotiations were lengthy, after which John P. Wilson, a Chicago lawyer, drew up a contract. When the committee reported on 10 January 1900, each member of the board was called on for an expression of opinion. The contract put the value of the property, equipment, and goodwill of the college at $217,000 and provided that the entire property be leased to the university for twenty-five years, or until the agreement was terminated, at $12,000 a year plus taxes and assessments. The net earnings were to be divided, two-thirds for the stockholders and one-third for the university with the latter

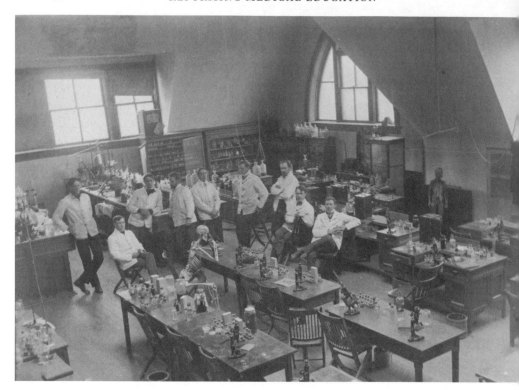

Physiology and Biophysics Laboratory, Urbana. Courtesy of the University of Illinois at Urbana-Champaign Archives.

going into a sinking fund to be used to purchase the property. During the pe-riod of the lease the university was to use the revenues of the college to advance medical science without being confined to any branch of sectarian medicine. The agreement did not bind the state in any way financially. Under the contract the executive faculty of the College of Medicine was to have an advisory rela-tion to university officials with respect to all matters pertaining to the college, and it was to have the right to nominate candidates to fill vacancies in the corps of instruction. The contract for a new lease for twenty-five years dating from 1 May 1900 to 30 April 1925 was executed on 9 February 1900. Thus the School of Medicine officially became the University of Illinois College of Medicine.[20]

The union of P&S and the university and the acquisition of the college's property by the university was hailed as a great accomplishment.[21] The board of trustees entered into the agreement believing that the university could real-ize annually the amount needed to pay off the purchase price in twenty-five years. But the medical school had outgrown its original quarters, and the cor-poration, with the approval of the university, purchased for $186,000 the West Division High School, a huge building standing back-to-back with the original

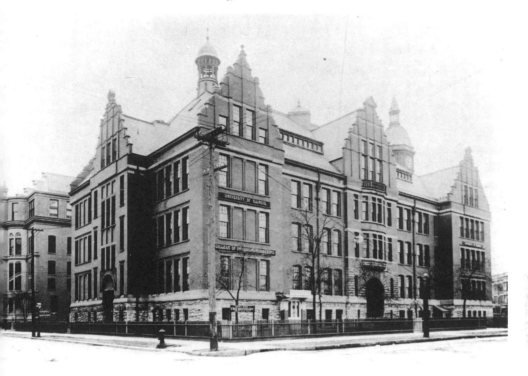

The University of Illinois College of Medicine building. Courtesy of the University of Illinois at Urbana-Champaign Archives.

P&S building and facing north at Congress and Honore streets. The authorities converted the school into a modern medical college at an anticipated cost of $70,000 to $100,000, confident that the facility would yield sufficient net income to cover the increased obligations. In addition, the corporation, with the approval of the trustees, acquired the Illinois School of Dentistry and converted the original medical college building into the College of Dentistry. In June 1901, however, the original building was partially destroyed by fire. Repairs, needed improvements, and expansion ran up the costs, and with the reform of medical education along scientific lines, expenses grew faster than income. The university was not receiving a sufficient annual return to be able to liquidate its debt in twenty-five years.[22]

Financial conditions in the medical school were deteriorating, but those close to the scene found this hard to admit. In 1898 and 1899 the corporation authorized payment of a 3 percent dividend twice each year. In April 1900 officials increased the capital stock to $217,000 and the number of shares to 2,170, valued at $100 each, and declared a dividend of two and two-fifths of a share for each outstanding share. Thus John B. Murphy, who had owned 70 shares, now owned 238 shares. Steele, Quine, Byford, and Newman, each of whom had owned 27

shares, now owned 92 shares each. In addition, the board declared a 10 percent dividend. In September, to husband their resources, the directors did not
declare a dividend. In 1900–1901 the college paid the stockholders $13,066 in
dividends. A year later the college suffered a net loss of $8,786, but the directors
paid $6,508 in dividends. In 1902 the authorities had to borrow $30,000 to meet
current obligations. In 1904 they paid no dividend, but a year later they declared
a 3 percent dividend twice.[23]

Although the financial condition of the college was worsening, prominent
faculty members were, to use Pusey's words, drinking cream rather than skim
milk. Most of them had lucrative practices, several were medical entrepreneurs,
and the loss of dividends from the college did not threaten their standard of living. Steele and Quine had homes in the Prairie Avenue district south of the Loop
where Chicago's mercantile and industrial titans lived (Steele was at 2920 Indiana Avenue, and Quine was at 3160 Indiana Avenue). T. A. Davis and Charles
Davison both lived on West Jackson Boulevard, and Davis had a summer place at
Delavan, Wisconsin. Pusey and perhaps Davison employed a chauffeur. John B.
Murphy, who was "probably making more money at the present time than any
other surgeon in the world," spent extravagantly. At a meeting in Chicago of
the American Gynecological Association, Murphy invited all the members and
visitors to an excursion on Lake Michigan. As reported, "fully two hundred and
fifty guests attended. The steamer was exquisitely fitted up for the reception—
music and flowers being most conspicuous until the gentlemen's smoking room
was reached; there a huge bank of flowers concealed a barrel of imported Wuerz-
burger beer with its silver spigot protruding from the mass of roses and forget-
me-nots—a barrel frequently replaced and never quiescent during the trip!" In
the ladies' cabin a similar fountain gave forth Mumm's champagne. At dusk the
banquet room was opened, and all feasted on good things prepared by "the chief
and his assistants." Murphy paid for it all. An intimate friend of Murphy thought
the affair would cost Murphy about five thousand dollars. Could he afford it? "I
should say so," the friend replied, "it's only a day's work for [Murphy]." Since he
had gained fame for appendectomies he had earned fifty thousand dollars in
three months for abdominal sections alone.[24]

By October 1902 the board of trustees was alarmed at the financial results of
the previous two years and the prospects for the current year. The board's Committee on the Medical School, declaring that the State of Illinois could not with
honor continue to employ a private corporation to educate the young men and
women of the state, recommended that the contract between the university and
the College of Medicine be fulfilled as early as possible.[25]

Several noteworthy appointments were made around the turn of the century. Charles Davison, who was born in 1858 in Lake County, Illinois, earned
a master's degree from Northwestern University and an MD (1883) from the
Chicago Medical College. A surgeon, he was an intern at Cook County Hospital

in 1883–84 and attending surgeon at several hospitals in Chicago in the 1890s. He began at P&S in 1897 as professor of surgical anatomy, became an adjunct professor of surgery in 1900, and became professor of surgery in 1904. Friends of P&S engineered Davison's election to the board of trustees in 1904 so that he could serve as liaison between the medical school and the university. He served on the board from 1905 to 1911.[26]

Albert J. Ochsner (1858–1925) was the child of Wisconsin pioneers who emigrated from near Zurich, Switzerland. Educated first in the county schools, he earned a BS from the University of Wisconsin in 1884, the honor man of his class. As an undergraduate he became greatly interested in the comparatively new subject of microscopy. Graduating from Rush Medical College in 1886, he spent two years studying in Vienna and Berlin and on returning home became a surgeon under the inspiration of Moses Gunn and in association with Nicholas Senn. Ochsner was a member of the Rush Medical College faculty from 1886 to 1895. E. Fletcher Ingals described him as an excellent surgeon and a superior teacher for small classes but not well fitted for lectures because he was a poor talker. In 1900 Ochsner became professor of clinical surgery at P&S. In that year he was elected to the chairmanship of the Section on Surgery of the American Medical Association, and in 1902 he was elected a fellow of the American Surgical Association. Ochsner served on the faculty of P&S until his death in 1925. He authored a number of valuable treatises on surgery and held high offices in various surgical societies. "One of the most eminent surgeons in the United States," Ochsner contributed to making Chicago a national surgical center.[27]

Bernard Fantus, who was born in Budapest, Austria-Hungary, in 1874, emigrated with his family to Chicago, where he worked in a drugstore and studied pharmacology. His family was too poor to pay the son's medical school expenses, so the father agreed to do all the printing for P&S in return for tuition. Fantus graduated from P&S in 1899 and interned at Cook County Hospital. In 1901 he began a practice on the West Side and accepted a faculty appointment at P&S as professor of pharmacology and therapeutics. For most of his professional life he was an attending physician and the director of therapeutics at Cook County Hospital. One of his notable accomplishments while there was the development of the world's first blood bank. Previously when blood transfusion was required, donors had to be called for, and a little blood had to be drawn from half a dozen volunteers to find one of the blood type to match that of the patient. Patients not infrequently expired before blood suitable for transfusion could be obtained. Visiting Russia, David J. Davis, then dean of the medical school, had been greatly impressed by some of the work he had seen there, particularly with cadaveric blood. He encouraged Fantus to study this new form of therapy, and in the scientific climate that Ludvig Hektoen had helped create the first blood bank in the United States was established at Cook County Hospital in 1927.[28]

George P. Dreyer was still another valuable addition to the faculty. Born in Baltimore in 1866, he earned a BA at Johns Hopkins University and then took up graduate work in physiology and chemistry, receiving a PhD from Johns Hopkins in physiology in 1890. Dreyer pursued pathology and clinical studies at the Johns Hopkins Hospital and matriculated at the College of Physicians and Surgeons of Baltimore. In 1900 he became professor of physiology at P&S, where he inaugurated laboratory instruction in physiology. He published a number of studies on physiology in various medical journals.[29] As dean of the junior faculty in the College of Medicine, Dreyer inspired confidence.

Charles S. Bacon was born in Spring Valley, Wisconsin, in 1856. He attended public schools and the Whitewater State Normal School and graduated from Beloit College in 1878. He taught high school for three years and then entered the Chicago Medical College, from which he graduated in 1884. He served as an intern for eighteen months at Cook County Hospital, where he focused on obstetrics. In 1886 he opened his own medical office, and in 1889 he became an instructor at the Chicago Policlinic, where he became a full professor in 1891. Bacon pursued gynecological studies in Berlin, Paris, and London and later studied obstetrics in Prague, Vienna, and Munich. In 1903 he became professor of obstetrics and head of the department of obstetrics and gynecology at P&S. His writings consisted of papers presented to medical societies. He worked closely with President James in the effort to raise funds to support the university's College of Medicine. Bacon was a member of the Ethical Culture Society and a man of principle. During World War I as an advocate of peace, he joined the Socialist Party.[30]

These new appointees were well educated, many had pursued advanced studies in Europe, and all but Dreyer had practiced medicine before casting their lot with P&S.

Women in medicine increasingly became a force to reckon with in the nineteenth century.[31] They had a difficult time in establishing their rightful place in American medicine, but they did so more easily and more quickly in the United States than in many but not all European countries.[32] Women gained a foothold in medicine in Chicago at an uneven pace.

Although the women's rights movement gained momentum in early nineteenth-century America, most medical colleges refused to appoint women to the faculty or admit them as students. In 1847 Geneva College in Geneva, New York, admitted Elizabeth Blackwell as a student, for some a shocking event. Blackwell finished the two-year course with honors in 1849, the first woman to graduate in medicine in the United States. In 1847 Harvard refused to admit Harriot K. Hunt as a medical student. A year later, in reaction, Samuel Gregory with his brother George established the New England Female College in Boston. It was the first medical college for women in the world. It began as an eclectic school, but in 1874 it merged with a homeopathic school, Boston

University School of Medicine. Other schools for women followed. In Chicago in 1870 Mary Harris Thompson with the help of William H. Byford and Norman Bridge of Rush Medical College, William G. Dyas of the U.S. Sanitary Commission, and Charles W. Earle cooperated in founding Woman's Hospital Medical College, incorporated in 1887 as Woman's Medical College. In 1892 Northwestern University absorbed the college, and it was renamed Northwestern University Woman's Medical School. Despite the optimism of all involved about the future of the school, the lure of coeducation led to falling enrollments. By 1899 six medical colleges in Chicago admitted women, and in 1902 the Northwestern University Woman's Medical School ceased to exist.[33]

In the late nineteenth century women began to gain greater opportunities in medicine. In 1870 the University of Michigan medical school admitted its first woman student, Amanda Sanford. But women attended some classes separately, and Sanford was not entirely welcome. At her graduation she was "hooted and showered with abusive notes" by male students. When the Johns Hopkins Medical School opened in 1893, it admitted women students because a few influential Baltimore women had raised an endowment for the school on the condition that women be admitted on the same terms as men.[34]

The three university-related medical colleges in Chicago perpetuated the traditional bias against women in medicine. In 1852 Rush Medical College admitted Emily Blackwell, who had been refused admission to eleven medical schools for one reason or another. Blackwell spent her first year at Rush, but the Illinois State Medical Society berated Rush for admitting a woman, so Rush refused to allow Blackwell to finish the two-year course.[35]

Years later Rush cautiously opened its doors to women. In the 1888–89 session Effa V. Davis was a clinical assistant professor of obstetrics, perhaps the first woman on the faculty.[36] Writing confidentially, E. Fletcher Ingals informed President Harper that P&S was trying to hire Davis. Rush was paying Davis fifty dollars, said Ingals, while P&S was offering her seventy-five dollars. Rush could not afford to lose her.[37] In 1898 Julia D. Merrill, an 1895 graduate of Woman's Medical College, was on the Rush faculty, and in 1905 she was an associate in the department that dealt with diseases of children.[38]

Rush apparently graduated its first women students, Ora Byrd Stanard and Pearl Hubert, in 1896.[39] A move to admit more women students was considered for practical reasons. President Harper thought that the best way to introduce quiet and order among rowdy Rush medical students was to "get hold" of women from Woman's Medical College. Ingals agreed. He wanted to recruit such women at Woman's Medical College as were qualified to enter Rush, even if Rush had to aid some of them financially. (Rush fees were higher than those at Woman's Medical College.) The majority of women at Woman's Medical College, Ingals was informed, wished to come to Rush.[40]

The Chicago Medical College, later the Northwestern University Medical School, admitted three women students in the autumn of 1869, but strong opposition to their presence ended the experiment in coeducation after a single year. Later, the Chicago Medical College was spared the need to admit or employ women because Woman's Medical College of Chicago provided opportunities for women in medicine. In 1892 Northwestern University took over the Woman's Medical College, which operated as the Woman's Medical School of Northwestern University, an entity separate from the Northwestern University Medical School, until it closed in 1902. Although Annette May McIntyre was a clinical assistant in neurology at Northwestern in 1917–18, Anna Ross Lapham, formerly on the P&S faculty, is considered the first female faculty member of the Northwestern University Medical School. In 1919–20 she was a demonstrator in operative obstetrics. She gradually rose in rank and served as an assistant professor of obstetrics from 1926 to 1946.[41]

In its early years P&S was traditional in its attitude toward women in medical education. When P&S affiliated with the university, the prospect of admitting female students was alarming. The faculty feared that a good many men would drop out if women were admitted. But as a land-grant institution the university was open to all qualified students, and Quine insisted that the college must admit women on equal terms with men. According to Steele, however, neither college officials nor the board of trustees favored such an innovation. On 8 June 1897 Pusey asked President Draper if the faculty could postpone admitting women for a year by saying that the instructors were not yet ready for them. Draper was willing to allow the present status to continue until the P&S board changed its policy. In late June, however, Lucy L. Flower, a forceful woman trustee and a champion of progressive causes, secured the board's approval of a resolution that women would be admitted starting in 1898.[42]

Women jumped the gun. During 1897–98 perhaps as many as twenty women were in attendance. The first female graduates, Eunice B. Hamill, Eliza A. Lyon, and Jennie Lind Phillips, apparently entered the fourth-year program and graduated MD in 1898. Hamill had studied at Woman's Medical College from 1895 to 1897. Lyon had an 1880 MD from Hahnemann Medical College. Phillips had completed three years at Woman's Medical College.[43]

Why did women transfer to P&S when they were well along in their medical studies elsewhere? The records of six of the seven women who graduated from P&S in 1899 help answer the question. Lora L. Beedy and Hannah L. Hukill had both studied at Harvey Medical College for two years before entering P&S. Marie A. Fellows had spent one year at Jenner Medical College and one year at Bennett Medical College before transferring to P&S. Helen T. Hisom had studied at the University of Southern California Medical College in 1895–97 and at Woman's Medical College in Chicago in 1897–98 before entering P&S. Mary G. Hunter had an MD from Cleveland University of Medicine and Surgery (1896) and Alberta V. McClung had an MD from the University of Minnesota (1897) before they became students at P&S.[44]

Personal considerations may have governed choices. Jenny Lind of Woman's Medical College, for example, married Frank A. Phillips, a faculty member at P&S. Dislike of faculty members or of the course of study may have prompted transfer. Did students from Woman's Medical College anticipate easier or harder going at P&S? Hamill was an excellent student at Woman's Medical College, and at P&S she ranked fifth in a graduating class of 106.[45] For Beedy, Hukill, Hisom, and perhaps others, it seems clear that the transfer to P&S was a step up qualitatively.[46]

When women were admitted, Quine recalled, they were treated "with undisguised hostility and contempt," but when persecution took the form of "positive vulgarity and personal abuse," the men themselves promptly repressed the offenders, although women would not inform on their persecutors. They met the situation with "tact, patience, and courage."[47]

Others viewed the historic event more favorably. *Plexus*, the college journal, observed without comment that two women from Woman's Medical College of Chicago had enrolled in P&S in the autumn of 1897. "We claim distinction," said the historian of the Class of 1901 (which entered in 1897), "for being the first class to which the ladies (bless them!) were admitted." The academic work of the first women "has shown favorable comparison with that of the men," *Plexus* reported, "and none of the possible difficulties that were apprehended in their admission has proven well founded." A year later a senior wrote that "the ladies appear like little oases in a desert of be-whiskered men." In 1899 a class historian, writing about female students, referred to "those airy, fairy creatures technically known as 'hens.'"[48] Despite condescension, the men soon learned to take female students seriously. For the ten years beginning in 1900, a total of 441 women students registered in the college. The number ranged from 36 to 75 a year, an average of 44.[49]

Harassment of women students was not tolerated. In February 1899 Twing B. Wiggin, a professor of physiology, made remarks to a mixed class that raised objections. The incident got into the newspapers. Quine suspended Wiggin from the faculty but later restored him. Draper thought the punishment sufficient. The public was very sensitive about such matters, he added, and it deserved assurance that such talk would be stopped. In April 1900 a female student charged various students and a faculty member with indecent conduct toward her. After investigating the matter, Quine dismissed six students whose conduct had not been satisfactory and warned five to improve their conduct or they would be dismissed. He expelled the woman who brought the charges.[50] The records are silent as to the reasons for Quine's action.

Women arrived at P&S in 1897 as faculty members as well as students. Two females joined the faculty in that year: Rosa Englemann as a clinical instructor in gynecology and children's diseases and Anabel B. Holmes as a clinical instructor in nervous diseases.[51] Holmes was an 1892 graduate of Woman's Medical College of Pennsylvania. We know little more about her.[52] Englemann was highly quali-fied. Born in Milwaukee in 1860 to immigrant German parents, she was edu-cated in private schools and graduated with a BA from Milwaukee College. She began the study of medicine with Nicholas Senn in Milwaukee and graduated from Woman's Medical College of Chicago in 1889. Prior to her faculty appoint-ment, she had gained experience in private practice and in various hospitals. In May 1900 Englemann was elected clinical instructor in pediatrics to work in the dispensary.[53]

Once the door opened to them, a number of women faculty entered. In 1898–99 Engelmann and Holmes were joined by Rachelle S. Yarros, an instructor in clinical obstetrics. A year later Yarros was an adjunct professor, while Engelmann and Holmes held their former positions. In 1900–1901 and again the following year the faculty included four women: Yarros, an adjunct professor; Holmes, now an adjunct professor of microscopical and chemical diagnosis; Corinne B. Eckley, a demonstrator in anatomy; and Alice Lois Lindsay-Wynekoop, an assis-tant in biology. Eckley and Lindsay-Wynekoop were faculty wives. All of these appointees except Eckley were MDs.[54]

In 1902–3 the faculty of 139 in all ranks included 12 women (8.6 percent). Four were holdovers: Yarros was now an associate professor, while Holmes, Eckley, and Lindsay-Wynekoop held the same positions as a year earlier. Three of the new appointees were in professorial ranks. Bertha Van Hoosen and Lucy Waite were both professors of clinical gynecology, and Jean M. Cooke was an adjunct professor of microscopical and chemical diagnosis. Five others were instruc-tors in various fields: Josephine E. Young and Mary G. McEwen, both in clini-cal gynecology; Rachel Hickey Carr and Anna Ross Lapham, both in surgery; and Henrietta Gould in clinical laryngology, rhinology, and otology. Lapham, as noted earlier, later went to Northwestern. She is regarded as the first female faculty member in the Northwestern University Medical College.

The number and percentage of female faculty members continued to increase. In 1903–4 the faculty of all ranks numbered 139, including 15 women (10.8 per-cent). It may well be that the University of Illinois College of Medicine had a higher proportion of women faculty members than any other medical college in the nation (except for women's medical colleges and those that taught some form of alternative medicine).[55] Among the women who had been appointed earlier, Yarros was now a professor, Holmes held her former title (microscopical and chemical diagnosis) to which "instructor in medicine" was now added, and Corinne Eckley was now an instructor. Among the new appointees, all MDs, Mary Jeannette Kearsley was an adjunct professor of medicine, while the other four were instructors: Frances M. Allen in pediatrics, Estella A. Horton in sur-gery, Marja Dowiatt in surgery, and Lora L. Beedy in orthopedic surgery.

The women in the lower ranks were well prepared. Frances M. Allen earned an MD at the University of Michigan in 1896.[56] Rachel H. Carr (1887) and Mary J. Kearsley (1888) had medical degrees from Woman's Medical College of Chicago.[57] Alice Lois Lindsay-Wynekoop (1895), Marja Dowiatt and Josephine E. Young (both 1896), Anna Ross Lapham and Mary G. McEwen (both 1898), and Estella A. Horton (1899) all had MDs from Northwestern University Woman's Medical School.[58] Lora L. Beedy (1899) and Henrietta Gould (1901) were graduates of P&S.[59]

Jean M. Cooke, one of the women of professorial rank, graduated from the University of Michigan Medical School in 1895. From 1900 to 1908 she was an associate professor of microscopical and chemical diagnosis at P&S.[60] Lucy Waite, clinical professor of gynecology extramural and clinical professor of obstetrics from 1900 to 1908, graduated from the old Chicago University in 1880 and obtained medical degrees from two homeopathic institutions in Chicago, Hahnemann Medical College and Harvey Medical College. She spent two years in Vienna and Paris studying gynecology and abdominal surgery. Returning home in 1887, she became an authority in her specialty and the author of several medical articles. For a number of years she was house surgeon in the Chicago Gynecological Institute and later professor of gynecology and abdominal surgery in the hospital connected with Harvey Medical College.[61]

Two of the early women faculty members merit special attention. The career of Rachelle S. Yarros illustrates the influence of P&S on the teeming life of the city of Chicago. Rachelle Slobodinsky was born to wealthy parents near Kiev, Russia, in 1869. At the age of thirteen she joined the Russian revolutionists. Fearing that the czar's police might imprison or exile her, at the age of seventeen she accepted money from her parents and fled to the United States. Arriving in New York in 1886, she worked in New York and New Jersey sweatshops and for a time lived among poor workers. Russian friends convinced her to seek a medical degree and provided financial help. She spent a year in the College of Physicians and Surgeons of Boston. In 1891 she moved to Philadelphia and graduated from the Woman's Medical College of Pennsylvania in 1893. In 1894 she married Victor S. Yarros, a radical exile from Ukraine and a journalist. They settled in Chicago. In 1895 after completing a medical residency at Michael Reese Hospital, Rachelle Yarros started an obstetrical and gynecological practice on the Near West Side.[62]

In 1897 Yarros became an unsalaried instructor in clinical obstetrics at P&S. We know nothing about the circumstances of her appointment. The 1898–99 *Annual Announcement* of P&S listed her as an instructor in clinical obstetrics, while the catalog for 1899–1900 described her as an adjunct professor of clinical obstetrics. In April 1899 the teaching faculty referred the question of her title to the dean. The following September the executive faculty agreed to pay Yarros six hundred dollars per year for services as superintendent of the obstetrical clinic.

She gave students practical training by having them help her with home deliveries and in the West Side Hospital. Yarros first attended a meeting of the teaching faculty on 6 April 1900 and again on 20 May 1901. She rose in rank, becoming an adjunct professor, an associate professor, and by 1904 a clinical full professor.[63]

In 1907 Rachelle and Victor Yarros became residents of Hull House. There, among the immigrant poor, she saw the horrors of venereal disease, prostitution, and abortion. In 1914 she helped found the American Social Hygiene Association, and a year later she became the general medical director of the newly founded Illinois Birth Control League. In 1923, aided by the league and Margaret Sanger, a crusader for contraceptive freedom, Yarros launched the second birth control clinic in the United States. She believed that constructive birth control must concern itself frankly with marital happiness and that apart from the rearing of a family, sex gratification was necessary to intimacy and tender affection between husband and wife. Yarros published *Birth Control and Its Relation to Health and Welfare* (1925) and *Modern Woman and Sex* (1933), her most important book. She provoked controversy over birth control, notably with Herman Bundsen, commissioner of health in the city of Chicago. Rachelle Yarros held her position in the College of Medicine at P&S until 1926.[64]

Bertha Van Hoosen joined the faculty in 1902. Born in 1863 on a farm near Rochester, Michigan, she graduated from high school in Pontiac, Michigan; received a BA from the University of Michigan in 1884; and despite parental disapproval enrolled in Michigan's medical department, graduating in 1888. Believing that her medical training at Michigan had been clinically inadequate, she devoted the next four years to clinical residencies in three different hospitals in Michigan and Boston.[65]

In 1892, although warned that she could not succeed in Chicago, she opened a private practice in the city. "Chicago impregnated me with its future possibilities," she wrote. "Chicago was not my decision. Chicago was my unescapable affinity." Rachel Hickey Carr signed Van Hoosen's application for licensure. Van Hoosen's practice developed slowly at first, but she kept active by teaching anatomy and embryology at the Woman's Medical College. During these years she also worked in gynecological and obstetrical clinics with Byron Robinson, a specialist in the field. In 1896 Van Hoosen was offered the position as chief of staff in Mary Thompson Hospital for Women and Children. She turned it down for personal reasons. Hearing that the position as head of gynecology and obstetrics in the University of Michigan Medical School was open, she rushed to Ann Arbor and told Victor C. Vaughan, the dean of the medical school and a friend, that she wanted the job. Vaughan turned her down because she was a woman. Returning home she learned that Woman's Medical College had closed, leaving her with no teaching or college position, no clinic, and no hospital appointment.[66]

Shortly thereafter she met Dean Quine. He asked how she would like to be professor of clinical gynecology in P&S and conduct a surgical clinic every week,

and he described the requirements for holding a clinical position in a coeduca-
tional medical school. "The students are a rough lot," Quine explained. "I have
known them to put a professor that they did not like right out of the window!"
Further, to hold a surgical clinic every week demanded recourse to a wealth of
surgical material. Could Van Hoosen operate so automatically that she could
give at the same time a systematic and instructive lecture? "Can you do all this?"
Quine asked. Van Hoosen raised her fist, brought it down on Quine's desk with
a thud, and swore, "I will!" Quine then "smiled one of his beautiful smiles," Van
Hoosen wrote, and said, "Now, isn't that remarkable? That is the only answer I
would have accepted, and I didn't even know it."[67]

Van Hoosen was not aware that the majority of the faculty were strongly against
her on the acknowledged ground of gender. Yarros informed Van Hoosen that
when Quine put up her name for appointment, it met with indifference and was
handed from committee to committee without recommendation. Yarros never
knew what was done to put it over, but Quine, she explained, was very clever.
He had once said when the faculty had turned down something he wanted very
much, "All right, gentlemen. Disgrace your dean, if you wish. You have that
privilege." A month later Van Hoosen received word of her appointment.[68]

Quine and Van Hoosen then planned a campaign to win acceptance for a
woman surgeon. Her course was to be elective so that any student need not
study under a woman, and the clinic was to be open to juniors, thus obviat-
ing comparisons, since older members of the faculty taught the seniors. Van
Hoosen recounted some harrowing experiences as she established herself in
the college. For her first surgical clinic she decided to shift the spotlight from
herself by presenting an unusual and rare case. She put the patient in the West
Side Hospital, adjoining the college, and when she prepared to operate not one
student was in the amphitheater. Later one or two students looked in, word
spread, and soon students from every class and members of the faculty came to
see the abnormal case. Van Hoosen never again lacked an audience through all
the years that she conducted the weekly surgical clinic.[69] Van Hoosen served on
the P&S faculty until 1912. On leaving, she became professor of obstetrics and
head of the obstetrics department at the Loyola University School of Medicine.
In 1917 Van Hoosen went to see James about getting back on the P&S faculty or
getting some other woman in place of Mary G. McEwen, an assistant professor
of clinical gynecology at the college. James had Van Hoosen to lunch. We know
nothing about what prompted the proposal, but we do know that McEwen was
not on the faculty the following year.[70] Van Hoosen was cofounder and first
president of the Medical Women's National Association (American Medical
Women's Association).[71]

The admission of women to medical colleges led some to ask if coeducation
was conducive to the best interests of medical schools and medical education.
That women were admitted as a matter of expediency was evident, but it could

not yet be claimed that they were admitted because it was in the best interests of medical education. The outcome was being watched. These were the comments of an editorial writer in a woman's medical magazine in 1901. But the issue had been settled, and there would be no turning back.[72]

We know little about African Americans at P&S because official records did not classify students by race. We can nevertheless identify at least three African American students in the period covered by this book. There may have been more. Perhaps the first was Isabella M. Garnett, who attended Harvey Medical College in 1897–99 and graduated from P&S in 1901.[73] Another African American is among a group of students in a physiology laboratory in a photograph taken about 1910 that is reproduced in this book. Still another African American was Robert N. Arthurton, a junior in 1914, who is discussed in a later chapter.

By 1904 the authorities at P&S had assembled a large and strong faculty. In quality it was perhaps neither better nor worse than the faculties of Rush and Northwestern. The college was proceeding under full sail in affiliation with the university when a new president assumed office. Before turning to President James and his efforts to reform medical education, we should familiarize ourselves with the Quine Library and the students at P&S.

CHAPTER 6

The Quine Library and the Students

The College of Physicians and Surgeons of Chicago (P&S) developed unevenly in its first fifteen years. Affiliation with the University of Illinois in 1897 marked a new beginning, and so too did the arrival in 1904 of Edmund J. James as president of the University of Illinois. Throughout these years and later, the Quine Library was taking shape as one of the best of its kind, and the student body had its own distinctive character.

The Quine Library

A good medical library is as necessary to a well-equipped medical college as are laboratories and clinical facilities, although at the turn of the century few medical faculties admitted as much. The P&S library began when the first president of the college, A. Reeves Jackson, left to the school at the time of his death in 1892 between three hundred and four hundred volumes as the foundation for a library. No immediate provision was made to care for the gift.[1]

When Bayard Holmes became secretary of the college in 1891, there were some fifteen hundred volumes locked up in black walnut bookcases and termed the A. Reeves Jackson Library. Holmes hired a graduate librarian, got carpenters to make open book shelves, and started a real library.[2]

Soon thereafter Holmes called attention to libraries for medical schools, likening them to the libraries of university graduate schools that emphasized the seminar method of study and research. A medical college library, said Holmes, should furnish the means of training students in medical bibliography and bibliographic research; furnish, through medical literature, material for the study of every medical science that formed a part of the medical curriculum; furnish material for the study of the sciences collateral to medicine; and make possible the proper pedagogic methods in medical schools. Years passed before the P&S library met the justifiably high standard set by Holmes.[3]

Some faculty members habitually searched the medical literature for help when faced with a challenging medical or surgical case, while the library grew by the gifts of friends, faculty members, and exchanges.[4] Quine took a deep interest in the library and at an early date began to donate books, texts, periodicals, and encyclopedias to the collection. The New York Academy of Medicine donated ninety-eight volumes, among them a large number of "medical classics" in French or German and some books from the library of the pioneer American gynecologist J. Marion Sims. The U.S. Surgeon General's Office sent some treatises dating back to the sixteenth century, hundreds of students' theses in Latin and foreign languages from leading European universities, British and American medical journals, and the *Index Catalogue* of the Surgeon General's Library in Washington, an alphabetical arrangement of author and subject titles in the vast field of medical literature. Dr. John Bartlett of Chicago presented the library the *Medicinische Jahrbücher* for the years 1845–87, the "Index Medicus" of the Germans.[5]

The library was for reference only. It occupied a room in the college building and was open daily from nine in the morning to five in the afternoon with the exception of Saturday, when it closed at noon. In 1896 five dollars of the annual student fees began to go to the library, and a year later the college employed a trained librarian. She classified the books according to the Dewey decimal system, compiled a card catalog, and affiliated the library with the American Medical Library Association, which enabled the library to benefit from the Library Exchange.[6]

Quine was a generous donor. Among his valuable gifts were the *Century Dictionary and Cyclopedia; Reference Handbook of the Medical Sciences;* John Ashurst's *International Encyclopedia of Surgery: A Systematic Treatise on the Theory and Practice of Surgery; Annals of Surgery, International Clinics, Index Medicus;* Sajous's *Annual of Universal Medical Sciences;* complete sets of the *Journal of the American Medical Association* and the *Chicago Medical Recorder;* and incomplete files of other leading medical journals. In addition, Quine provided three hundred dollars a year for the purchase of medical periodicals and new editions of textbooks. *Plexus,* the college magazine, called Quine the "patron saint" of the library. In 1897 in recognition of his generous benefactions, the faculty named the college library the Quine Library.[7]

By 1900 the library held 3,316 bound volumes, 400 unbound volumes, about 5,000 pamphlets, and hundreds of unbound journals. In the number of its volumes and the amount of its working material the library stood first in Chicago after the medical department of the Newberry Library. The average daily attendance of ninety at the Quine Library exceeded that of the Newberry Library. In 1899 the librarian compiled more than fifty reference lists.[8]

In 1901 the library moved to the new college building, where it occupied rooms on the second floor. The two largest were a reading room and a stack room. There was also an office for the librarian, a room for shelving duplicates, and a small workroom. The reading room contained reference works, textbooks, and indices. On the walls above the molding were photographs of faculty members, a bronze bust of A. Reeves Jackson, and a bronze bust as well as an oil painting of Quine. The faculty had a small reading room. Next to it was a stack room with fourteen thousand volumes in 1907. In 1911 the library had a daily attendance of 185.[9]

Quine remained a generous benefactor. In February 1905, observing that he owned $22,600 in the bonds and $2,200 in the stock of P&S, he informed President James that he wished to donate these securities to the university "on the annuity plan" for the maintenance of the library of the College of Medicine. The following December, noting that the university owned the Quine Library absolutely, Quine said that he had been trying for years to get the trustees to accept an endowment of $25,000 for the support of the library but to no avail. If the board did not formally accept his offer by 1 January 1908, Quine added, it would be withdrawn. James and the board's Committee on the School of Medicine then interviewed Quine. Presumably they settled the matter satisfactorily.[10]

President James, who was determined to create a great library for the university in Urbana, took an active interest in strengthening the medical school library. In 1911, a newspaper reported, James requested David H. Galloway, an 1893 graduate of the medical school and a prominent physician in Roswell, New Mexico, to make provision in his will to give the university his library of five hundred bound volumes and a thousand pamphlets that covered every branch of science and technical knowledge. According to the newspaper, the request would be granted.[11]

In 1913 when the German bookseller Fock wanted to sell the university the Saemisch library on ophthalmology, James consulted Casey A. Wood, a professor of ophthalmology at the College of Medicine, about the purchase. Wood, who had spent twenty years assembling for himself an outstanding collection of literature on the eye and its diseases, owned most of the books in the Saemisch library. But the Quine Library was very weak in ophthalmic works of reference, Wood observed, and he advised James to purchase the Saemisch library for about $800 and to make it complete by buying missing items secondhand. A year later a small collection of German and French works on the eye, the Krämer library, became available. A price of $200 would be about one-fifth of the market value, Wood reported. James approved the purchase for $175 if Wood would guarantee that the books were in good condition.[12]

By 1916 the Quine Library contained 17,625 bound volumes and was receiving 230 annual periodicals, of which 160 represented standard scientific journals, and 98 of those had complete or approximately complete files on the shelves.[13] Four years later the library included 21,000 bound volumes as well as reprints and separates. The Quine Library was taking its place as one of the best medical school libraries in the country. It was justly considered the pride of the medical school.

The Students

At the turn of the century medical students came to P&S with varied expectations. Their lives in a professional school were intense. Some were teenagers with no more than a high school education, while others were graybeards with a medical degree upon matriculating. Affiliation with the university stimulated enrollment. In the seven years from affiliation in 1897 to 1904 when James became president of the university, attendance trended upward. Much of the total enrollment in the four-year course of study was in the clinical years. Some of the transfers came from schools that offered only a two-year course, while many had been conditioned by other colleges, especially the American Medical Missionary College and the University of Iowa.[14] Over the years the number and percentage of students in the clinical years gradually evened out, as shown in Table 3.[15]

During these seven years an average of 55.9 percent of the students were in the clinical program, and an average of 7.7 percent of the students were women. In these same years the number of graduates also had an upward trend, as illustrated in Table 4.[16]

Table 3. Composition of the student body, 1897 to 1904

Year	Enrollment			Clinical Years		Percent of Female Students
	M	F	Total	No.	Percent	
1897–1898	391	17	408	229	56.1	4.1
1898–1899	479	35	514	238	46.2	6.7
1899–1900	539	41	580	302	52.0	7.0
1900–1901	625	48	673	375	55.7	7.1
1901–1902	658	50	708	429	60.5	7.0
1902–1903	616	73	689	402	58.3	10.5
1903–1904	641	53	694	435	62.6	7.6

Table 4. Graduates of P&S, 1898 to 1904

Year	Number
1898	106
1899	115
1900	136
1901	165
1902	222
1903	218
1904	216

Table 5. Composition of the student body, 1904 to 1913

Year	Enrollment			Clinical Years		Percent of Female Students
	M	F	Total	No.	Percent	
1904–5	613	40	653	425	65.0	6.1
1905–6	522	43	565	353	62.4	7.6
1906–7	469	36	505	303	60.0	7.1
1907–8	440	36	476	280	58.8	7.5
1908–9	480	40	520	273	52.5	7.6
1909–10	493	33	526	244	46.3	6.2
1910–11	480	38	518	248	47.8	7.3
1911–12	500	37	537	276	51.3	6.8
1912–13	516	35	551	258	46.8	9.9

In the period from 1904 to 1913 the composition of the student body remained much as in the years from 1897 to 1904, as illustrated in Table 5.[17]

During these years an average of 54.5 percent of the students were in the clinical years, and an average of 7.3 percent of the students were female. Both averages were slightly lower than in the earlier period. By way of comparison, from 1890 to 1913 female enrollments in the nation's regular medical schools averaged 4.05 percent of total enrollment.[18]

The medical college was located on the Near West Side of the city, which was known as Chicago's Latin Quarter. P&S was surrounded by other medical and educational institutions. In addition to the Cook County Hospital, the region embraced Marquette School, Rush Medical College, the Chicago College of Dental Surgery, Woman's Medical College, Bennett Medical College, the Illinois Training School for Nurses, the Chicago Homeopathic College, the Hospital for Women and Children, and the Cook County Detention Hospital for the Insane. This midwestern equivalent of the Parisian student quarter was vibrant with physicians, surgeons, and aspiring doctors. And since the Chicago Cubs played at a ballpark just south of Cook County Hospital, crowds of fans often swelled the numbers in the area.

On arrival at P&S new students were an undifferentiated aggregate of males and females from widely scattered places with a great diversity of ages. They lacked cohesion, and sophomores made the lives of freshmen miserable.[19] An instinct for unity manifested itself in the class system.[20] The election of class officers gave freshmen their first sense of a common enterprise, and each class maintained its identity through four years of medical school. In the senior year the class historian wrote an account of the class's adventures as medical students. *The Illio,* a yearbook sponsored by the junior class in Urbana, published the class history. A representative of *The Illio* at the medical school provided coverage of activities at P&S for the Urbana publication.

P&S was a professional school, and the life of a medical student differed from that of most undergraduates working for a bachelor's degree. Medical students worked hard with little cessation. They were perhaps more industrious than the average undergraduate. They had made a career choice and knew that success in life depended on what they learned and their academic record. Nevertheless, a distinguishing feature of the life of medical students was the extent to which it resembled that of college undergraduates.

Traditional college customs, recreations, and amusements were popular at the medical school, but because of the diversity in the age of medical students, participation in some college activities may have been highly selective. One class at P&S adopted a motto, "Ut Prosimus" (That We May Be of Service), a color (purple), and a yell that went:[21]

> Hobble Gobble! Razzle Dazzle!
> Siz! Boom! Bah!
> P. & S. of '99
> Rah! Rah! Rah!

It is hard to imagine fifty-year-old students joining enthusiastically in the class yell.

The instinct for unity led in 1896 to the adoption of a new college button. The device combined the colors red and yellow, "blood and iodoform," in an artistic cross of red resting upon a circle of orange. On the arms of the cross was "P. & S." in gold. The red cross typified a medical man's life work (female students had not yet been admitted when the button was adopted), while the orange circle was emblematic of the endless work and usefulness of the college. The golden letters stood for "Pure Science, Patient Study, and Permanent Success."[22]

Formal college ceremonies resembled those on American college campuses. Class Day opened and closed with prayer. The program, interspersed with musical selections, included an address by the class president, the class history, the presentation and acceptance of a gift from the class, the class poem, and the class prophecy. At Commencement Exercises on the following day an orchestra played while the audience was being seated (in 1896 in the Grand Opera House). A local clergyman opened the ceremony with an invocation and closed it with a benediction. A faculty member delivered the doctorate address (in 1896 John B. Murphy used the occasion to describe the advances in nineteenth-century medicine), the president of the university or of the board of directors conferred degrees and announced honors, and a faculty member gave the charge to the class (in 1896 Quine's charge demonstrated his high-mindedness), which was followed by the response of the class and a valedictory.[23]

In 1898 Samuel C. Garber's valedictory address had as its theme "scientific medicine is before us." The field is broad, Garber avowed; it touched almost every other science. Its corners were yet untilled; its waters were deep, often

unfathomable. "Today," Garber declared, after giving medical sectarians a drub-
bing, "we launch our little barks upon the uncertain sea of life. Success is the
port we all desire to make. . . . Gently but firmly, we have been inducted into
the intricacies and details of scientific medicine. . . . The parting moment has
come. . . . May God speed the day of your prosperity, and may Fortune shower
upon you her choicest blessings."[24]

Despite the uplift (and the prospect of riches), medical students were not
goody-goodies. Some indulged in the contemporary practice of chewing to-
bacco and expectorating indoors, and there were isolated acts of misbehavior. In
November 1899 a disturbance between the sophomore and junior classes led to
the appointment of a new Committee on Discipline.[25] And in 1900 a freshman
who placed a ring on a table in the dissecting room and was absent momentarily
returned to find the ring was gone. His posted notice offering a reward of $2.50
for return of the ring elicited no response. When he raised the reward to $5 a
sophomore returned the ring, demanding the $5 before handing it over. Asked
why he had not returned the ring earlier, the sophomore replied that the reward
was too small and he needed the money.[26]

Disciplinary cases reveal much about student life and college standards. In
1901 when three junior students were caught cheating on an examination on
obstetrics, Quine informed them that they would be given no credit for the term
of work in which they were caught cheating.[27] Also in that year Quine informed
a student who had been proved guilty of drunkenness on several occasions that
he would receive no credit for one term of instruction and would be granted his
diploma in May 1902 only if not guilty of drunkenness at any time before then.
The student did not graduate.[28]

In the spring of 1908 three members of the junior class, each of whom had
an excellent academic record, were enrolled in a class in surgical pathology in
which they turned in surgical drawings belonging to a classmate rather than
their own. College authorities suspended each of them for a year. All three men
offered essentially the same excuse. They held jobs to pay their way through
school; overworked and crowded for time and not having their own drawings
completed, they handed in the drawing of another person on the spur of the
moment, not deliberately. They believed that the punishment imposed was too
severe. The junior class took up their case. A spokesman for the junior class,
writing to President James, asked the University Council of Administration to
reverse the penalty imposed by the college and added that the junior class was
prepared to petition the Illinois legislature and others for relief. James replied
that unless new evidence about the case could be presented, the facts would
stand. The publicity given by a petition to the legislature would harm the three
men for years to come, no matter how the case was settled. And if the council
reversed the penalty and reinstated the men, the fact would come to the attention of state medical examining boards, which would rule out an institution that

condoned such an offense. James would be glad to talk with any member of the junior class. Only one of the three penalized juniors graduated from P&S (in 1913, a year late).[29]

A monthly magazine, *The P. & S. Plexus,* later *The Plexus,* usually known simply as *Plexus,* was the official publication of P&S. Established in January 1894, it began publication in October 1895. Its object was to promote the advancement of the institution, to increase relations between the faculty and the student body, and to acquaint the medical scholar with the latest advances and researches in the profession. Management of the magazine was under the control of an elected faculty committee, which chose the student editor. Each class was represented on the editorial staff. The senior class had two editors, and the other classes had one each. *Plexus* included editorials, book reviews, a feature titled "Cook County Hospital Examination Questions," and photographs of faculty members.

Plexus also published articles by faculty members on medical topics. John B. Murphy, for example, wrote on an operation for strangulated hernia; John A. Benson wrote on the value of physiological study; Adolph Gehrmann wrote "Bacteriology: A Popular Science"; Carl Beck wrote "Our Methods of Studying Surgical Pathology"; Quine wrote "Aortic Aneurism—A Clinical Lecture"; and Charles S. Williamson wrote on Hodgkin's disease.[30] The magazine also published faculty articles on topics of general interest. Among them were William T. Eckley, "Facial Expression"; Weller Van Hook's tribute to the famous surgeons Theodore Billroth and Jules-Emile Péan; Steele's 1898 doctorate address "Character As an Element of Success"; and Andrew S. Draper's 1903 doctorate address "The Personal Equation in the Medical Profession."[31]

Two faculty articles in *Plexus* are especially noteworthy. One was Henry P. Newman's "Berlin Letter" of 8 December 1898. Newman had gone to Berlin to study twenty years earlier, he observed, when a young man had to go there to complete his medical education. Now the tables had been turned. Americans had been perfecting their medical schools while Europe had stood practically still. The method of instruction was more concise and systematic here than there. It was better for an American medical student to stay at home for his education than to go to Europe. And before long, Newman believed, the tide of seekers after knowledge would set "toward our live western institutions."[32] Newman testified to the fact that the center of medical research and education was shifting from Germany to the United States.

A second important faculty article was by George P. Dreyer. In an address at the opening exercises of the college in October 1903 titled "The College of Physicians and Surgeons: A Retrospect and a Forecast," Dreyer offered a brief history of the college and went on to say that the position of the modern medical school placed its faculty on a level with the philosophical and other professional faculties in a university and carried with it an obligation on the medical faculty to teach and to cultivate in students the habit of thought and also to enlarge the boundaries of human knowledge. In sum, said Dreyer, the proprietary medical college was now the University of Illinois College of Medicine, and medical faculty members should act accordingly.[33]

Plexus served a useful purpose. With a circulation of twelve hundred monthly and with special issues of two thousand per month, it was also profitable. One year the student editor who leased the journal made a profit of $545. But the possibility of the student editor to behave irresponsibly was a faculty concern. In February 1899 the faculty appointed a committee to look into the condition of *Plexus* and to determine its financial status with a view to recommending such support as the committee saw fit. The committee apparently found some disturbing things. In December the faculty decided that the college journal should always remain under faculty control, so it appointed a committee to secure ownership and control of *Plexus*.[34] The committee found that Guy G. Dowdall, the editor who graduated in 1900, had left an unpaid printer's bill. His successors, Emil J. Merki (a 1902 graduate) and Herbert C. Waddle (a 1903 graduate), did not get along well, and they had incurred debts. So to ensure honest management of *Plexus* and to counterbalance any possible indebtedness at the expiration of the lease of Merki and Waddle, the committee bought *Plexus* for $400. Thus the college was protected against debts and could set the terms of the lease.[35] The journal continued to operate.

Relations between students and faculty were not entirely harmonious. A student who suggested that student voices on teaching be heard with a view to improving the medical college was no doubt dissatisfied with some of his courses.[36] In 1898 a student-faculty conflict led to an impasse that the dean resolved. Students were charged with indulging in "improper conduct" in a class in genitourinary diseases. Those who failed to sign a paper disapproving of the conduct were told that they would not pass the course. After the faculty heard a committee representing the class, the matter was referred to the dean. When the students who had refused to sign the note of disapproval had satisfactorily explained their conduct to him, the dean decreed, they would be accepted into the class.[37] "We know we are not afraid," the Class of 1906 boasted, "to leave the class room when a Prof is late."[38] Students sometimes occupied a classroom in advance of a scheduled lecture, closed the windows, and lit pipes, cigars, and cigarettes to "smoke out" an unpopular or boring teacher. On one occasion students refused to attend the lectures of a young physiologist brought to the college from Johns Hopkins.[39] Another time, Quine recalled, students put a faculty member out of a window.[40]

Among themselves, students may have severely criticized their instructors, but negative comments rarely made their way into surviving records. Rather, students fulsomely praised both the faculty in general and individual faculty members. Their instructors, they avowed, included some of the brightest and most prominent medical men. They singled out George P. Dreyer, whose scientific demonstrations and well-given lectures made a lasting impression;

Charles S. Williamson, whose natural brilliancy and work in Europe made him peculiarly fit for an ideal teacher; William A. Evans for making pathology a reality; Jean Cook, a valuable instructor in clinical microscopy; and Bertha Van Hoosen for profitable gynecology clinics. Willliam T. "Pop" Eckley and his wife Corinne, acclaimed for their able supervision in the dissecting room, were student favorites.[41]

Students extolled John B. Murphy. His clinics, they reported, with his invitation to those in the amphitheater—"'Come down, please, what is the matter with him?'—are justly regarded as a rare treat among our boys." Murphy's clinics were extremely interesting owing to the number of cases presented together with their treatment, and they attracted a large audience. As a teacher Murphy was considered unexcelled. Murphy was "*the* true clinician among clinicians."[42]

William E. Quine received accolades from both colleagues and students. While on the faculty at the Chicago Medical College, wrote William E. Harsha, professor of surgery at P&S, Quine was regarded as "the greatest teacher of materia medica Chicago had ever had." And he was immensely popular with students. Two of the greatest medical schools in the country had offered him a tempting salary to unite his future with theirs. At P&S Quine was regarded in the medical profession as one of the foremost teachers in the country. Students admired and honored him. As a family physician he had an enormous following, and for years he was one of the busiest practitioners in Chicago.[43] The senior class gave a reception and ball in honor of Quine that became an annual event. On 8 February 1904 more than five hundred attended the ball in Illinois Hall, which closed with the presentation of a loving cup as a token of esteem. Dancing and games were provided for all those present.[44]

Medical students had a reputation for being rough and rowdy. In 1896 the journalist A. L. Benedict declared that the modern type of medical student was "probably better behaved than the average of any other body of men or boys."[45] He had not visited P&S, where medical students found an outlet from "the unceasing grind so characteristic of medical schools" by breaking up chairs, ejecting a disliked professor from a classroom, and engaging in the sport of "passing him up."[46] In this common practice, huskies in the front row of an amphitheater would grab a fellow student by the armpits and start him on his way up to the top row, with stout hands speeding the body along from one tier of seats to another. If the victim did not resist, he might reach the top row only slightly worse for wear. The real excitement came when some well-muscled victim resisted.[47] On occasion students who were determined to avoid taking an examination and to prevent others from taking it involved the whole class in a riot. A free-for-all ensued, with destruction of clothing, shrieking and howling, and breaking of furniture.[48]

In June 1900 Quine reported that relations between the men and women medical students were less discordant than they had been the previous year.

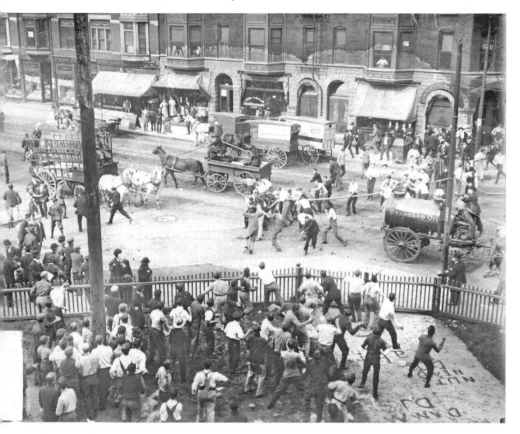

College of Physicians and Surgeons Class Rush, Ogden Street, 1908. Courtesy of the Chicago History Museum.

Moreover, five men had been suspended for misconduct, and one woman was "privately expelled" for serious offenses. Quine described relations between the male students and the young women of the West Division High School, which was adjacent to the college building, as "extremely unwholesome."[49]

Rites of passage mark important transitions in life, and American colleges adopted the practice of European universities in subjecting new students to some form of initiation. "Hazing" was the term employed in America to describe the familiar ritual of initiating and disciplining freshmen. Hazing was a product of the class system whereby all students who entered at the same time were considered members of a single class throughout their college course. Medical students perpetuated this feature of collegiate life.[50]

Sophomores considered themselves superior beings and exhibited their contempt for freshmen by calling them D.J.s (Damned Juniors) and in more disagreeable ways. They tried by brute force, for example, to occupy a classroom that the freshmen had not yet vacated. According to Dean Quine, one class of sophomores distinguished themselves as "hoodlums and rowdies and as nothing else."[51] Freshmen suffered such indignities, but not happily. "In a few more weeks," a freshman gloated in April 1898, "we will cease to be D.J.'s, and will then begin to swell up, and will not any longer dodge an upper classman when we meet him on the stairs."[52]

Freshmen devised ways to retaliate. The Class of 1907 took credit for establishing the Class or Color Rush, an annual fall encounter in which freshmen challenged the physical supremacy of sophomores by trying to capture their flag.[53] This "primitive barbarous warfare" in which the "green, ignorant, uncouth, pestiferous" freshmen accepted the challenge of the sophomores was capable of turning violent. On 1 October 1908 the conflict raged from 10:00 a.m. to noon, when the "weary, muddy, egg bespattered, shirtless, bruised and torn [freshmen] were forced to beat a retreat," carrying their wounded heroes off the field in "inglorious and bitter defeat." The encounter was so hotly contested that it led to a riot and caused a blockade of streetcars and intervention by the fire department. No one was killed, but several required surgical attention.[54] And yet the Class Rush gave both freshmen and sophomores a sense of class unity.

Athletics provided a more acceptable outlet for robust animal spirits, and on the medical campus the pattern of athletics closely resembled that at the university. In the 1890s when baseball was the main collegiate sport, P&S had a baseball team, and when football replaced baseball in favor, P&S acquired a football team. The Athletic Association (AA) managed athletic activities and rapidly incurred debts. In March 1897 the board of trustees agreed to pay the indebtedness of the AA, not exceeding eight hundred dollars, from any surplus funds of the medical school. Hereafter, the board decreed, officials at the School of Medicine were to see that students conducted their athletic matters wholly upon their own financial responsibility, with the approval of the faculty athletic committee and the Athletic Advisory Board.[55]

The P&S football eleven usually played five or six games a year with neighboring schools. In October 1897 the medical faculty authorized the actuary to spend up to one thousand dollars annually to support and encourage athletics. It was understood that if the university refused to assume the expense, the faculty would individually assume their pro rata share of the costs.[56] A month later about one thousand rooters attended the annual game between P&S and Rush for supremacy of western medical colleges on the gridiron.[57] By December the AA had a deficit of about seven hundred dollars. Each faculty member was honor bound to pay his share, the faculty ruled, and if the university would not furnish funds for athletics, the faculty would have nothing more to do with athletics in a formal way. So the games went on, and in February 1899 the medical faculty voted to continue their support of athletics by direct appropriation if necessary.[58]

FOOT BALL TEAM OF '97.

Husk, R. E.   Blayney, R. H. B.   Majors, F. B.   Kohler, F. B.   Flippin, R. T.   Wells, Mgr.
McCormick. L. T.   Krotter, L. G.   Meyers, C.   Dowdall, L. E.
Wynekoop, R. H. B.   Turner, Q. B.   Weakley, L. H. B.   Carr, R. G.

College of Physicians and Surgeons football team, 1897. Courtesy of Special Collections
and University Archives, University of Illinois at Chicago.

Students controlled the AA. Their ideas about athletics were in accord with
the practice of American universities, but they proved to be costly. In 1898–99
football cost the college $1,068. In November 1899 the college provided an ad-
ditional appropriation of $500 for expenses of the AA.[59]

The faculty belatedly realized that the AA was irresponsible. In the spring of
1900 the faculty Committee on Athletics looked into matters. It found numerous
problems, many of which the committee quickly rectified. The team was without
equipment, which the committee had to buy; the committee had to rent a new
training ground; the AA was operating a training table at a cost of $354 a year
and defending it as an established university custom; there was no accounting for
funds turned over to the AA by the football manager; and there was considerable
dissatisfaction with the scheduling of games. Six games had been played in 1899;
nine others had been arranged but not played for various reasons.[60]

If athletics were to be maintained, the committee concluded, the AA should
be under faculty control. The college should adopt an athletic policy, appoint
a faculty manager of athletics and a subordinate student manager, discontinue
the training table, employ a coach, pay off the current debt, and provide five
hundred dollars a year for athletics. These measures were implemented. The

committee was "fully convinced that the maintenance of athletics in medical colleges, while it is a medium of advertising and a means of engendering the college spirit, is, as presently conducted, detrimental to the interests of medical education." The Executive Faculty declared that the college would not recognize or support any baseball or football team and that no special privileges would be granted members of any such team, but in the near future the college would establish a gymnasium and a chair of physical culture.[61]

Thus reformed, at least in intent, the games continued. In the autumn of 1900 the P&S eleven played a motley assortment of teams, including the St. Charles, Illinois, Athletic Club; Lake Forest University; the Northwestern University Dental College; the Chicago Dental College; Notre Dame University; and the University of Chicago. P&S won four games, lost one, and tied one.[62]

Women introduced basketball into American colleges in the 1890s, and men followed. In 1903 basketball was inaugurated at P&S. During 1904–5 the basketball team played twelve games in and around Chicago.

As college students did elsewhere, medical students organized an assortment of special-interest groups. Those musically inclined formed both the Glee Club and the Mandolin Club, each of which performed in venues in Chicago. William M. Harsha, a professor of surgery, may have brought the Masonic Society to the campus. In 1902 he requested a room for its use one evening a week, and the faculty agreed to provide a room where all such clubs could meet. Some students formed the Medical Society. The P&S AA held an annual reception. In February 1899 it was held in the West Chicago Club. The patronesses were faculty wives, the wife of Governor John Tanner, and the wife of President Andrew S. Draper. Among the highlights of the social year was the Junior Promenade, given by the junior class to honor the senior class, and the Senior Ball.[63]

The Young Men's Christian Association (YMCA) had a strong presence in the United States, and especially on college campuses, in the late nineteenth and early twentieth centuries. The YMCA of Chicago, which was affiliated with the State Association of Young Men's Christian Associations of Illinois, had offices on La Salle Street. With the cooperation of the faculty it worked for the benefit of medical students on the West Side. The YMCA of Chicago maintained social rooms with newspapers and magazines for members. With a membership card, which was recognized by all Chicago YMCA buildings, one could use the gymnasiums in the Ys of the city.[64]

The P&S YMCA had its headquarters on the first floor of the college building. The Y's Committee on Management consisted of five faculty members. The YMCA of Chicago appointed a medical student as executive secretary of the YMCA of the medical school. The college granted the secretary a scholarship in lieu of paying its dues to the Chicago YMCA. At the opening of the school year the secretary assisted students in finding desirable rooming places. "Special attention," the secretary reported in 1914, "was given to the men of the colored race who find it extremely difficult to obtain desirable homes on this side of the city." The secretary also helped students find employment as truckmen, guards, waiters, furnace tenders, and salesmen. The secretary compiled a complete directory of the students. The directory had a by-product: it was the basis upon which requisition was made to the State Board of Health by the anatomy department for dissecting material.[65]

Members of the faculty and student body who belonged to some evangelical church were eligible for membership in the P&S YMCA, while any college man of moral character might become an associate member. All students were welcome at the YMCA. Members held religious meetings once a week on Thursday from 12:30 to 1:00 p.m., and Bible study classes met once a week. In February 1904 in the YMCA assembly hall the Reverend Dr. C. B. MacAfee, pastor of the Forty-first Street Presbyterian Church in Chicago, gave a speech titled "The Claim of Christ on the Young Man of To-Day."[66]

The YWCA also had a presence in the medical college, and the Student Volunteer Movement for Foreign Missions was represented at P&S. Members of the latter were guided by the movement's watchword, "The Evangelization of the World in This Generation." In 1905 ten students, including four women, were active in the evangelical organization, and by 1914 the number had risen to fourteen medical students, who held regular meetings on Sunday afternoons in the Second Baptist Church at the corner of Lincoln Street and Jackson Boulevard.[67]

In 1914 James, having gone through the medical school district on the West Side, was much discouraged by what he saw. He wondered if the YMCA of Chicago could not take up the problem of erecting a great building in that part of the city primarily for the use of students. A modern building, James informed the general secretary of the Chicago YMCA, could be made to carry its own expense by combining a sufficiently large dormitory feature. The Cook County Hospital was going to be the center of one of the greatest medical school districts in the world, said James, and the students in the area would be served by the YMCA. The acting general secretary replied that the YMCA of Chicago had been giving earnest consideration to such a building; it was one of the pressing problems of the city. He hoped to confer with James on the matter. No more came of the proposal.[68]

Greek-letter social fraternities were an important feature of American college life, and when P&S was founded medical fraternities began springing up around the country. Nu Sigma Nu, the first fraternity to admit medical students, was founded at the University of Michigan in 1882. Within a decade four others followed: Alpha Kappa Kappa at Dartmouth in 1888; Phi Chi, a union of two local medical societies, in 1889; Phi Rho Sigma at the Chicago Medical College in 1890; and Phi Beta Pi at Western Pennsylvania Medical College in 1891. These societies offered the advantages of fraternal affiliation and the benefits that accrued from membership with others in the same profession.[69]

The West Side campus provided fertile soil for social fraternities, and over a period of years male students established at least eight chapters of national medical fraternities in the college. In February 1892 the Eta chapter of Nu Sigma Nu came into being at P&S. Large and prestigious, Nu Sigma Nu initially had eighteen "Fratres in Facultate," fourteen "Fratres in Urbe," and twenty-three "Fratres in Universitate" (including eleven seniors, eight juniors, and four freshmen). Some years later twenty-eight prominent faculty members along with twenty-seven students (seven seniors, eleven juniors, six sophomores, and three pledges) made up the society.[70]

Phi Rho Sigma established its presence at P&S with the Beta chapter in October 1894. In its early years the chapter included twenty-eight faculty members, twenty-two members in the city of Chicago, and twenty-three students (ten seniors, four juniors, seven sophomores, and two freshmen). Early in 1896 the members acquired their own fraternity house at the corner of Paulina and Congress streets. There, close to the college, they held their meetings and conducted their social activities.[71]

In December 1899 the Eta chapter of Alpha Kappa Kappa was formed at P&S. A year later the local chapter had seven members in the city and thirty in the college. In 1903 Alpha Kappa Kappa had eleven honorary faculty members, six honorary nonfaculty members, eleven seniors, twelve juniors, seven sophomores, and six pledges, for a total of thirty-six student members. In 1910 the fraternity had twenty-six student members (seven seniors, one junior, eleven sophomores, six freshmen, and one pledge).[72]

Although little is known about the Beta chapter of Pi Psi Theta, it had fourteen members and its own attractive house when the 1902 yearbook first noticed it. The Illio included a photograph of the house.[73]

Phi Beta Pi established its Iota chapter at P&S in 1902. At the time it had twenty-six active members and two pledges. In 1910 the thirty members consisted of five seniors, eleven juniors, eight sophomores, and six freshmen. Many students desired a fraternity affiliation, so the fraternity grew larger. In 1914 the local branch of Phi Beta Pi included nine faculty members and forty students (eight seniors, twelve juniors, twelve sophomores, six freshmen, and two pledges). Phi Beta Pi also had its own fraternity house.[74]

Sigma Phi Epsilon was founded at Richmond College (later the University of Richmond, Virginia) in 1901, and two years later the Beta Alpha chapter of the national fraternity arose at P&S. By 1910 the local group had a total of forty-three members (sixteen seniors, four juniors, fifteen sophomores, one freshman, and seven pledges).[75]

A chapter of Phi Delta, which had been founded in 1901 at Long Island Hospital College, existed at P&S by 1908.[76] Phi Chi, founded at the University of Vermont in 1886, established a local chapter in December 1909. Three years later the chapter had forty-two student members (twelve seniors, fourteen juniors, nine sophomores, and seven freshmen). And by 1914 it possessed its own fraternity house.[77]

Although most of the fraternities at P&S were branches of national groups, Alpha Phi Sigma was a native growth. When formed in 1910 it had four faculty members, six city members, and twenty student members (six seniors, four juniors, three sophomores, and seven freshmen). Alpha Phi Sigma proved to be contagious. Chapters were soon established at Northwestern University Medical School and at Rush Medical College.[78]

Greek-letter societies attracted a significant proportion of the male students. Students may have joined a fraternity with a chapter house for the sake of board and room and mutual assistance in study, but the long hours of hard study would have left little time for sociability. Fraternities became a divisive force in the college, especially when chapters occupied their own fraternity houses. Thus, Greeks had a built-in advantage over Independents (so-called Barbarians) in campus affairs. In 1906 one student viewed the competition between "frats" and "barbs" for election of officers for the sophomore class as exciting because victory went to the "barbs."[79]

Medical fraternities for women may have been especially important to females as a means of affirming their authenticity in the medical profession. Nu Sigma Phi, a fraternity for women, was founded at P&S in 1898, a year after women were first admitted to the college. At its inception the fraternity included sixteen city members, all but four of whom were MDs, and twelve student members in three different classes. Although numerically small, as a proportion of the female medical students the membership was large. In 1902 the local chapter of Nu Sigma Phi had twenty-three alumni and associate members, mostly MDs, and sixteen active members. In 1911 the local chapter of Nu Sigma Phi consisted of three "Sorores in Facultate," fifty-six "Sorores in Urbe" (thirty-six of whom were MDs), and twelve "Sorores in Collegio" (ten actives and two pledges).[80]

In 1899 a chapter of Alpha Epsilon Iota, which had been founded at the University of Michigan in 1890, was established at P&S. At its inception the local fraternity had graduate members, associate members, honorary members (Emily Blackwell, Mary Putnam Jacobi, and three others), affiliated members, one faculty member (Rachelle Yarros), and nine active student members. The Alpha Epsilon Iota colors were black, white, and green; the flower was the white carnation; and the pin was a five-pointed star. A year later the fraternity had thirteen active members (three seniors, eight juniors, and two sophomores). As females took a more prominent place in medical colleges, Alpha Epsilon Iota grew. By 1906 there were ten chapters around the country. The Delta chapter at P&S included eight faculty members, all MDs; twenty city members; and fourteen college members. Van Hoosen and Yarros were among the faculty members. Thirteen of the twenty city members were MDs, while most of the others

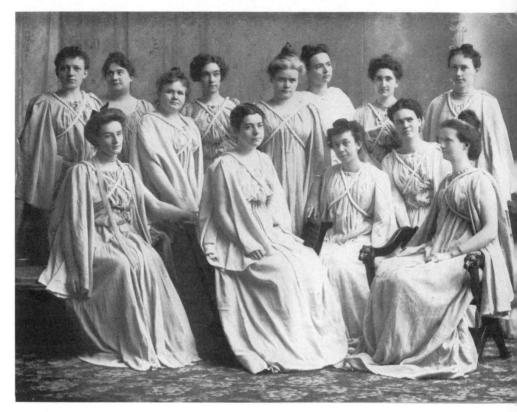

Nu Sigma Phi. This photo was published in the *Illio 1901*. Courtesy of the University of Illinois at Urbana-Champaign Archives.

were faculty wives. The college members included eight seniors, two juniors, two freshmen, and two non-graduate students.[81]

Alpha Omega Alpha, an honorary medical fraternity, originated at P&S. William W. Root was its founder. A Cornell University BA, he had taken advanced work in chemistry at Cornell and at the University of Chicago and had taught in secondary schools for several years before entering P&S. The rough and ready, hurly-burly atmosphere of the school shocked him, but he was impressed with the number of men with brains and character in the senior class. The idea of an honorary society as a means of uplift in the student body appealed to him. Early in August 1902, at the end of his third year in the college, Root asked Ernest S. Moore, a junior, if he would help form an honor fraternity for the medical profession similar to the Phi Beta Kappa society. It was to be nonsecret and would be made up of juniors and seniors who would campaign for higher medical standards and a higher standard of scholarship. Moore agreed to help, others considered the proposal, and a number of seniors met in

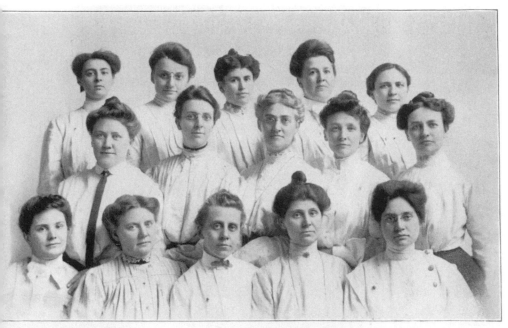

GEORGIANA DEVORAK   CLARA SEIPPEL   DR. HELEN GREIG   MARTHA HAYWARD   MARY SCHWARTZ
         MRS. HILL   LENA HATFIELD   XENIA BOND   NELLIE BAKER   LOUISE ABBOTT
DR. NOLAN   DR. VAN HOOSEN   DR. COOKE   DR. YARROS   DR. HAGANS
ALPHA EPSILON IOTA

Alpha Epsilon Iota. This photo was published in the *Illio 1906*. Courtesy of the University of Illinois at Urbana-Champaign Archives.

the library and elected officers. On 25 August Root met with several students in the bacteriological laboratory and founded an honor fraternity. Its motto was "To Be Worthy to Serve the Suffering." Turned into Greek, the motto gave the initials Alpha Omega Alpha, the name of the new fraternity. Undergraduate membership was based entirely on scholarship, personal honesty, and potential leadership. The number of student members could not exceed one-sixth of the total number expected to graduate in that class. In his senior year Root transferred to Rush Medical College, and chapters of the fraternity were quickly formed at Rush and Northwestern. In less than a decade seventeen chapters had been formed, and Alpha Omega Alpha was still spreading to other medical schools.[82]

The Alpha chapter of Phi Delta Kappa, also an honorary medical fraternity, was formed at P&S in 1916. It was overshadowed by Alpha Omega Alpha, and little more was heard of it.[83]

Perhaps most P&S students would have endorsed the statement of a classmate who complained, "To the medic all is medicine. . . . His life is with few exceptions a monotonous though interesting grind over bones and powders and bandages. No Junior Prom's [*sic*], or Senior Balls enliven his existence for the simple reason that for him 'medicine, medicine, only medicine' is the thought and if success is to come in the future, present opportunities must be utilized."[84] Surely the complaint failed to acknowledge that there was another side to the life of a medical student. To be sure, medical students pored over "bones and powders and bandages," but they also found time for many of the entertaining and sometimes rowdy activities that made up the American collegiate experience.

CHAPTER 7

Early Years of the College of Medicine under President James

After opening in 1882, the College of Physicians and Surgeons of Chicago (P&S) developed unevenly. Torn by internal dissension and financial insecurity during the 1880s, it became more stable in the early 1890s and began anew in 1897 when it affiliated with the university. But the leasing arrangement worked less well than envisioned, and Andrew S. Draper, the president of the university from 1894 to 1904, lacked understanding of the nature of a university, which emphasizes scientific research and the discovery of new knowledge. Edmund J. James, who took office in 1904, was determined to create a genuine university for the people of Illinois and was equally determined to make a high-quality medical school an integral part of the University of Illinois. This chapter analyzes the development of the College of Medicine up to 1912, when P&S and the University of Illinois severed their tie and each briefly went its own way.

Edmund J. James

Edmund J. James (1855–1925), who served as president of the University of Illinois until 1920, was superbly qualified for the office. A native of Illinois who grew up in Normal, Illinois, he had briefly studied the classics at both Northwestern and Harvard universities. In 1875 he went to Germany, where he earned a doctorate in political economy at the University of Halle and gained a strong reverence for German institutions, especially the nation's devotion to scholarship and the conviction that the government should take an active role in advancing public welfare. Returning to Illinois in 1877, he served as principal of high schools and published a crusading educational journal until 1883. Having won a national reputation with articles that criticized the prevailing doctrine of laissez-faire in public policy, he became professor of public finance and administration at the University of Pennsylvania where, beginning in 1883, he was for thirteen years the dominant force in the newly established Wharton School of Finance and Economy. In 1896 James went to the University of Chicago as

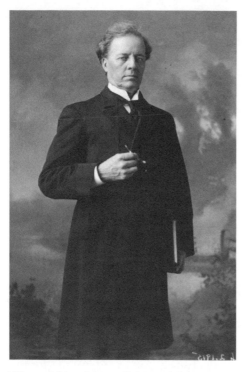

Edmund Janes James. Courtesy of the University of Illinois at Urbana-Champaign Archives.

professor of public administration and head of university extension. President Harper praised him fulsomely, telling James that "among all the men who have worked with me within twenty years, there is no man whom I have esteemed more, and with whom I have worked more affectionately than yourself."[1] In January 1902 James became president of Northwestern University, but his hope of transforming the Methodist liberal arts college into a university proved to be premature, so he moved on.[2]

James was highly qualified to preside over the immature University of Illinois. It had tremendous potential, he realized, but had not yet found its true identity. He boldly proclaimed his determination to create a great university on the prairie in east-central Illinois. Accordingly, he set out to invigorate the graduate school, to build a library adequate to research needs, to recruit a faculty whose members were successful teachers as well as productive scholars, to develop professional training, and to make the university's presence felt in Chicago. A highly disciplined man of medium stature, James drove himself hard and expected full commitment from members of the faculty. In politics he was a progressive Republican. He kept a diary, and his entries on the medical college are invaluable in understanding the reform of medical education in Chicago. In this book his diary is drawn on for the first time in studying the medical scene in Chicago. A man of principle with a healthy ego, James took risks in promoting his views. He had the ability to differ sharply with others while remaining on good personal terms with them. He bred deep loyalty in the overwhelming majority of the faculty. James married Anna Margarethe Lange, the daughter of a German Lutheran clergyman whom he met while in Germany. A cultivated woman, she was a devoted helpmate. On Friday, 13 November 1914, when she breathed her last, James wrote, "Peace came to her dear soul! Help me, O God!"[3] A devoted Methodist, James regularly attended church on Sunday. For recreation James, whose health was never robust, rode Maje, his favorite horse.

James was a pioneer in the reform of medical education in the United States. His commitment is best seen in context. Reform movements of many kinds gathered strength in the late nineteenth century as Americans became aware of the social and economic dislocations that attended the rise of an urban and industrial society, and in the early twentieth century a progressive impulse began to transform the nation. In politics, that impulse was evident in the efforts of the political parties to curb monopolies, revitalize democracy, and promote the public welfare. In religion the progressive impulse manifested itself in the Social Gospel movement, which sought to apply the teachings of Jesus to curbing abuses and reforming the socioeconomic order. In the intellectual realm, loyalty to old and rigid moral certainties gave way to pragmatism as a way of understanding reality. The world was seen as fluid and plastic, open by experimentation to marvelous possibilities.

In addition, devotion to science as a panacea permeated American thought at the turn of the century. Science, it was widely believed, could be harnessed in the service of ameliorating a wide range of problems and promoting social, intellectual, and technological advance.[4] James believed that science was the way forward. The most striking peculiarity of a true university, he declared in his inaugural address as president of the University of Illinois in 1905, was "the scientific character of the training which it affords."[5]

James had been committed to the reform of medical education since 1875. As a student of public administration in Germany he had studied the function of the state in relation to the life of its citizens under Lorenz von Stein (1815–90). Stein's lectures on public administration included a survey of the relation of the state to medicine because Stein believed that the health of citizens, which was the basis of good health in the body politic, depended to a large extent on a sound sanitary policy on the part of the state. To promote public health, the state needed to encourage the advance of medical knowledge and to train practitioners who applied this knowledge in the treatment of disease. In working out a sanitary code, the state had to depend on the advice of its medical men, and the sanitary code had to be adapted to the conditions of the society and time in which it was to apply. Thus the medical men who were called on to advise the government on its sanitary policy must be statesmen as well as physicians and men of liberal education, whether the education was acquired in school or in the practical experience of life.

James had his first opportunity to apply his views on medical education while he was a professor at the University of Pennsylvania. In 1885 William Pepper Jr., provost of the university, appointed a general committee to study the better integration of the professional schools of the university with the college and the technical schools. James was a member of the subcommittee on the medical school. Drawing on Stein's teaching and his own study of the existing state of medical education in different modern countries, James recommended that the university require for admission to its medical school the completion of the sophomore year in the college of liberal arts; that a medical course of five years, counting from that time, be inaugurated, the first two of which, corresponding to the last two of the college course, should be given to the study of the underlying sciences of medicine (anatomy, biology, chemistry, physics, and physiology); and that the last year should be given practically to the hospital work and the two intermediate years to clinical instruction. James defended his recommendation on three grounds. The physician should be an educated and cultured gentleman with a liberal education, should have a thorough scientific training, and should have acquired the practical knowledge that makes him an efficient practitioner.[6]

The history of medical education in the United States, James once declared, was not one of which the country had reason to be proud. The great mistake from the point of view of public interest was the commercialization of medical education. Physicians found sources of profit in the system: fees from students, the reputation from being connected with a medical school, and a consulting practice from referrals of former students.[7] At the same time James believed that medical education occupied the most strategic position in the domain of professional training that was an attribute of the new American universities. And Chicago, James asserted, was destined to become the leading center of professional education in the United States.[8]

Since its founding the city had grown dramatically. Between 1850 and 1860 the population had nearly quadrupled. By 1880 Chicago contained 503,185 souls. The World's Columbian Exposition of 1893 gained the city international attention, and by 1900 the population stood at 1,698,575. A decade later it reached 2,185,283 and was still growing. Strategically located, Chicago was the entrepôt for the grain and cattle of the Midwest and the hub of a splendid railroad network that gave the city access to eastern markets.[9] In 1903 James published an essay titled "The Opportunity of Chicago to Become a Great City."[10] However dynamic, Chicago was widely seen as a raw and raucous metropolis controlled by corrupt politicians who looked tolerantly on the uglier manifestations of rampant vice. Despite its flaws, none doubted that Chicago had a great future.

The Medical College That James Took Over

James assumed responsibility for a big and complex medical college with a brief but reputable history. From the beginning of his presidency he thought that the contract between the university and P&S to conduct medical education had to be abolished because it prevented either party from taking a very advanced or progressive stand in the development of higher standards of medical education. He did not realize this goal until 1910.[11]

In 1904 Daniel A. K. Steele was president of the college. Since 1886 he had been professor of the principles and practice of surgery and clinical surgery. He had never studied abroad, but in 1888 the American Medical Association (AMA) accredited him as a delegate to a meeting of the British Medical Association at Glasgow. On this occasion he visited the principal medical institutions and hospitals of England, France, Germany, and Switzerland.[12]

William E. Quine was dean of the faculty. Quine had never studied abroad, and he wrote little for publication. But by force of character he exercised immense power within the college. Many regarded him as one of the best medical instructors in the city of Chicago. Frank Billings, a former student, described Quine as an ideal teacher as well as a "living example of a Christian gentleman." John B. Murphy, a surgeon and colleague, described Quine as the highest of the ideal type of the old school, a connecting link between an older and a new generation of Chicago medical notables. As a didactic and descriptive lecturer he had few equals. James B. Herrick of Rush Medical College portrayed Quine as a splendid family physician whose patients loved him as a man and friend. Students had deep affection for Quine.[13]

And yet Quine did not escape criticism. He was agnostic as to bacteria in disease, wrote Bayard Holmes, a faculty member at the college, and his instructional method was sermonizing. After a formal entrance into the amphitheater, Holmes recalled, Quine began his lecture in a low voice by giving

> a synopsis of his last sermon. He gradually raised his voice as he approached the sermon of the day. He then gave in short terse sentences definitions and descriptions and the onset and progress of the disease in the most didactic and authoritative manner. The sentences grew in length and magnificence and the voice in resonance and force until the crisis was reached and the critical discharge of the disease and of the sermon came in a frenzy of word painting. Then . . . his voice fell to a whisper, the glaring white handkerchief was drawn from its concealment in the semi-clerical garb, . . . and the indications for treatment which would thwart the fatal crisis were vouchsafed in the remnants of strength left after this artistic performance. The impression made upon the student was lasting. The picture was complete. It was not exactly photographic, it was rather a painted bas-relief. It seemed to say "As it was in the beginning, is now and ever shall be, world without end. Amen."[14]

The picture drawn, Holmes insisted, was of a condition that never existed. "The notion that typhoid may be thus didacticly [*sic*] described is a fiction of the authoritatively presumptuous mind."[15]

Quine's admirers and critics both possessed part of the truth. Quine, along with many other physicians of the time, was a transitional figure. He began his career when didactic lectures and rational theories as to disease prevailed, and he continued to teach as scientific medicine and laboratory instruction became paramount. Fortunately, Quine moved with the times.

In 1904 the faculty of P&S numbered 129, most of whom were practitioners as well as part-time teachers. The roster included 41 professors, 7 associate professors, 25 adjunct professors, 5 assistant professors, 4 clinical professors, 3 associate clinical professors, and 44 instructors.[16] For several years thereafter the faculty ranged from about 144 to 155 members, with approximately the same proportions in different academic ranks.

Some recent appointees took a prominent role in the life of the college. Casey A. Wood was born in Ontario in 1856 and was the son of a well-known physician. He received his elementary and higher education in Canada, graduating in 1877 with an MD from the Faculty of Medicine of the University of Bishop's College, Montreal. He quickly retired from general practice to devote himself to the treatment of diseases of the eye and ear. He studied ophthalmology and otology first in New York and then for two years in Berlin, Vienna, Paris, and London. In 1889 he settled in Chicago and acquired a large practice while also holding many medical positions. In 1898 he became professor of clinical ophthalmology at P&S. Wood was assistant editor of the *Annals of Ophthalmology and Otology;* translated treatises in his field from German, French, and Italian; and was the author of medical works.[17]

Charles S. Williamson, appointed in 1901, was a valuable addition to the faculty. Born in Cincinnati in 1872, he graduated with a BS (1893) and an MD (1896) from the University of Cincinnati and shortly thereafter went to Europe for postgraduate medical work and original research. He spent three years abroad mainly in Leipzig, Berlin, and Vienna with short stays in Paris and London. Returning to America, he started a practice in internal medicine in Chicago. Williamson began at P&S as an adjunct professor of medicine and became professor of clinical medicine a year later.[18]

In the years from 1904 to 1912 some twenty women MDs held positions as instructors or assistants. Only a few rose in rank. Five of this group had medical degrees from P&S, four had medical degrees from Woman's Medical College of Northwestern University, three had medical degrees from the University of Michigan, two had medical degrees from Harvey Medical College, and one had a medical degree from Hahnemann Medical College. A large number of these women taught obstetrics or gynecology.[19]

James Seeks Legislative Aid

As president, James was responsible for many interrelated medical matters. His main objective was to bring the medical college under the control of the university and to reform it in line with modern medicine. His experience in Germany, where medical education was an integral part of the universities, predisposed him to take this view. In addition, leading authorities at P&S realized that the sun was setting on the proprietary medical college. To gain control of P&S James needed to obtain an appropriation from the legislature. He was indefatigable in this quest, which dragged on for years. James also pursued another important goal. In his effort to reform medical education, he sought to consolidate the three university-related medical schools in the city in order to make Chicago a center of medical research and education. He pursued these two goals simultaneously, but for the sake of clarity it is best if we discuss them separately, beginning with his effort to secure a legislative appropriation.

The First Round

Soon after taking office in 1904, James persuaded his board to declare that no institution be affiliated with the university unless entire control of it be turned over absolutely to the trustees, and in mid-December James informed P&S officials of his desire to transfer the property of the college to the university at once, without waiting on the maturity of the lease.[20]

The P&S directors secured an opinion from William J. Hynes, a Chicago lawyer, as to the validity of the contract and what obligations, if any, the university could give in lieu of the provisions of the lease without asking the legislature for an appropriation.[21] Hynes concluded that any action closing out the existence of P&S for an amount less than that stated in the contract would require the consent of every stockholder.[22] P&S officials thought that a considerable majority but not all of the stockholders would favor such a recommendation.[23] Since the contract could not be broken, James concluded that it was necessary for the university to make the college a department of the university. The university would then be able to get a legislative appropriation and develop a high-class medical school.[24]

Oscar A. King, vice dean, proposed that the legislature appropriate $217,000 to purchase the stock of the college. James called the proposal unreasonable. The directors of P&S had made a contract with the university in the belief that the school would be profitable and in time would become a department of the university without expense to the state, said James, but the whole thing was a speculation, and the legislature would refuse to make good on it. Since the school could not be maintained on fee income alone, James advised P&S to give the university its property, estimated to be worth $217,000, for $63,500 in 4 percent bonds. This would make a virtue of necessity, returning to stockholders the actual cash value of their investment and ensuring the establishment of the leading medical school in Chicago on a solid foundation.[25]

When the board of trustees dealt with these matters on 17 January 1905, members agreed that it would be futile to go to the legislature with King's proposal, and they reiterated the suggestion that P&S donate its property to the university for $63,500 in 4 percent bonds. The trustees also declared that "medical education should be incorporated as an integral part in the work of the University in the same sense as agriculture and engineering education." Only Leonidas H. Kerrick, a cattle breeder who thought that the university should not engage in medical education, voted no.[26] James informed Kerrick that the university was "irrevocably tied up" with P&S and had to conduct medical education as efficiently as possible.[27]

James drafted a bill to authorize the trustees of the university to acquire the property of P&S. As he explained, the stockholders were willing to turn over the property and goodwill of the college valued at $217,000 for $63,500 in return for which the university would assume the mortgage indebtedness of the college to an amount not exceeding $86,000 and the floating indebtedness of the same to an amount not exceeding $28,325. For payment of said mortgage and other indebtedness and property, the bill authorized the university to issue 4 percent bonds secured by a mortgage on the property acquired from P&S and payable at the will of the university. The authority to do all this was given on condition that the university acquire "the absolute, uncontrolled ownership in the real estate, buildings, equipment, good will, and other property and rights of every kind whatsoever" of P&S, including its charter and other privileges. James composed a long argument in favor of the bill.[28]

It would help to secure the consent of the legislature, James told the stockholders, if they would donate their holdings to the endowment of the medical school. Quine and Steele had each agreed to donate securities valued at twenty-five thousand dollars; another fifty thousand dollars would bring the total to one hundred thousand dollars, a sum that would help persuade the legislature to give the trustees the authority they requested.[29]

At a meeting on 24 February every stockholder present except one agreed that if the transfer were consummated, each stockholder should subscribe at least 25 percent of the par value of his stock to the endowment of the medical school. James then sent the stockholders a letter asking them to contribute to the fund. With the letter went a summary of the work of the college since its affiliation with the university.[30]

In April Republican legislators introduced the appropriations bill in both the Senate and the House, and Senator Henry M. Dunlap, a Republican from Savoy and the university's spokesman in Springfield, lined up support for the bill in the General Assembly. On 27 April a motion to give the bill a second reading and refer it to the Senate Committee on Appropriations was passed by a vote of 36 to 4, but no more was heard of the bill.

Observers assigned many reasons for the failure. One was that it was introduced so late in the session. In choosing a time, James explained, he had followed the advice of friends of the university. The real difficulty, said James, was that members of the legislature did not think the state should buy a private corporation, and some thought that the university should not undertake medical education. As a result the university was compelled to conduct the college under the existing contract for another biennium. James recommended that P&S make an effort to raise the medical standards of the college, reduce its debt, declare no dividends, and make a clearer financial statement for the next biennial appeal to the legislature.[31]

The Second Round

In 1906 James returned to the pursuit of state aid. Knowing that he needed a good plan to present to the legislature, one that was simple, easy to understand, and fair, he mulled over the arguments for and against the state purchasing the medical college. Why should the state pay for it, he asked, when the trustees of Chicago Medical College gave their property to Northwestern and when the University of Chicago refused to take over Rush Medical College unless Rush offered a million dollars to endow the medical school? If those who founded the college wanted to advance medical education, they already had their reward in setting up a service to the community. If they meant to make a profit, why should the state make their speculation good? The university had no obligation to purchase P&S, but if the university was going to operate a medical school, the cost-effective way to begin was to buy it, and it was only fair to give the men who began the college their original investment plus interest.[32]

Thus James and the board's Committee on the College of Medicine, chaired by Charles Davison, and a committee of P&S agreed that the contract between the two schools should be terminated; that the notes given by the college corporation under the contract, amounting to $19,600, be abrogated; and that the university purchase the property of P&S at a price to be determined by appraisal of the value of the tangible property. Two architects appraised the buildings at $213,000, a realtor appraised the land at $57,200, and two physiology professors appraised the equipment at $115,314.25. The total came to $385,514.25.[33]

On 11 December the board of trustees agreed to ask the legislature for $386,000 to enable the university to erect or acquire its own buildings and equipment for the conduct of medical education, provided that in case the trustees saw fit to purchase the property and equipment of P&S they should pay no more for it than the actual value of the tangible property of the college. (The board also requested $1,468,500 for the operating expenses of the university plus $1 million for buildings for the university for 1907–9, bringing the total asking to $2,468,500 in addition to the $386,000 in the medical bill.) Governor Charles S. Deneen, who attended the meeting of the board as an ex officio member, voted in favor of the requests.[34]

On 26 December the Executive Faculty of P&S met with university trustees William L. Abbott, president of the board, and Charles Davison to outline a campaign to support the bills. Steele emphasized the need to create a strong sentiment in favor of the measure in the minds of legislators, prominent public men, and the Chicago press and then "bombard the Governor with demands from all parts of the State for its [the bill's] passage."[35]

To ensure passage of the bills it was essential to have the support of leaders of the medical profession in Chicago and throughout the state. Publicly recommending in mid-January that the legislature grant the funds requested were Frank Billings, dean of Rush Medical College and a former president of the AMA; Nathan S. Davis Jr., dean of the Northwestern University Medical College; Arthur D. Bevan, professor of surgery at Rush and chairman of the Council on Medical Education of the AMA; George W. Webster Sr., president of the Illinois State Board of Health and of the Chicago Medical Society; William E. Quine, dean of the College of Medicine of the University of Illinois; and J. F. Perry, president of the Illinois State Medical Society. The appropriation would help elevate the standard of medicine in Illinois and the West, these worthies declared, and would put the University of Illinois on a plane of equality with such other state universities as Michigan, Minnesota, Iowa, and Missouri.[36]

In early 1907 Henry M. Dunlap of Savoy and Peter P. Schaefer of Champaign introduced appropriations bills in the General Assembly.[37] A campaign then began to enlist support. James knew that both David E. Shanahan and Corbus P. Gardner, the chairmen of the appropriations committees in the House and Senate, respectively, opposed the bill. To change their attitude, James thought, local physicians would have to persuade them. Steele worked at getting favorable coverage in the press and talking to men to whom Governor Deneen listened.[38]

James sent a statement about the medical school to members of the legislature. Quine sent a circular letter to P&S alumni who lived in Illinois. Abbott, Davison, and Steele called on Fred A. Busse, a Republican saloon keeper, machine politician, and ethnic German who served as mayor of Chicago from 1907 to 1911. Busse promised to back the bill and to influence his friends in its favor.[39]

James was aggressive in seeking the endorsement of Chicago editors and publishers for his plans. In mid-February the *Chicago American,* an evening newspaper owned by William Randolph Hearst, observed that the alternatives were either to accept lower standards in the medical school or for the university to take it over. Fourteen other state universities, the newspaper added, had medical schools. The city had a number of second-rate medical schools, which gave Chicago a bad name both at home and abroad. They had to be wiped out.[40]

The *Inter Ocean* was prepared to publish an editorial opposing the bill, but Steele intervened with one of the editors, and on 20 February the newspaper declared in favor of the bill. To the charge that the purpose of the bill was to unload upon the state an unprofitable enterprise for the relief of the present owners, an editorial said that the pending bill gave authority only to purchase tangible property at its market value and that the University of Illinois needed to keep pace with other universities. Iowa, Wisconsin, Michigan, and California were doing considerably more for their state universities than Illinois, and none of the other states had half the population or wealth of Illinois.[41]

With support for the bill evident, in mid-February J. Newton Roe publicly opposed the measure. Roe was dean of the School of Pharmacy at Valparaiso University and secretary of the corporation that operated the Chicago College of Medicine and Surgery (Valparaiso) and the Chicago College of Dental Surgery. The largest enrollments at the Indiana-based university were in the Chicago departments; medicine had 600 students, and dentistry had 449. According to the Reverend H. S. Spalding of Loyola University, the Chicago College of Medicine and Surgery "although nominally" affiliated with Valparaiso University was in fact "owned and dominated by Mr. Roe."[42] Establishment of a medical and dental college in Chicago conducted at the expense of the state, Roe charged, would be to the disadvantage of the Chicago College of Medicine and Surgery (Valparaiso). The Valparaiso college would agree to withdraw its opposition to the appropriation, Roe offered, provided that the university cease to operate its dental college and allow Valparaiso to take the equipment of the university's dental infirmary and pay for it an amount to be determined by appraisal. Roe wanted his proposition considered as a compromise. If the bill to acquire the P&S failed and the university wished to continue its department of dentistry, Valparaiso would be willing to leave matters as they were.[43]

Archie J. Graham, a 1902 graduate of P&S, observed that an element of the P&S faculty had always opposed university control of the medical school because they used the clinics to feed their own practices and let in poorly prepared students to swell the dividends on their stock. All of this was common knowledge. Graham wondered if this element was behind the opposition of the Valparaiso college or if the P&S element opposed the appropriation on their own behalf.[44]

Some of the other proprietary colleges asked Hahnemann Medical College of Chicago to join them in opposing the bill; alternately they offered to ally with Hahnemann in doing so. George F. Shears, the senior professor of surgery at Hahnemann, spurned the suggestion. Hahnemann favored the university purchasing the property of P&S, Shears avowed, and Hahnemann had made its views known to Governor Deneen. Hahnemann's support of the bill was based on the expectation that the university would give homeopathy every consideration in the medical college should the bill pass.[45]

James seemed willing to incorporate a homeopathy department at P&S, but Quine demurred. In 1899 he had stated his views on homeopathy in an address titled "The Medical Profession: The Causes of Its Division into Discordant Elements and the Reasons I Am Not a Homeopath" and given to the faculty and students of Dunham Medical College, a homeopathic school. His remarks were published that year.[46] The university had a right to teach in P&S any of the systems of medicine it pleased, Quine admitted, and James could appoint as many homeopaths or sectarian teachers as he wished but not at the expense of P&S. The appointment of sectarians would not be accepted because such practitioners could not compete with nonsectarian medicine.[47]

In early March the House Appropriations Committee held a hearing on the bill. Steele sent his "committee on propaganda" to Springfield to be able to answer questions. He wanted two prominent doctors from both Rush Medical College and the Northwestern Medical School and some prominent physicians not connected with any of the medical schools in Chicago to speak in favor of the bill. According to Steele, legislators from Chicago and northern Illinois were practically unanimous in support of the bill, but downstate legislators would presumably require encouraging. Ezekiel P. Murdock of Bennett Medical College, who had attended organizational meetings of P&S in 1881, was prepared to appear before the committee advocating the measure. Shears and others from Hahnemann planned to go to Springfield to urge passage of the medical bill.[48]

The hearing in Springfield was tumultuous as supporters of the bill squared off against opponents. "War of Pills Is Waged" wrote the prestigious *Chicago Tribune*. Patrick H. O'Donnell, an attorney who represented the Chicago College of Medicine and Surgery (Valparaiso), thought that the bill had "a contagious disease which would put fourteen independent and thriving medical schools out of business if it were passed." The Valparaiso-based college insisted that the bill was "designed to work as an injury to other schools." When P&S denied the charge, O'Donnell's clients offered to drop their opposition in return for surrender of the P&S dental school. Steele had this proposition in writing. According to the *Tribune*, both the homeopaths and the eclectics opposed the bill because of the alleged advantage it would give to an allopathic school. When the hearing ended, David E. Shanahan of the appropriations committee did not know whether the bill had "appendicitis or fatty degeneration of the liver."[49]

The hearing did not go well for them, James and Steele admitted. Frank J. Heinl, a member of the appropriations committee, told James that the bill was "a dead dog." But James and Steele looked forward to another hearing. Meanwhile, both those for and against the measure had the Chicago Real Estate Board value the medical college property, and Steele compiled figures showing that up to 1897 a total of $217,000 had been put into the enterprise. To plead his case, James prepared an account of the history and status of the university's relation to P&S. He sent copies to Governor Deneen and others.[50]

The trustee Charles Davison knew that Corbus Gardner, chair of the Senate Appropriations Committee, would have the say as to appropriations for the university and that his sentiment toward the university was all right. Davison also knew that the state treasury had two million dollars less than was supposed, so he advised James to quickly get an understanding with Gardner about money that should go to the university.[51]

On 4 April James presented his case in a brief appearance before the Committee of the Whole House and a longer appearance before the Senate.[52] He made a favorable impression. Shanahan said that originally he was rather opposed to the bill, "but every 'darned' doctor in his district had been camping on his neck in favor of it so that he had now made up his mind to support it."[53] Yet in both chambers sentiment against the bill was strong. If the university wished to establish a medical school, opponents argued, it should start with much finer equipment and much more complete buildings than the university would get by purchase. James wondered whether this was an argument or an excuse. His attitude was "Never say die."[54]

On 7 May the Senate Appropriations Committee passed the bill by 30 to 6 and asked the House to concur. On 9 May the House Appropriations Committee refused to recommend the bill by a vote of 18 to 17. The bill appeared to be dead. Shanahan said that he would fight the bill but would not prevent its friends from rescuing it if they had the strength. According to the *Chicago Post,* an evening newspaper owned by Herman H. Kohlsaat, James was active on behalf of the bill and was considered "one of the most effective of the legitimate lobbyists" in Springfield.[55]

On 11 May the House dealt with the bill during a session that lasted from 10:00 a.m. to nearly midnight. As reported by the *Chicago Examiner,* Hearst's morning newspaper, disorder swept the House the moment Shanahan called up the bill. Lobbyists crowded the aisles. Democrat Lee O. Browne of Ottawa raised a storm by demanding their ouster. "This is a gold brick," declared Emil O. Kowalski, a Republican from Chicago who chaired the House Committee on Public Buildings and Grounds. "Too much for ramshackle buildings," said Michael J. Daugherty, a Democrat from Galesburg. The opposition was said to come from foes of Governor Deneen, who feared that the medical college, under state control, in connection with backers of the West Side Park System would make the executive branch of the state government supreme on the West Side of Chicago. At 11:30 p.m. the medical bill passed the House by 91 to 40.[56]

The initiative now lay with Governor Deneen, so the medical profession of the state appealed to him. At the annual meeting of the Illinois State Medical Society in Rockford on 21–23 May, President J. F. Perry, alluding to the 11 May hearing, criticized legislators for paying attention to "spectacle peddlers" and other forms of quackery while practically laughing Frank Billings, president of the Illinois State Board of Charities, out of the State House. Members of the society instructed Charles S. Bacon, Everett J. Brown, and J. Whitefield Smith to urge Deneen to sign the bill giving P&S to the university.[57]

Brown and Smith called on Deneen, who explained that he had made up his mind to veto the bill because the money could not be appropriated without a special tax levy and because the university was already getting too much. Moreover, Deneen had received a letter from Chicago stating that the bill was a "bought up one." The writer offered to send proof, which the governor requested. In addition, Deneen did not like the position that James had placed him in before the medical profession of Illinois by flooding him with five hundred letters from physicians in the state. Although Deneen thought that acquisition of the medical college would be a grand thing for the university, he thought that the price was too high and that Hahnemann Medical College had been offered to the university free of expense and free from debt.[58]

According to the *Chicago Examiner,* Deneen's opposition "resulted partly from a privately conducted investigation and partly from data placed in his hands to indicate that a boodle fund, said to be $10,000, was used to pass the bill." When the charges of graft reached him, Deneen declared that there was "basis for taking out a warrant or going before the grand jury." Opponents of the measure said that they were willing to initiate such prosecution, but they noted that a link in the chain of evidence was missing. The governor discovered that the West Side Hospital, which was located just west of the medical building on Harrison Street and was operated in connection with P&S, was owned largely by stockholders who owned the college. Deneen was well informed. As noted earlier, the West Side Hospital had been organized as a private corporation. If the college plant were sold, Deneen was told, the hospital owners would be able to hold up the state either on a sale of the hospital or by placing a price on its privileges. There was no nearby ground that could be acquired by the state for a hospital. In view of these facts Deneen said that he would veto the bill, and he did, explaining that appropriations for 1907–9 were greater than the state could afford without an increase in the rate of taxation.[59]

Deneen had not treated either the university or P&S fairly, Bacon protested. "Had he not given us reason to believe that he was favorably inclined to our measure," wrote Bacon, "we should not have spent so much time and energy in passing the bill through the legislature. Had we supposed that he required a free gift of the School . . . or we had known that he would not trust the University Trustees, we never would have begun our agitation." Deneen had "evidently listened to advisors unfriendly to the University as well as to the School." It was not improbable, Bacon thought, that the legislature would be willing to pass the bill over the governor's veto, but the attempt to do so would require delicate handling.[60] No one made an effort to override the veto, so relations between the university and P&S remained essentially as they had been since 1900. Years later Walter C. Jones, a state senator in 1907, said that it was found impractical to appropriate the sum requested for the stated purpose without taking money that was necessary for caring for the insane and other dependents of the state and for the operating expenses of the university and other educational institutions.[61]

James expressed disappointment over failure to get an appropriation bill passed to acquire P&S for a medical college. He had worked as hard as he could for the bill, and he thought that no influence whatsoever was used except that which was perfectly legitimate.[62] Thus the university and P&S had tried twice to obtain a state appropriation to support a medical school, but the Empire State of the Midwest was not yet ready to shoulder the responsibility.

The Third Round

During the James administration the university at Urbana-Champaign grew rapidly, and on 15 January 1909 the administration responded by requesting larger appropriations than ever before. For the biennium 1909–11 the board asked for a general appropriation of $2.773 million plus $3.25 million for new buildings, including $500,000 for housing the medical school, a special grant of $1 million for buildings on the Urbana campus, and $395,160 for the College of Agriculture. The total request came to a sum enormous for the time: $7,418,160.[63]

The subject of university appropriations excited unusually active discussion during the sessions of the Forty-sixth General Assembly.[64] On 17 February Charles Adkins, a Republican from Bement, introduced a bill for the general appropriation for the university. The bill sailed through the House, and with amendments the Senate concurred on 18 May. But Adkins's bill included nothing for the College of Medicine, and the college got nothing.[65] As King Lear told his daughter Cordelia, nothing would come of asking for nothing.

The reason for omitting medicine in the appropriations request is hard to fathom. James promoted many university interests at the time, including the Graduate College, a school of education, ceramics, and mining engineering, and he may have decided to let medical education rest briefly. The income of the state was relatively very small then, he explained, and state officials did not favor increasing the tax rate. As a result the legislature drastically reduced the amounts asked for by the university. The state provided $1,642,500 for the biennium in the general university bill, $250,000 in the building bill (for Urbana), $381,000 in the agricultural bill, and $15,000 for mining engineering, for a total of $2,288,500.[66]

By 1909 the university had been at bat twice for the College of Medicine and each time had struck out. The university did not even go to the plate the third time.

The College of Medicine in Comparative Perspective

Ever eager to know the full dimensions of the problems he encountered, in 1909 James asked George P. Dreyer, a physiology professor, to gather information about the medical schools of the state universities of Michigan, Wisconsin, and Minnesota.[67] Dreyer compiled data that compared these medical schools with that of Illinois for the academic year 1909–10. His report provides a valuable comparative perspective on the University of Illinois College of Medicine.[68]

As entrance requirements were concerned, Dreyer noted that Michigan, Wisconsin, and Minnesota all required two years of college work in addition to a high school diploma or equivalent, while Illinois required only the latter. In enrollment, Minnesota had 172 students; Wisconsin, with a two-year program, had 44 students; Michigan had 408 students in 1908; and Illinois had 514 students. The average in tuition and fees per annum was Minnesota, $110; Wisconsin, $70 to $120; Michigan, $90 to $200; and Illinois, $157. The budget for the entire medical department for salaries and supplies, not including heat, light, buildings, and grounds, ranged widely. For Minnesota it was $108,654; for Wisconsin, $30,470; for Michigan, $156,991; and for Illinois, $40,000. Putting his data in tabular form, Dreyer showed that Minnesota and Michigan had the largest and best-paid staffs in the scientific departments and that Wisconsin was proportionately better off than Illinois. One example will illustrate the point. In the pathology and bacteriology departments, Minnesota had $17,720 for salaries, $4,976 for supplies, and $30,000 for equipment; Wisconsin had $7,200 for salaries, $1,870 for supplies, and $7,000 for equipment; Michigan had $17,100 for salaries, $7,850 for supplies, and $30,000 for equipment; Illinois had $4,510 for salaries, $750 for supplies, and $2,500 for equipment.

It was impossible, Dreyer contended, to portray the real conditions in the four medical schools by statistical measures, because taken at face value the figures were misleading. So Dreyer commented on the quality of the instruction at the College of Medicine. Despite the small percentage of paid full professors and assistants in the scientific departments, he wrote, the teaching work was as intensive as it was extensive. All the branches included in the curriculum of the best schools were embraced, and the entire energy of the teaching force was concentrated on undergraduate instruction, whereas the schools with salaried teachers throughout made advanced work and original research an important feature of their programs. Research work in a university medical school was necessary, Dreyer believed, but the average undergraduate medical student had no time for advanced courses or original work. At P&S relations between faculty members and students were "intimate and continuous" for whatever fraction of his time each teacher might give to the college, and the fact that the medical sciences were taught mainly by clinicians engaged part-time in medical practice did not necessarily imply inferior instruction.[69]

Except for physiology, Dreyer admitted, the laboratory equipment at P&S had excited unfavorable criticism from outside inspectors. Dreyer defended matters by contending that the entire equipment available was directed to undergraduate work and that the available equipment was used with the utmost efficiency. Neither rooms nor microscopes, for example, stood idle the greater part of the day, as in the other schools.

Although the instruction in most departments was satisfactory and the equipment fairly adequate, Dreyer wrote, the students did not grade up to the standard set by the other great state university medical schools. The result might

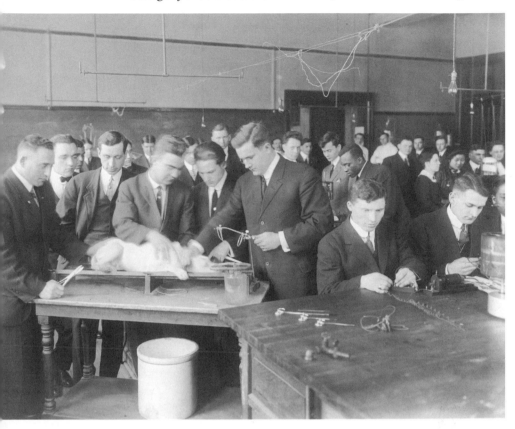

Physiology Laboratory, University of Illinois, Urbana, circa 1910. Courtesy of the University of Illinois at Urbana-Champaign Archives.

seem paradoxical, but the explanation was not difficult. The matriculants at P&S were largely high school graduates, and the course of study had to be arranged to suit this grade of student. Instruction in physics, chemistry, and biology had to be supplied indirectly or incidentally. Even so, all the branches of medicine taught elsewhere were presented at P&S to about the same extent and thoroughness. As a result the course of study was unreasonable and practically impossible for the average student. The freshman year consisted of 540 didactic and 648 laboratory hours, a total of 1,188 hours; the sophomore year consisted of 594 didactic and 604 laboratory hours, a total of 1,198 hours. The demands made upon the ability of the student were pedagogically unjustifiable, and the effect was to encourage superficiality and shallowness. Students developed a habit of working merely to pass examinations and get through, losing all appreciation of scientific training that they were unable to acquire in the time allotted.

Dreyer's report underscored the situation that James portrayed in his campaigns to secure a legislative appropriation to support the P&S and to upgrade the quality of medical education at the school. P&S was at a disadvantage compared

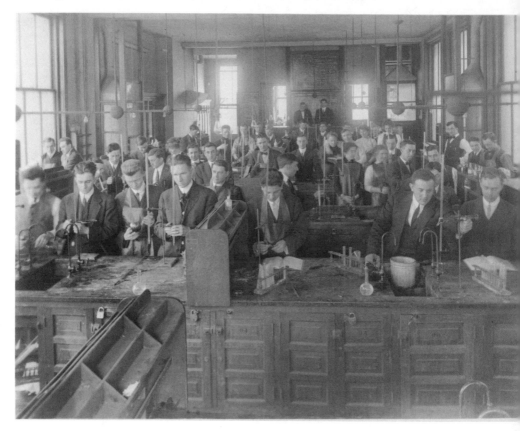

Chemical Laboratory. Courtesy of the University of Illinois at Urbana-Champaign
Archives.

to the medical schools of three neighboring state universities, but it made the best
of the handicaps under which it operated.

The disparity in the support of the medical schools of the universities of Minnesota, Wisconsin, and Michigan on the one hand and Illinois on the other was
highlighted by statistical data that compare the state of Illinois with the other
three states. Illinois had a larger population and was wealthier than any of the
other three states. In 1910, for example, Illinois had a resident population of 5.639
million, while Michigan's resident population was 2.810 million, Wisconsin's was
2.334 million, and Minnesota's was 2.076 million. Data on personal income by
state in 1910 are not available, but the figures for 1929 help in reconstructing the
relative standing of each state in 1910. In 1929 personal income in Illinois was
$7,291, compared to Michigan at $3,809, Wisconsin at $2,007, and Minnesota
at $1,548.[70] The data demonstrate that James faced an enormous problem in his
battle to reform medical education in Illinois.

CHAPTER 8

Advancing the College of Medicine

While seeking legislative appropriations and digesting Dreyer's report, Edmund J. James continued his multifaceted campaign to reform American medical education. This involved him in an attempt to consolidate the university-related medical schools in Chicago in order to make the city of Chicago a world center of medical research and education while at the same time trying to improve the quality of the academic work in the College of Medicine. While thus engaged, James got caught up in the conflict over the medical situation in Chicago and Abraham Flexner's report *Medical Education in the United States and Canada*, also known as the Flexner Report.

James Seeks Consolidation

According to Harry Pratt Judson, president of the University of Chicago, Henry S. Pritchett, president of the Carnegie Foundation for the Advancement of Teaching, proposed a union of the medical departments of Northwestern, Rush, and the University of Illinois.[1] On 30 April 1909 over lunch, the presidents of these institutions, Abram Harris, Judson, and James, reached an understanding as to how to proceed on Pritchett's proposal.[2] Judson reduced their agreement to writing and sent copies to the others. His draft outlined the creation of a new corporation for instruction and research in medicine with a board of trustees consisting of two persons each from the University of Illinois, Northwestern University, and the University of Chicago, with these six choosing three others. The three named medical schools were to be put under the control of a new creation, the Chicago School of Medicine. The faculties of the three medical schools were to tender their resignations, after which the board was to constitute a new faculty, guided solely by scientific merit. The new school was to have such arrangements with existing hospitals in Chicago as might be practicable. The first two years of medical instruction were to be offered in the colleges of the three named universities, and the clinical instruction was to take place in the new school of medicine. A plan was to be formed for the erection, equipment, and endowment of a research hospital under the charge of the Chicago School of Medicine. Adequate provision was to be made for an endowment.[3] James submitted the proposition to the authorities at the College of Physicians and Surgeons of Chicago (P&S), and he returned to the matter later.[4]

In June James gave the commencement address, titled "Governmental Function of the Medical Profession," at Rush Medical College in Chicago. No copy of the text can be located, and newspapers did not report the speech. Most likely James advanced a favorite theme: that the education of qualified doctors was costly and could not be done without state support and that the state had an obligation to promote the public health. Later that month James spent an evening discussing the medical school situation with close colleagues David Kinley, dean of the Graduate School and vice president of the university, and Eugene Davenport, dean of the College of Agriculture.[5]

In July, knowing that admissions requirements in the university's College of Medicine came under criticism, President James and university registrar William Pillsbury met with the Committee on Admission of the College of Medicine. James also conferred with Francis G. Blair, state superintendent of public instruction, about medical college certificates.[6]

On 28 October James spent the early afternoon discussing the medical school with university trustees Abbott and Davison and with P&S faculty members. Davison took James to inspect University Hospital, at the corner of Ogden Avenue and Lincoln (later Wolcott) and Congress streets. Davison, Steele, and Bacon were among the founders of the hospital. James also conferred with P&S officials and others about the budget and lease of the medical college and the university's contract with P&S.[7]

On 23 November James "worked on material to be presented to the Carnegie Foundation in re Medical School." Presumably the subject was the union of Northwestern, Rush, and the university's medical school. Three days later James had lunch with Governor Deneen, Pritchett, and Abbott of the board of trustees. James conferred with Pritchett again the next day, and in early December he and Abbott discussed the medical school situation.[8]

On 3 February the College of Medicine dominated the agenda when the board of trustees met at the Grand Pacific Hotel in Chicago. James explained that on 15 January Nathan P. Colwell, secretary of the Council on Medical Education of the American Medical Association (AMA), had informed him that at its meeting on 28 February the council expected to present a report showing which medical colleges of the United States and Canada were acceptable or not acceptable. After "a very careful" investigation of P&S the council had found three defects that were of too serious a nature to permit the council to include P&S in its acceptable list.

First was an apparent failure to enforce entrance requirements. Even the modest requirement of a high school education or its equivalent was overlooked. The council understood that James had already taken up this matter with the college. Second, advanced standing was sometimes granted for work done in low-grade medical schools. Students matriculated in one of the weaker Chicago medical schools and later transferred to P&S. Third and most serious, six members of the P&S faculty were also on the faculty of Jenner Medical College, a night school and one of the five or six lowest grade and poorest equipped medical colleges in the United States. Some of these men were among those in chief control of Jenner and therefore responsible for its existence. Knowing of James's personal interest in higher educational standards and desiring to aid in building up the nation's medical schools, the council hoped to receive assurance that the university would correct the defects described.[9]

James had sent Colwell's letter to Quine, asking him to lay it before the Executive Faculty of the medical school and ask for their recommendations. Illness prevented James from attending the meeting of the Executive Faculty on 28 January, but he sent Quine extracts from a letter dated 24 January from Pritchett of the Carnegie Foundation. Since seeing James, Pritchett wrote, he had sent James the report of the Carnegie Foundation on the medical school (an advance copy of the Flexner Report), and had had the medical department of the university reexamined (by Flexner). The reexamination had confirmed the facts brought out by the first examination. The Carnegie Foundation was willing to aid the university in this matter, wrote Pritchett. "At the same time I am bound to say that as the situation now stands it seems to me that the University of Illinois is injuring medical education in the State, not helping it, by the continuance of its medical school."[10]

In his letter to Quine James had added that the Association of American Medical Colleges had found the standards of the university's medical school "decidedly lower" than the minimum standards accepted by the association. All these things taken together, said James, pointed to "a very serious" condition with which the medical faculty "ought to wrestle in earnest."[11]

Quine replied that the Executive Faculty had voted to recommend that henceforth every applicant for admission to the College of Medicine be required to furnish proof of a satisfactory high school education and that no member of the teaching force be permitted connection with any other institution. James's demand for more and better teachers and better equipment for the freshman and sophomore courses of instruction had been referred to the Committee of University Relations chaired by Pusey. "It is my opinion," Quine concluded, "the College of Medicine ceased to be self-supporting last night [28 January 1910] and that it will never be self-supporting again. In my opinion the college cannot furnish better teachers and more of them and better equipment, out of its earnings. It has already gone beyond its powers in trying to satisfy the demands of the University."[12]

Meanwhile, the P&S faculty and the board of directors had considered the criticisms of the Council on Medical Education and those in the advance sheets of the report of the Carnegie Foundation (the Flexner Report). In general they regarded the criticisms as inaccurate or unjust, but they agreed to repair some of the defects noted. To the charge that six members of the faculty were also members of the faculty of a night school, they admitted that they had four teachers to whom such criticism applied. We know from his own testimony that Samuel A. McWilliams, a founder of and professor at P&S, taught at Jenner from 1901 to 1903, at Dearborn Medical College in 1903 and 1904, at Reliance Medical College from 1907 to 1911, and at Bennett Medical College in 1910–11.[13] The faculty and directors agreed that the present relations between P&S and the university were untenable. The university demanded a higher quality of medical education than was possible on the basis of tuition income, and it could not provide funds for the purpose.[14]

The board of trustees approved the recommendations of the P&S Executive Faculty as to the points at issue: admission to the medical school, admission to advanced standing, and no member of the medical faculty should be connected with any other medical school. The university registrar was to supervise the admission of students to the medical school and to secure strict enforcement of the stated regulations.[15]

James had prepared himself for the second item on the board's agenda, "Discussion of Medical Situation," by outlining the following talking points:

1. Present Condition untenable
   (2) Must be changed now
   (3) Either the Medical Faculty & College of Physicians & Surgeons must provide funds to improve the School to the standard of the better State University Medical Schools or
   The University must do so
   or
   The affiliation should be dissolved
   (4) If the University is to do it, it can undertake the task only with the consent of the Legislature & by the help of legislative appropriations
   (5) Practically speaking it can get no help from the legislature as long as the present so called contract exists.
   (6) The only possibility of getting legislative aid is to convert the present so-called contract into a simple lease for a definite period terminable yearly at the option of the Univ & at such a low rental & under such other terms as will satisfy all reasonable people that the interests of the State are fully safeguarded.
7. This can be done on the following terms:
   (a) ten year lease, terminable yearly on notice by University.

    (b) Rental based on 4% interest on the legitimate, clearly ascertained, present indebtedness of the College of Phys. & Surgeons.

    (c) Option of purchasing for the present indebtedness at any time within ten years.

    (d) Control of stock in hands of University.

8. If the Legislature refuses to make adequate appropriation for the support of the School at its next session the lease will be terminated one year from Sept. 7, 1910, & the College of Physicians & Surgeons will take over the Medical School.

9. Any other plan seems full of difficulties.[16]

James probably presented his case to the trustees, but the record of the meeting shows only that the board discussed "the relations between the University of Illinois and the College of Physicians and Surgeons of Chicago and conclusions drawn therefrom." The board referred matters to its Committee on the College of Medicine for consideration and report at its next meeting.[17]

As was his practice, James consulted others about his course. On 8 February he called on "Flexner, ag[en]t of Carnegie Foundation," at the La Salle Hotel in Chicago. They had lunch and talked over the medical school situation. James also conferred with both P&S officials and prominent Chicago doctors, including both Bevan and Billings of Rush Medical College. Bevan was also chair of the Council on Medical Education of the AMA. Billings agreed to support the university's application for legislative aid. In Springfield James discussed the medical problem with Francis G. Blair, state superintendent of public instruction, and Governor Deneen, who agreed to approve of a temporary lease.[18]

James continued to envision the creation of the Chicago School of Medicine. In mid-February he reminded Judson that they had conferred about the medical situation and that Flexner and others had suggested that a union should be brought about among P&S, Rush, and the Chicago Medical School. James asked Judson if there was any use in trying to effect such a union.[19] Judson did not see why they should not move on the matter of medical instruction at the present time. "If we can get a suitable basis of union," he wrote, "it seems to me that we shall have a substantial ground on which to build up a strong Chicago School of Medicine, which will commend itself to men of means in the city."[20]

In February, as we saw above, the board had talked about relations between the university and P&S without coming to a conclusion. On 12 April James and members of the board met informally with members of the board of directors of P&S. They discussed matters and appointed a joint committee to confer. At the time the difficulties over the medical school situation weighed heavily on James. The main problem, said James, was how the stockholding interest in the medical college could be compensated. James was quite sure that any proposition that involved the state paying anything for the stock was doomed to failure.[21]

On 26 April the joint committee reached an understanding that became the basis for a contract that was to supersede the existing contract between the two parties on 1 July 1910. The agreement made several provisions. First, the existing contract had to be terminated. Second, the college would give the university a two-year lease of its real and personal property and of its name and goodwill. The lease was to be renewable at the end of two years for a like period and again at the end of that extension for another two-year period, all at an annual rental of $18,500. Third, the college was to turn over its plant to the university in a good state of repair. The university was to pay all taxes (not including assessments for local improvements) and to maintain the property in good condition and keep it insured in the name of the college. The university was not to be responsible for repairs necessitated by fires or by other causes not incident to the occupancy of the property as a school building. Fourth, all notes and any accrued interest on them, owing to the university by the college, were to be converted into a convenient form of non–interest-bearing indebtedness, which could be applied as 5 percent of the purchase price of the property of the college should the university make such purchase at any time. Fifth, any funds belonging to the college and held by the university were to be returned to the college and used by it to reduce its floating debt.[22]

James submitted the memorandum of agreement to Governor Deneen, who suggested a few changes of language and endorsed it.[23] The whole board then considered the matter and appointed a committee with authority to negotiate a contract for a new lease. At the request of James, Oliver A. Harker, the board's legal counsel, drafted and redrafted a new lease, which was presented to the board. Governor Deneen, having consulted the attorney general of Illinois about the term of the lease, proposed that it extend to 30 September 1911, that is, one year instead of two. The board approved these arrangements.[24]

The board also took steps to ascertain the extent, condition, and value of what it was leasing. On 29 July James M. White, the university's supervising architect, reported to the board on the condition of the physical buildings belonging to P&S, and Henry B. Ward, a zoology professor at the university and former dean of the University of Nebraska medical school, reported on the condition of the apparatus and equipment in the buildings. Working from an inventory list furnished him, Ward found that most of the items were old, tattered, often dirty, not of much use, and overvalued.[25]

So the university had gained ultimate control of P&S. As James later informed Henry S. Pritchett of the Carnegie Foundation, the university had taken over the medical school and had become "as distinctly responsible for it as it is for the engineering and agricultural schools." The university had leased the property of P&S for the use of its medical school and was going to ask the legislature for an appropriation of one hundred thousand dollars a year to support it. If the university obtained this sum, James wrote, "we shall be able . . . to put our medical school by the side of the best schools in the country. If we fail in our attempt it is my present intention to recommend to the board that the University give up the attempt to do any work in the field of medicine and to continue that policy until the legislature is willing to endow the work properly." Pritchett read James's letter "with great satisfaction."[26]

No doubt negotiations regarding the lease were much on James's mind on 6 June, the day that the Carnegie Foundation issued the Flexner Report. That evening James answered a toast at the P&S banquet to the "Carnegie Foundation and Medical Education in Chicago."[27]

James, the Reform of Medical Education, and the Flexner Report

While attempting to obtain a legislative appropriation and to consolidate the university-related medical colleges in Chicago, James remained actively engaged in the reform of medical education both within the University of Illinois and in the city of Chicago. On taking office in 1904 he had encountered a problem related to medical education. In addition to the four-year medical course in Chicago, the university offered the Course Preparatory to Medicine in Urbana. This was a six-year continuous course in general science and medicine. Students in the course took three years of prescribed work plus ninety-seven hours of electives in Urbana and then went to the medical college in Chicago, where they received a BA upon completion of one year's work in medical subjects and an MD after two additional years of medical study.

In October 1904 the Minnesota State Board of Medical Examiners ruled that it would no longer recognize medical colleges that granted advanced standing and would not admit graduates of such schools to Minnesota examinations for a license to practice medicine. This raised the question as to whether the university should insist upon the seven years combined course instead of the six-year combined course. Early in 1905 the medical faculty decided that candidates for graduation in the medical school be required to attend four full years in a medical institution and that P&S would not admit to advanced standing students who had done their scientific work in a liberal arts college. This ruling would abolish the combined six-year course, and the governing board of the university did not approve it. James suggested that the P&S decision might cost the college more students than it would gain, but if P&S thought that this was the better thing to do, he authorized it. The admission of students who had completed the three-year medical course offered at the university to the third year of P&S, James said, would not violate in spirit or letter the P&S announcement that it did not give advance standing to graduates of liberal arts colleges.[28] His reasoning was a bit too clever.

Although the Northwestern University Medical School accepted the Minnesota ruling, both Rush Medical College and P&S opposed it. The secretary of the Minnesota board invited representatives of both Rush and P&S to appear before the board in April if they wished but with no prospect of the decision being changed. Dean Quine informed the Minnesota State Board of Medical Examiners that P&S would, after the present session, discontinue time credit on degrees from scientific and literary colleges.[29]

The dean of the university's College of Science appointed a committee to study the situation. Reporting on 10 October 1905, the committee declared that the combined six-year course in science and medicine unquestionably afforded a much better general education and a materially better preparation for the practice of medicine than the four-year course of the medical college and "that any discrimination against it as compared with this four-year course is unjust to the University, unfair to the student, and detrimental to the progress of medical education."[30]

The committee advised that henceforth the six-year course be called a medical course and that students who registered in it with a view to graduating from a medical college be classed as medical students. The committee also advised that university instructors who taught in this medical course in subjects required for the medical degree be regarded as instructors in the medical college and listed accordingly in university publications. The committee recommended that a new circular on medical education in the university be prepared in accordance with the views in the report and sent to every physician in the state and to every member of the current graduating class of Illinois high schools.[31]

The faculty of the College of Science adopted the report, and on 27 October the dean of the College of Science, E. J. Townsend, communicated the resolutions in the report to Dean Quine with the request that the P&S faculty formally adopt the resolutions. The faculty of the College of Medicine did so on 4 November, and in December the university senate approved the new statement.[32] Thus the university continued to offer the six-year medical course.

But the question arose as to whether it was sound educational policy for the university to decline to give its bachelor's degree to students who had taken three years of the university's medical course and then fulfilled the requirements of the fourth year of that course at some medical college other than P&S. A committee that studied the matter concluded that it would be injurious policy to limit the university's action in regard to this degree. The six-year course was designed to induce a large number of prospective physicians to take a sound scientific training in connection with their professional studies, and the suggested restriction would defeat in a measure the purpose of the offering. A student who took three years of medical work at Urbana and a fourth year equivalent to that prescribed by the university at a medical school of high standing should be given his bachelor's degree by the university.[33]

Far more important than the issue posed by the Minnesota ruling was the problem of the reform of medical education in America. James's activities along this line preceded but paralleled those of the organized medical profession. The AMA, established in 1847, viewed medical education as the area then in greatest need of reform, but it was not until 1904 that the AMA made its greatest contribution to the advancement of medical standards with the creation of its Council on Medical Education. The members were Arthur D. Bevan (surgery, Rush), chairman; W. T. Councilman (pathology, Harvard); Charles H. Frazier (surgery, Pennsylvania); Victor C. Vaughan (dean, Michigan); and J. A. Witherspoon (medicine, Vanderbilt). The council was intended to be a permanent national bureau on medical education. During 1904–5 the council assessed the quality of medical education in the United States. The results showed that the quality of American medical education was far inferior to concurrent medical training in Germany, France, and England. Notable deficiencies were low admissions requirements, poorly trained teachers, inadequate facilities, and insufficient financial support.

On 20 April 1905 the council held its first annual conference in Chicago. It was attended by delegates from state and territorial licensing bodies and committees

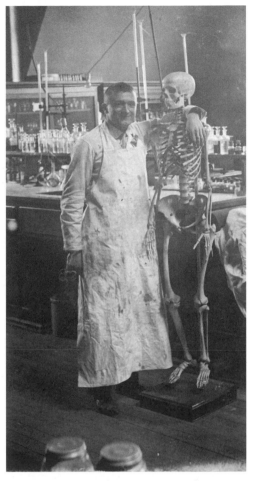

Medical student, University of Illinois, Urbana. Courtesy of the University of Illinois at Urbana-Champaign Archives.

of both the Association of American Medical Colleges and the Southern Medical College Association. The council formulated two standards designed to make American medical education equal to that in Germany, France, and England. An "ideal standard" envisioned for eventual adoption comprised a preliminary education sufficient for entrance to an American university; five years of medical work, with the last two years devoted to the clinical branches; and a sixth year as an intern in a hospital. This "ideal standard" was revolutionary at the time and not practical as an immediate goal. So the council recommended an interim standard for immediate adoption. It called for a preliminary education of four years of high school, a four-year medical course, and passing an examination before a state licensing board.[34]

The council had no legal authority, but it determined to ascertain the facts and to give them to the public, believing that inefficiency and fraud were best suppressed by exposure. At its second annual conference, on 12 May 1906, the council divided the medical schools of the nation into four classes based on the showing that their graduates made in the examinations held by the state boards of health. The first class had rejections of less than 10 percent, the second class had rejections of 10–20 percent, and the third class had rejections of more than 20 percent. The fourth class included schools that did not offer sufficient data to be classified. Bevan concluded that fifty-four medical schools in five different states were especially "rotten spots" that were responsible for most of the bad medical instruction. Not more than six of the fifty-four could be considered acceptable. Illinois, with fifteen medical schools, led the list of states that were especially "rotten spots."[35]

These results led the council to inspect the 160 medical schools in the country. A member of the council or its secretary, Nathan P. Colwell, a Rush MD of 1900, or in most instances both the secretary and a council member visited each of the schools and graded them on 10 points on each of 10 items, making a possible score of 100. The council then arranged the schools into six classes: A, B, C, D, E, and F. The A class had a score of 90 to 100, the B class had a score of 80 to 90, and the C class had a score of 70 to 80. The three classes above 70 formed an acceptable list; therefore, the council recommended that the state boards recognize these schools as being up to standard. Schools in the D and E classes, with scores from 50 to 70, should be recognized, said the council, provided they made improvements that would bring their work up to the grade of 70. Schools in the F class, scoring 50 and below, should not receive the recognition of the state boards. The inspection found schools that were "absolutely worthless," some of which were no better equipped to teach medicine than was "a Turkish-bath establishment or a barber-shop." The study revealed that of the 160 schools, 81 (50.6 percent) received markings above 70, 47 (29.3 percent) received markings between 50 and 70, and 32 (2 percent) received markings below 50.[36]

The report prompted a great wave of improvement in medical education in the country. As the work of the council developed, some council members thought that it would aid their cause if the Carnegie Foundation for the Advancement of Teaching would approve and publish its work. The Carnegie Foundation had been set up in 1905 to grant retirement pensions to college professors, a task that required the foundation to define exactly what a college was. In 1909 Henry S. Pritchett, president of the foundation, persuaded its trustees to conduct studies of professional education with a view to its reform. Pritchett wished to start with the legal profession, but apparently the organized lawyers rebuffed him. When the Council on Medical Education asked Pritchett to make their evidence the subject of a special report on medical education to be published by the Carnegie Foundation, Pritchett immediately accepted.[37]

Pritchett selected Abraham Flexner to make the special report. Flexner, born in Louisville in 1866 and raised by poor immigrant Jewish parents, studied the classics at Johns Hopkins University. In 1886 he graduated with a BA, after which he organized a private preparatory school in Louisville that won him a reputation. After graduate study at Harvard, where he earned an MA in 1906 despite his dislike of the place, he went to Europe and studied comparative education in Berlin. His first book, *The American College* (1908), severely criticized the elective and the lecture systems of American colleges. Thus Flexner's qualifications for investigating medical education were general, a plus for Pritchett, who wanted a layman, not a medical man, for the task. Pritchett had to fight hard to get his board's

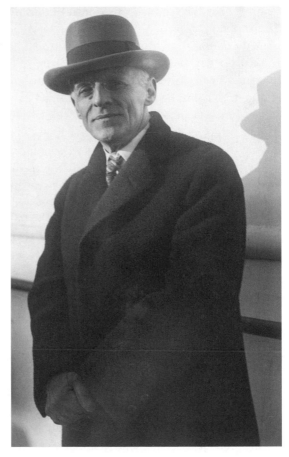

Abraham Flexner. Courtesy of the Bernard Becker Medical Library, Washington University School of Medicine.

approval to hire Flexner. Beginning in 1909, Flexner spent a year and a half investigating medical schools and preparing his report. He worked closely with the Council on Medical Education.[38]

Flexner's study of medical education was the first stage in a distinguished public career. He described himself as a humble servant of the people who directed major philanthropic organizations. In his own words he was "an aggressive, articulate, uncompromising intellectual who was deeply involved in activities of considerable importance." He was often abrasive and intransigent. After he visited the medical school of Washington University, for example, Pritchett admonished him for lacking the courtesy to call on officials of the institution.[39]

When Flexner visited Chicago to investigate the medical situation, he stepped into a conflict that had intensified since 1906, when Arthur Bevan reported that the Council on Medical Education had found that Illinois led the list of medical schools in different states that were especially "rotten spots" of medical education. The charge provoked a battle between the Illinois State Medical Society and the Illinois State Board of Health. The society had led the campaign that resulted in the establishment in 1877 of the Illinois State Board of Health Act and the Illinois Medical Practice Act, viewed by contemporaries as the most advanced at the time. The State Board of Health, seven unpaid members and a paid executive secretary, was charged with the dual task of promoting the public health by sanitary, quarantine, and hygienic measures and with ensuring good doctors by regulating medical education and practice. In 1879 John H. Rauch, an MD from the University of Pennsylvania and the first president of the board, became its executive secretary, a powerful administrative post. Under his dynamic leadership the board substantially strengthened the public health program in Illinois while also raising the standard of medical practice to the highest possible level. Between 1883 and 1889 Rauch issued reports on the results of examining medical schools in and beyond Illinois. The board exposed fraudulent and incompetent medical schools and improved medical education by establishing minimum admissions requirements, lengthening the curriculum, and setting high academic standards. Rauch was "the John the Baptist of reform in medical education in this country," but the medical schools he caused to close used their political influence to retaliate, and in 1891, under pressure, Rauch resigned.[40]

In July 1897 James A. Egan, who earned an MD from Chicago Medical College in 1893, became the executive secretary of the Illinois State Board of Health. His main interest was expansion of the public health service, and since regulating the practice of medicine took about 80 percent of the time and energy of the board, he wanted to get rid of it. He saw large possibilities for growth in the field of sanitation and hygiene.[41] Many Illinois physicians blamed the State Board of Health under his direction for low educational standards in the Chicago medical schools and for the overcrowding of the medical profession. The Illinois State Medical Society made its opposition to Egan and the Board of Health known through their official organ, the *Illinois Medical Journal*. The editor, George N. Kreider, an 1880 MD from New York University Medical College (the University of the City of New York), repeatedly used Bevan's "rotten spots" characterization to spearhead an attack by the medical society and the Council on Medical Education of the AMA on the Illinois State Board of Health and its ally, the Chicago Medical Society, whose head was George W. Webster Sr., also president of the State Board of Health.[42]

In April 1909 Abraham Flexner, the agent of the Carnegie Foundation, investigated medical schools in St. Louis and then went by train to Chicago. In talking with people he apparently fed their dissatisfaction with local conditions in medical education. In early November Carl E. Black of Jacksonville, an 1887 graduate of Rush and a former president and current chairman of the Judicial Council of the Illinois State Medical Society, was an invited guest at the annual meeting of the Southern Illinois Medical Society in East St. Louis. On the last day of the meeting the members permitted Black to introduce a resolution. It had been brought to the attention of the members of the Southern Illinois Medical Society by several sources, Black observed, that Illinois had become one of the "rotten spots" of the United States in medical education and licensure, whereas in former years the state had been ranked among the five highest in these matters. The Southern Illinois Medical Society had always demanded a high standard of medical education and of admission to practice. Therefore, it resolved "that the Southern Illinois Medical Society without prejudice toward our Board of Health, but solely for the information of its members and other physicians interested, do hereby request the Secretary of the Illinois State Board of Health to explain through the official *Bulletin* of the Board or through the columns of the *Illinois Medical Journal* why Illinois should bear the stigma of being one of the plague spots of this country in medical education, medical examination and medical licensure."[43]

In December, under the heading "Illinois and 'Rotten' Medical Education," the *Illinois Medical Journal* printed the resolution and opened its column for discussion of the question. Editor Kreider hoped that the secretary of the Illinois State Board of Health would explain the causes that had "conspired to give our fair state its very undesirable position and reputation in medical education, medical licensure and medical practice."[44] Thus, by late 1909 Bevan's characterization of Illinois as one of the "rotten spots" of medical education in the country was linked with Flexner's later charge that Chicago was the "plague spot" of the nation in medical education.

Egan received the text of the resolution before December 1909, when it appeared in the *Illinois Medical Journal*. After discovering who was responsible for it, he defended himself in the *Bulletin* of the Illinois State Medical Society. No responsible source had ever called Illinois the "plague spot" of medical education, said Egan, who added that the resolution was obviously unfounded and of notoriously questionable origin. He challenged Kreider and Black "to point out any responsible utterance or writing, except the resolution above referred to, in which Illinois has been alluded to as 'one of the plague spots of this country in medical education, medical examination and medical licensure.'"[45]

From February to April 1910 members of the Illinois State Medical Society and officials of the Illinois State Board of Health carried on a bitter dispute in the *Illinois Medical Journal*. Doctors criticized Egan and Webster for betraying the medical profession by doing nothing to protect the public health and to regulate medical colleges. Egan and Webster replied that they had tried to change the law setting the requirements for admission to medical schools, but the profession had not supported them. Black and others characterized Illinois as one of the "rotten spots" and Chicago as a "plague spot" in medical educa-tion. Egan and Webster wanted them to cite their sources. Although Bevan had referred to Illinois as one of the "rotten spots" in 1906, Flexner had not yet pub-lished the report in which he characterized Chicago as the "plague spot" of the nation in medical education. Flexner and Black had probably used the term in conversations.[46]

Patricia Spain Ward, a historian who has written about P&S, contends that "given all the circumstances as we now know them, Flexner (who was without doubt one of the 'sources' mentioned in the resolution) could scarcely do other-wise than respond by writing that Illinois was in fact 'the plague spot of the country.'" Although Flexner stigmatized medical education alone without refer-ence to examination and licensure, he charged that Chicago medical schools "flagrantly violated" the "fairly adequate" Illinois law with the "indubitable con-nivance of the state board." Ward defends Egan and argues that in his famous re-port Flexner displayed antagonism toward Chicago medical schools. To be sure, Egan was obligated to follow the law, which required only a high school diploma or equivalent for admission to medical schools. But the question remains as to Flexner's accuracy in characterizing the medical schools of Chicago.[47]

Flexner investigated carefully before writing his report. He suspected the hon-esty and sincerity with which the Illinois State Board of Health administered the medical situation in Illinois because it had first suspended and then recognized five or six wretched medical schools and further because of the discrepancies between the results of the state board's examinations and those conducted by the Civil Service Commission. So while in Chicago in April 1909, he engaged John L. Fogle, an attorney in the office of the Bar Association of Chicago, to look into the matter at fifty dollars an hour. Pritchett authorized the expenditure.[48]

Fogle indicted the State Board of Health and its officials. First, he reported, between July 1907 and March 1908 the state board had suspended seven schools, three of which it later reinstated and three of which it did not reinstate, while it suspended, reinstated, and again suspended one. These actions were taken upon report in each case of the secretary or of a committee of the board. The colleges were reinstated after making representations that the defects by which they were suspended had been remedied and after examination and report by a committee of the board or the secretary. Fogle charged that the reformation of these colleges had not been real.

Second, Fogle presented evidence to show the discrepancy between the men who had been licensed as physicians upon examination by the state board and the low scores of those men in the civil service examinations in Chicago for interns in the County Hospital. One reason for the discrepancy was the op-portunity for leakage of the examination questions of the state board before the examination occurred. But the principal defect was the appointment of careless and incompetent monitors who had charge of the papers and students during the examination. In the last examination held by the state board, two sons of George W. Webster Sr., president of the state board, were among the monitors. George W. Webster Jr., about twenty-five years of age, was "thoroughly incompetent and irresponsible," Fogle declared, while Ivan B. Webster was not yet of age. Moreover, at a recent examination Fogle had been impressed by the apparent youthfulness and inattention of the persons acting as monitors.

Fogle also reported that the State Board of Health was not a responsible agency in handling its funds, and he found that osteopaths were not investigated for exceeding the limitations of their licenses under the statute as the law required.

Fogle's exposure of James A. Egan, the secretary of the State Board of Health who was vested by statute with broad powers and discretion, was unsparing. Egan had graduated from Northwestern University Medical College, Fogle reported, but his contemporaries had never considered him either capable, efficient, or trustworthy. Although a majority of the better element of the medical profession in Illinois had charged Egan with incompetency and graft and had condemned him, Egan had been reappointed and kept in office by the governor, the reason being that he was a political protégé of Mayor Busse of Chicago. Fogle credited Egan with several accomplishments while in office but said that Egan was "not only inefficient and corrupt but a positive menace to the people of the State."[49]

Flexner himself investigated the medical schools in Chicago before issuing his report. At his request, for example, in October 1909 Quine submitted a statement on the composition of the faculty of P&S. The faculty of 153 included 52 professors (9 alumni of P&S and 43 others), 36 adjuncts (12 alumni of P&S and 24 others), and 65 instructors (33 alumni of P&S and 32 others). The inbreeding was noticeable only at the level of instructor.[50] The budget for the college for the year 1909–10 showed an estimated income of $75,000 and expenses of $73,497, leaving a balance of $1,503. The major expenses were salaries for instruction, $14,055; salaries for service, $16,940; building ground and rent, $12,000; and interest on the high school property, $11,052. Heat and light were budgeted at $5,000, laboratories at $4,000, and the library at a modest $250.[51]

Flexner also discussed the medical situation in Chicago with James. At lunch in Chicago on 17 April 1909, Flexner, James, and Quine "went over the whole ground." Quine was "completely convinced both as to the necessity and the feasibility of the scheme," Flexner informed Pritchett. "He [Quine] called it 'a noble project', offered to give up at once his chair, his stock & his bonds and ventured to say that others would be similarly minded." The meaning of "the scheme" will become clear as we proceed. "President James," Flexner continued, "was at first non-committal, waiting, I think, partly to see how the cat [his medical faculty] would jump, and partly because he has had some vague hope that the state would give him his own medical school." And yet James was "clearly anxious not to let the present school stand between him and the Foundation. At the close he expressed himself as convinced of the feasibility of the plan and as willing to meet with Presidents Harris and Judson to discuss it." Flexner said that he would convey this information to Harris, who was to take the initiative in calling the three together. "James strikes me as rather canny," Flexner observed, "but, if as I believe, the faculty of the P. & S. favor the thing, he will not oppose it." Subsequently Flexner saw Bevan, Billings, and Pusey, whom he described as "all increasingly eager." For the present, Flexner thought, the momentum of the scheme would carry it along some distance.[52]

In February 1910 James expressed an urgent desire to see Flexner. To prepare for meeting him, Flexner dined with William A. Pusey of P&S "who," as Flexner informed Pritchett, "talked freely, after a little preliminary skirmishing." Flexner gained the impression that James was the obstacle to any concerted action. According to Pusey, James's view was that "the State University ought to have its own medical school, it ought not to go partnership with anyone." Flexner assured Pritchett that in talking to James he would confine himself to the line that Pritchett had followed in talking with Henry B. Ward of the University of Illinois. Flexner had no idea why James should be so keen to talk about the matter further.[53]

The next day Flexner spent three hours with James and Ward going over the local situation.[54] Flexner immediately sent Pritchett the gist of their discussion. First, James had reviewed in detail the development of the university situation with the evident intent of vindicating his ambition to build a state-supported medical school in Chicago. Flexner conceded that medicine might profit immensely by the state's interest in it. James thought that he could get seventy-five thousand dollars from the state to spend in Chicago. Flexner asked if James expected to use the city and county hospitals. James replied yes, so Flexner asked if that did not involve a continuation of competition with those institutions that had resulted in restricting school privileges within them. James admitted that it was not probable that the state could get more out of municipal hospitals than the local institutions had gotten. Therefore, Flexner argued, unless the state built James a hospital in Chicago, there could be no future for his clinical situation. "I believe," wrote Flexner, "that impressed him as a real obstacle."[55]

Flexner then asked James whether the legislature might not object if he asked for large sums to outdo the local schools and if, in that event, a comparatively slight obstacle could not halt his whole scheme. He appeared to grant that he would need the cooperation or at least tacit consent of other local school interests to get his appropriation through. Now, then, Flexner said, "Suppose you try cooperation, instead of competition? That puts the State in the position of supporting medicine; it also enables the other schools to help you get your appropriation and to welcome you into the City and County hospitals."[56]

James quite amazed Flexner by granting that this was possible, that by some subdivision or apportionment of departments an arrangement might be feasible that would combine state and endowment institutions. "While he did not commit himself to this as a program, he went further towards a definite expression as to its feasibility than ever before with me." Later, at lunch, James reverted to the topic in some such words as, "It's a great work the Foundation is doing in this line. You have interfered with me by taking my efforts and attention from other matters and compelling me to concentrate them on this, but, on the whole, I really believe that has been best—and I don't even regret it now." The words struck Flexner as marking progress. "I feel pretty sure that the contractual relation won't last much longer, though, of course, I should not say that he will attempt a cooperative enterprise until he has actually found a strictly University enterprise impossible."[57]

Flexner's letters to Pritchett offer additional perspective on the medical situation in Chicago. They reveal James as single-minded in his determination to establish a state-supported University of Illinois College of Medicine in Chicago but only gradually convinced that cooperation with the leading medical schools in the city was essential to realize his objectives. But Flexner either exaggerated or misjudged the situation. James had always wanted the university to gain control of P&S and to obtain an appropriation from the state to support it. He had also worked with Harris and Judson to create a new Chicago School of Medicine. After 1910 James intensified his efforts to realize this goal. Flexner was an astute observer, but his reports would have given Pritchett an erroneous view of the medical situation in Chicago.

Abraham Flexner's *Medical Education in the United States and Canada,* published as Bulletin Number Four of the Carnegie Foundation on 6 June 1910, is a classic in the literature of medical reform in the United States. The impact of the report has been widely disputed. It has been called both a landmark and a piece of muckraking journalism. One author declared that "the report has received attention far out of proportion to its actual contribution to medical education."[58] Another author, asserting that the report was largely catalytic rather than innovative, adds that it achieved its "mythic proportions" because it came at precisely the right time; that money was forthcoming to bring a number of medical schools up to the standards of Johns Hopkins, which Flexner held as a model; and that Flexner's report stood alone in saying what other would-be reformers wanted to say but could not.[59] In any case, the report stirred up a tremendous controversy.

Flexner first described the proper basis of medical education and outlined an ideal four-year course of study. For Flexner, the Johns Hopkins medical school set the standard. He went on to discuss the financial aspects of medical education, medical sects, the state boards of examination, and the medical education of women and blacks. In noting the faults of medical schools Flexner did not spare P&S, which he described as among the schools that were "shrewdly and more or less outspokenly commercial." Often such schools had elaborate plants and on a routine level were pedagogically effective, but they were scientifically inert.[60]

Flexner investigated the medical schools of the country and evaluated them in light of his theoretical framework. He examined entrance requirements, student records, the size and training of the faculty, laboratories, teaching hospitals and other clinical facilities, and finances. In light of what he discovered he proclaimed "the utter contemptibility of the vast majority of proprietary schools unconnected with universities."[61] As for the city of Chicago, it was "in respect to medical education the plague spot of the country."[62]

His scathing criticism was not only about the medical schools in Chicago but also about the Illinois State Board of Health. With the indubitable connivance of the state board, Flexner asserted, ten of the undergraduate medical schools in Chicago admitted and prepared candidates for the Illinois State Board of Health examinations in contravention of the law and the rules of the state board, and the state board had deprived only one of these of good standing. In Flexner's view, efficient and intelligent administration of the law would reduce the number of medical schools in Chicago to three: Rush, Northwestern, and the University of Illinois.[63]

As for P&S, Flexner wrote that the entrance requirement, a high school education or its equivalent, had been "more or less nominal," and advanced standing had been "accorded to students from decidedly inferior schools, some of them among the worst institutions in the country." The physiology laboratory was well equipped, the pharmacology and chemistry laboratories were mediocre, while the anatomy, pathology, and bacteriological laboratories were adequate. For clinical facilities P&S relied on the Cook County Hospital, on the staff of which it held eleven appointments, and on a number of other institutions to which its students were admitted under the usual limitations. Prominent among these was the so-called University Hospital, which was a university hospital only in the sense that students from other schools were not admitted at all to the "existing opportunities, restricted as they are." On investigation the "clinical advantages" of the hospital shrank to three weekly amphitheater clinics of slight pedagogic value and four ward clinics in obstetrics.

In discussing how to modernize medical education in Chicago, Flexner said that if Rush, Northwestern, and the University of Illinois all went to the two-year college standard for admission, a single school adequately equipped with laboratories and hospital could care for all of the medical students in Chicago. But since none of the three universities teaching medicine in Chicago was likely to abandon the field to the other, Flexner recommended that each of the three universities continue to provide the instruction of the first two years and that all three combine to form a clinical department under joint management, "the first step towards which would be a concerted effort to procure a proper hospital for the use of third and fourth year men." It would be too expensive and "sheer extravagance" to equip properly three hospitals, but the Cook County and other hospitals could play the part for which they were suited in furnishing illustrative material for advanced students and make possible the development of instruction in all the specialties, for which American physicians were still forced to go abroad. "A great opportunity is thus fairly within the grasp of Chicago: the conditions to its realization are honesty and intelligence on the part of the state authorities, and cooperation between the three great universities of the state."[64]

The Flexner Report produced "an immediate and profound sensation. . . . The medical profession and the faculties of the medical schools, as well as the state boards of examiners, were absolutely flabbergasted by the pitiless exposure." So said Flexner, who received anonymous letters warning him that he would be shot if he showed himself in Chicago.[65]

Indeed, the report generated strong opposition, especially in Chicago. Egan denounced Flexner and his report (inspection of so many schools in such a short time was "farcical") and defended himself. J. Newton Roe of the Chicago College of Medicine and Surgery (Valparaiso) described the report as "medical politics." Arthur R. Edwards, dean of the Northwestern Medical School, characterized it as "pretty harsh."[66] The Reverend Henry S. Spalding charged that Flexner, the Carnegie Foundation, and the AMA had decided that there were to be only three medical colleges in Chicago—the state university, Rush-Chicago, and Northwestern—but when Loyola took over the Bennett School, the AMA realized "that the great influence of the Catholic Church would be behind the institution, so it was decided to crush the school at once and before it had gathered strength."[67]

James had anticipated Flexner by several years in evaluating medical education in and beyond Chicago. James read the report before it was published, and the end of the academic year provided him an opportunity to comment on it. On 6 June, the day the Flexner Report appeared, James made one of the "most severe indictments" of the medical schools ever heard in the city in "a broadside of condemnation tempered by sorrow." Speaking at the P&S alumni banquet in the Auditorium Annex, James described Flexner's criticisms as "in essence just and true." Chicago was indeed the "plague spot" of America in medical education, said James; one should not defend the indefensible. Chicago did not now have and had never had a first-class medical school, James declared. Unlike Flexner, James made no exception for the University of Chicago. The city of Chicago, James added, had a larger number of "inferior and false enterprises" than any other city in the United States. The presidents of Northwestern, the University of Chicago, and the University of Illinois had tried to develop a university medical school, James noted, but their efforts had not yielded even one properly equipped and organized first-class medical school. James called on people of wealth and people of the state to provide for medical education. When he stated his intention to ask the legislature for a greater appropriation for the University of Illinois medical school, five hundred banquet guests vigorously applauded.[68]

At the P&S commencement exercises the next day, James gave the annual address. His topic was the scientific medical school. He "scathingly arraigned" the general public for criticizing the quality of the medical schools without aiding them in any way. The City of Chicago and the State of Illinois gave nothing, said James, whereas all the states that bordered Illinois supported medical schools in their state universities.

James received many letters condemning his response to the Flexner Report.[69] C. A. Harkness of the Hahnemann Medical College, who described the Flexner Report as uncalled for, accused James of endorsing it in order to extract money from the state legislature. James was likely to get himself disliked, a reporter wrote, by some of the doctors who criticized the Flexner Report.[70]

To be sure. At the annual banquet of the Alumni Association of the Barnes University Medical Department in St. Louis, Missouri, G. Frank Lydston, a member of the University of Illinois medical school faculty since 1882, criticized Flexner as not being in a position to make fair and just comparisons between heavily endowed and independent institutions. Flexner viewed medicine as a science and emphasized the importance of the laboratory, said Lydston, who thought that the pendulum was swinging too far in the direction of the laboratory and pure science instead of the practicing physician.[71]

The most severe criticism of both Flexner and James came from Charles McCormick, president of McCormick Medical College in Chicago.[72] McCormick had read accounts of James's remarks in the newspapers and described them as "the outlines of what is evidently a conspiracy on the part of three Illinois Universities to attempt once more the outrage tried in 1898" by the presidents of Northwestern (Henry Wade Rogers), the University of Chicago (William R. Harper), and the University of Illinois (Andrew S. Draper). At that time the independent colleges had not only "whipped the scoundrels" but had punished the state university by reducing its appropriation for the next two years.[73]

According to McCormick, newspapers reported James as saying that he was going to seek public money to put P&S "on a certain alleged 'basis.'" McCormick wanted to serve notice that he would fight James to the finish. "You and your gang," he wrote, "are like a lot of old women gossips who are notoriously irresponsible, you go about making slanderous insinuations about everything, except university schools, in the belief that with public moneys, endowments, and the backing of a lot of snobs represented in the newspaper trust, you can push your way into a monopoly."[74]

McCormick then charged that all the "orthodox" schools, including the University of Illinois, accepted in their medical departments children seventeen years old and graduated them at twenty-one years old, whereas McCormick's

school took nobody under twenty-one. McCormick Medical College had survived seventeen years and had always been self-sustaining, McCormick boasted,
and its diplomas were recognized by the public as guarantees of competence.
McCormick provided some unsavory details about "old-fogy" schools such as
Rush, Northwestern, and P&S, which had admitted and graduated students who
were unqualified to be doctors. McCormick went on to write, "As to the measly
Jew, Abraham Flexner, of the 'Carnegie Foundation,' whose 'report' was printed
in the Tribune of yesterday [6 June], which should bring libel suits against the
Tribune and Flexner, by the colleges named as unworthy, I have only to say that
he is probably a reincarnation of Judas, the Iscariot, and will no doubt receive
his twenty pieces of silver."[75]

After rebutting Flexner's description of the Johns Hopkins medical school
as the "ideal" one, McCormick concluded, "McCormick Medical College runs
on its merits. It has no use for beggars, nor slanderers, and will fight them until
dooms-day by that master of all weapons, 'Publicity.' It will expose persons, con-
spiracies, gangs, and will fight in the courts if necessary to maintain its constitutional rights."[76] James politely replied that he had read McCormick's letter with
much interest.[77]

McCormick confirmed the charge that the city of Chicago was "in respect to
medical education the plague spot of the country." In 1902 and 1903 city directories listed the McCormick Optical College at 84 Adams Street. In 1903 Mc-
Cormick began calling himself an MD and president of the college. In 1904
he relocated to 2500 Prairie Avenue. On May Day 1907 he moved into the historic John B. Sherman dwelling at the corner of Twenty-first Street and Prairie Avenue with what was now called the McCormick Neurological College,
"consisting of twenty students, a blackboard and several van loads of apparatus,
books on ophthalmology and neurology, and pieces of mission furniture." He
had moved in without saying a word to his millionaire neighbors. When he
started nailing up a couple of large signs in front of the building, the wealthy
residents of the invaded district panicked. McCormick had signed a five-year
lease with the trustees of the Sherman estate. He agreed to put up only a small
sign in front and to take in no patients, especially no drunkards or crazy people.
Earlier that day he had chased away two delegates from an electrical workers'
union with a revolver. For several years McCormick ran his college from 2100
Prairie Avenue.[78]

During the summer the storm aroused by the Flexner Report subsided. James
continued to campaign for a legislative appropriation to support and maintain
the medical school and to urge a union of the College of Medicine with Northwestern Medical College and Rush Medical College, especially with Rush.

In early December at a meeting of the Physicians' Club of Chicago, James
began the evening with a talk titled "The Relation of the University of Illinois
to Medical Education." After noting how he came to believe in the need for the

state to support medical education and his efforts to reform medical education at the University of Pennsylvania and later, he said that the lease arrangement between the university and P&S had demonstrated that a modern medical school could not be maintained on the basis of student fees. Thus the university had decided to ask the legislature for one hundred thousand dollars a year for the equipment, maintenance, and extension of its school of medicine, and the outcome of the request would mark the beginning of new things in medical education in the University of Illinois, the city of Chicago, the state of Illinois, and the entire Mississippi Valley. The *Illinois Medical Journal* ran his remarks as a special article in January 1911.[79]

James B. Herrick, a professor at Rush, presided over the lengthy discussion that followed James's address. If the Flexner Report's conclusions were in the main "sane and judicial," said Herrick, which he believed to be the case, then Chicago had a heterogenous mass of medical schools, and medical conditions were such that Chicago was a plague spot in medicine.[80] As Herrick observed, James ought to know what was going on in the leading university-related medical schools because he had been on the inside of things at the University of Chicago, he ran Northwestern University at one time, and he was now running the University of Illinois.

In the lively discussion that followed, Arthur D. Bevan observed that modern medicine was a science that required a thorough training in a medical school and an internship in a hospital. Drawing on data compiled by the Council on Medical Education, Bevan noted that 38 of the 130 medical schools in the United States accepted this standard, but many American medical schools did not. In Chicago there were 16 institutions that turned out graduates who bore the title of doctor. Of this number, 5 schools turned out doctors who were legally permitted to diagnose, if they could, and to treat any cases that came to them, but they were not supposed to do surgery or to prescribe or administer drugs, and they were not entitled to call or advertise themselves as physicians or doctors.

The remaining eleven schools turned out doctors of medicine who, on passing the state license examinations, were permitted to practice medicine in any or all of its branches. Only six of the eleven, Bevan reported, were included among the colleges in Class A and Class B by the Council on Medical Education: Rush Medical College, Northwestern Medical School, the College of Physicians and Surgeons (University of Illinois), Hahnemann Medical College of Chicago, the Chicago College of Medicine and Surgery (Valparaiso), and Loyola University. Only the first three were accepted by the report of the Carnegie Foundation. The council placed five medical schools in Chicago in Class C, meaning that they were so poor that it would require a complete reorganization to make them acceptable. What Illinois needed in medical education, Bevan believed, was fewer and better medical colleges, a more strict enforcement of the requirements, and a thorough and practical examination of every candidate for license. "All of this is not so much an indictment of the state board, which is shown by existing conditions to be inefficient," Bevan said, "as it is an indictment against the entire educational system of our state which makes such conditions possible."[81] The great universities of the state had to provide educated medical men for Illinois, according to Bevan, and an efficient state board should protect people against the worthless commercial medical colleges and the diploma mills. Bevan was entirely right in his indictment of the entire educational system of Illinois and by implication the failure of the legislature to provide for the funding of the medical school of the state university.

Arthur H. Wilde, who spoke for Northwestern University, said that the university's request for an appropriation of one hundred thousand dollars for medical education was too small. Northwestern would support a request for more. Harry Pratt Judson, president of the University of Chicago, observed that the reforms in medical education that James envisioned a quarter of a century earlier were coming now. The time to put the new requirements for medical education into effect was this very day. "I believe that Chicago is to be, I hope early," Judson concluded, "a great center of advanced medical education in this country."[82]

The Reverend Henry S. Spalding reminded those present that "our new University of Loyola" was part of a old and extensive system of Jesuit education. If those present were going to raise the standard of medical education in Chicago, Loyola would cooperate, "but you must not think we are going to sit idly by and let Mr. Flexner, or Mr. Carnegie, or anybody else crush us out of business for the sake of the three schools that may surpass us in numbers." Loyola would work with the others; "all we ask is that you work with us and not work against us."[83]

George W. Webster Sr., president of the Illinois State Board of Health, defended his agency by saying that the legislature established by law a high school certificate as the entrance requirement for medical school, and the board had no power to change the law. James A. Egan defended his administration of the State Board of Health by noting a discrepancy between the Carnegie Foundation's report and the report of the Council on Medical Education. Four of the schools in Chicago unreservedly condemned by Flexner were pronounced acceptable by the Council on Medical Education. So who was right? Egan exculpated Illinois to the extent possible by saying that the conditions reported by Flexner as existing in Illinois were more than duplicated in other states.[84]

CHAPTER 9

Medical Politics, Reorganization, and a Retrospect

In mid-January 1911 the Board of Trustees of the University of Illinois decided to request $2.201 million from the General Assembly for the biennium 1911–13 for ordinary running expenses and maintenance of the plant, $1.150 million for buildings, and $200,000 for the College of Medicine, a total of $3.551 million. In addition the board asked for $1.570 million for agriculture, $75,000 for ceramics, and $230,000 for mining engineering. The total request came to $5.426 million.[1]

James hoped that a vigorous campaign to obtain the appropriations would succeed. Based on that hope he began to reorganize the College of Medicine before the appropriations bills passed. He juggled the pursuit of a legislative grant and reorganization of the college simultaneously, but it will help to describe these efforts in the sequence noted and provide a retrospect on the College of Physicians and Surgeons (P&S).

"Medical Politics of the Most Virulent Sort"

On 15 October 1910 the university's board had agreed to ask the legislature for one hundred thousand dollars per annum for the College of Medicine for 1911–13.[2] Knowing that E. Fletcher Ingals of Rush Medical College was jealous of the university's medical advance in Chicago, James sought to make him an ally in the effort to win legislative approval for the request. The trustees were asking the legislature for one hundred thousand dollars per annum for the university's medical school for the coming biennium, James informed Ingals on 25 October, and if the General Assembly granted the request, James would take it as notice that the state had decided to support medical education as thoroughly as it supported engineering and agricultural education. There would be little hope of obtaining such an appropriation unless Ingals and men like him who were interested in a large way in this great problem were willing to assist the university, James added, and he went on to ask if Ingals would be willing "to support such an enterprise to the extent of saying that in your opinion it would be a good thing, and letting me to quote you to that effect."[3]

Ingals replied brusquely. James had the opportunity to make the University of Illinois "of the greatest possible service to medical education and the science of medicine, and through these, to the public," Ingals wrote, but the scheme James outlined was "not calculated to produce such a result." A man in his position, James countered, often had to do the best that could be done under practical conditions. It would take the cooperation of men interested in large things to bring them about in a reasonable time. He craved the assistance of Ingals. Ingals said that he would be pleased to talk with James, but he added, cryptically and without committing himself, "I feel that we should do the best practical thing under the circumstances confronting us."[4]

James then prepared to bring pressure to bear upon the legislature. On 1 December he called on the editors of leading Chicago newspapers "in re the Medical School appropriation." Promising to help were Andrew M. Lawrence, editor of Hearst's newspapers the morning *Chicago American* and the evening *Chicago Examiner;* Leo S. Hinman of the *Chicago Journal;* Herman H. Kohlsaat, publisher of the *Record-Herald;* and the editor of the *Chicago Journal* (probably John E. Eastman). James also called on prominent Chicago physicians and medical educators, including Nathan S. Davis Jr., Frank Billings, Arthur D. Bevan, and John D. Murphy of Northwestern Medical School. James drafted a letter to the physicians of the state about P&S, which Abbott approved and Billings signed, and made a case for the appropriation in a letter to members of the legislature.[5]

On 9 February 1911 Republican legislators introduced identical appropriations bills in the Senate and the House. In the interest of public health and sanitation, the bills read, the state should assist in medical research and medical instruction in the same way as it did in agricultural, engineering, or legal research and instruction. An adequate medical school could not be conducted on the basis of fees alone.[6]

The Council of the Chicago Medical Society endorsed the university's request for one hundred thousand dollars a year and petitioned the governor and the legislature to make the appropriation. The document was signed by George W. Webster Sr., president of the Illinois State Board of Health; Frank Billings, president of the State Board of Charities; John B. Murphy, president-elect of the American Medical Association (AMA); Arthur Bevan, president of the Council on Medical Education of the AMA; Alfred C. Cotton, president of the Illinois State Medical Society; and William K. Newcomb, president-elect of the Illinois State Medical Society.[7]

The Illini Club of Chicago appointed three of its members to lobby for the appropriation in Springfield. James sent a circular letter to 9,744 physicians in Illinois describing the need for state support, asking them to talk to their legislators, and asking if they would allow their names to be appended to a petition that urged the General Assembly to endorse the appropriation. He then sent a letter to the 2,960 physicians who had signed the petition. He sent a letter pleading the cause to 203 members of the legislature, 180 daily newspapers in Illinois, 1,107 weekly newspapers, and 37 semiweekly newspapers, a total of 1,527 letters. He sent the members of the General Assembly a sixty-page pamphlet containing the names of the physicians who had signed the petition. Quine sent a letter to the physicians in Illinois who were alumni of P&S asking them to support the request. James also mailed a letter to 385 homeopathic physicians in Illinois explaining that the university had sole control over P&S and that it would conduct a medical school that knew no sect in medicine. In addition, he mailed a pamphlet, *Why the State of Illinois Should Appropriate $100,000 a Year for the Biennium 1909–11 for the Maintenance of the Medical School of the University of Illinois*, to all of the state legislators and to 1,324 Illinois newspapers. The pamphlet described the progress made in the promotion of public health since the time of Pasteur, Lister, and Koch; noted some things remaining to be done in the cause of public health; and depicted the position and opportunity in medicine awaiting Illinois. Twenty-four state universities had medical schools, James observed, and both Michigan and Minnesota generously supported theirs. A properly equipped medical school would supplement the work of state charitable institutions, James added, and the one hundred thousand dollars requested was not a large sum.[8]

On 29 March at the hearing on the bill before the House Committee on Appropriations, opposing forces squared off. George W. Webster Sr., president of the Illinois State Board of Health, and Alfred C. Cotton, president of the consulting staff of Cook County Hospital, headed a delegation from the Chicago Medical Society that supported the bill. "Dill Robertson headed the army of the aliens," James observed.[9]

John Dill Robertson spoke not only for the medical department of Loyola University but also for proprietary medical schools that feared the competition of the state university. Robertson was an unusual physician. In 1903 he had denounced bathing as hazardous to health. "When people leave off bathing," he told a meeting of the Chicago Eclectic and Surgical Society, "there will be little or nothing for the doctors to do. Pneumonia, colds, and a hundred other ills result from the foolish habit of washing the body." He himself, he boasted, had not taken a bath for two years. He kept clean by changing all his clothing once a day. Years later he told a gathering of brewers that people who drank beer, especially bitter beer, never had malarial fever. His medical knowledge was exceeded by his keen political instincts. In April 1915 William H. "Big Bill" Thompson, mayor of Chicago, appointed him commissioner of health of Chicago, at which time Robertson announced new views on cleanliness. "I stand for baths, plain soap, and water," he now declared.[10] Robertson served as commissioner of health until 1922.

Gilbert Fitzpatrick, who represented the Chicago Homeopathic Medical Society at the hearing, said that P&S could not be made the recipient of state aid because the school was $280,000 in debt and the $100,000 per annum appropriation carried the assumption that the state must take over the debt. The statutes recognized four systems of medicine—eclectic, allopathic, homeopathic, and physio-medical—he argued, and to aid any one alone discriminated against the others.

James and Quine were willing to make concession to sectarian medicine. James agreed that it would be unwise to spend any money on reorganizing the clinical years until he was able to put in one or two professors of homeopathic medicine, which he hoped would satisfy the "saner portion of the outfit." Quine, who had previously warned James not to appoint homeopaths to the P&S faculty, now advised James to offer to put in as many teachers of homeopathic materia medica and therapeutics and of the practice of medicine and clinical medicine as they wanted and on terms of equality with the corresponding teachers of regular medicine.[11]

Opposition to the appropriations bill for the College of Medicine prompted James to meditate on the problem of reforming medical education. James identified John Dill Robertson as the main opponent of the bill. "Robertson's appeal at bottom is that he has invested money which would become useless if the State took up the support of Medical Education," said James. "This is the same old plea which would bar all progress." James cited historical examples: turnpikes and stagecoaches versus railroads, buses versus automobiles, and academies versus high schools. In the era of scientific medicine, should private interest stand in the way of public benefit?[12]

In any event, the General Assembly made appropriations for the University of Illinois amounting to $3,489,300, a generous sum but considerably less than the $5.426 million requested. The legislature cut the request for the College of Medicine from $100,000 to $60,000 per annum.[13] Though this was less than anticipated, James proceeded with his plans to reorganize the college.

In late June 1911 James received word that certain eminent citizens of Chicago proposed to sue for an injunction against the state treasurer preventing him from paying to the trustees of the university any money appropriated for support of the medical school. "Of course it is possible to get some fool judge or other upon any fool proposition to issue an injunction," James said, but if people succeeded in tying up the university's funds it would make it impossible to reorganize the medical school for the coming year and might result in closing the school.[14]

In late July Edwin M. Ashcraft of Ashcraft and Ashcraft, a Chicago law firm, informed Oliver A. Harker, the university's legal counsel, that certain of Ashcraft's clients intended to apply for an injunction to forbid the state to turn over to the university any of the funds appropriated by the legislature for medical education on the ground that the constitutional provision relating to the passage of bills had not been observed, that is, a revision of the proposed bill had not been printed before it went back to legislators to be voted on. The board of trustees had concluded that it could not lawfully give a pledge not to use the money appropriated for the medical school during the coming biennium, and even if it could, it ought not do so.[15]

James asked Ashcraft to tell him the terms on which his clients would consent to withdraw their opposition so that he could make a recommendation to the board on the subject. If the contention of the clients was correct, an injunction would lead to an extra legislative session and probably to a declaration by the Supreme Court of Illinois of the invalidity of all laws passed under similar conditions by legislatures during the past few years. This would affect the interests of the City of Chicago in several different ways.

Ashcraft replied that he had talked with Harker, who had advised the board to allow the appropriation to lapse. Because the trustees could not afford to do so, Harker advised Ashcraft to proceed with the bill for an injunction. According to Ashcraft, his clients believed that if members of the Senate had known that the bill as amended had been printed it would have been defeated. To enjoin the paying out of this appropriation might affect the validity of other acts of the legislature, Ashcraft admitted, but he did not consider this a sufficient reason to disregard the plain provisions of the constitution. He planned to apply for an injunction in a day or two.

James learned that Henry J. MacFarland, the president of M. W. Wells and Co., a wholesale boots and shoes firm, and secretary of the Hahnemann Medical College Corporation, was the man who was to apply for the injunction. James wanted a chance to plead his case with MacFarland or with the officers and trustees of Hahnemann Medical College.[16]

Ashcraft replied that if the board of trustees was willing to agree not to withdraw the appropriation until he had, say, ten days' notice, he would be willing to defer applying for an injunction until James could be fully advised in the matter. He asked James to inform him by telegram of how he wished to proceed. Ashcraft hoped that the whole matter would not get in the newspapers.[17]

On 28 July Ashcraft and Ashcraft, acting on behalf of W. E. Neiberger of Bloomington, Illinois, notified the state auditor, the state treasurer, and the university's board of trustees that on 31 July the complainant would apply to James A. Creighton, a judge of the circuit court in Sangamon County, for a temporary writ of injunction in the cause. (Neiberger was an 1882 graduate of the Chicago Homeopathic College of Medicine.)[18] The bill of complaint signed by Neiberger on 29 July and submitted to Judge Creighton rehearsed the history of the legislative act that appropriated sixty thousand dollars for the maintenance and extension of the College of Medicine and concluded by asking that the auditor of public accounts and the treasurer of the State of Illinois be temporarily enjoined from paying the money to the university, "by means whereof the amount of said alleged appropriation will be illegally diverted from the Treasury of the State of Illinois and your orator [Neiberger] and other citizens and tax payers of the State of Illinois will be wronged and injured thereby."[19] The bill asked that on final hearing the injunction be made perpetual. The attorney general of Illinois applied for a postponement of the hearing until 2 August. Pending the outcome of the hearing, the board decided to act as if there were no injunction. Governor Deneen agreed with this plan, adding that if the injunction were granted, the General Assembly would cure the defect in the law by passing the appropriation of sixty thousand dollars per annum.[20]

Anticipating that the university would receive one hundred thousand dollars per annum for the College of Medicine for 1911–13, James had begun planning the reform of medical education at P&S. In early June he conferred with leading figures at the school while also discussing the union of the College of Medicine and Rush Medical College with James B. Herrick of the Rush faculty. James asked Ludvig Hektoen, a P&S alumnus who was a pathologist at both Rush and the University of Chicago, to become dean of the work of the first two years in the medical school. Hektoen declined and recommended Edward F. Wells, a professor of clinical medicine and associate professor of medicine at P&S. Pusey told James that with forty thousand dollars plus in salaries for new men "you would have by next Fall the medical school that would be accepted at once as the probable dominating influence in medical education in the West. Its effect on the situation in Chicago would be magical."[21]

In mid-June James informed Pusey that William H. Welch of Johns Hopkins, described by a biographer as "the single greatest reformer of medical education in the United States," was coming through Chicago in a few days. Since James could not be there, he asked Pusey to contact Welch at the University Club, talk over the medical situation and available men with him, make careful notes, and send James the benefit of the discussion.[22]

Pusey had an unhurried interview with Welch, who "assumed at once that the situation was potential of great things and that it would attract the best grade of men." His views on the subject were the same as those of Pusey and James. The first step was to develop the fundamental years, said Welch; it was hardly as important to get first-class heads of the departments as it was to get a collection of first-class young men who would grow up in the work.[23]

Welch mentioned some possibilities. They afford a good view of the state of the profession. In pathology, Welch regarded nine men highly: David J. Davis of Rush Medical College; Charles W. Duval, a professor at Tulane University since 1909; Edward Lecount, at Rush Medical College since 1892; Frank B. Mallory, an associate professor at Harvard since 1901; Eugene L. Opie, then of Washington University, formerly at Johns Hopkins, and a member of the Rockefeller Institute for Medical Research from 1904 to 1910; William Ophuls, who earned an MD at Göttingen and had been at Cooper Medical School in San Francisco since 1898; Richard M. Pearce Jr. at Pennsylvania, formerly of Bellevue; Edward F. Wells, a professor at P&S since 1886; and George H. Whipple of Johns Hopkins. Welch would hate to lose Whipple, who was his assistant. With the possible exception of Whipple, said Welch, Wells was perhaps the most eligible of the group.

In anatomy Welch advised James to get the advice of Franklin P. Mall, professor of anatomy at the Johns Hopkins School of Medicine since it opened in 1893. Mall, Welch added, would not mention the most brilliant and eligible man, Herbert M. Evans, an assistant professor of anatomy at Hopkins who worked with Mall. Welch also highly recommended Warren H. Lewis, another of Mall's assistants, who earned an MD at Johns Hopkins in 1900 and had been an associate professor of anatomy there since 1904. Welch viewed Charles Bardeen, professor of anatomy at the University of Wisconsin, as "a very high class man" and a born organizer.[24]

Welch thought that bacteriology should be combined with pathology or hygiene, preferably hygiene, and not be a separate department. Adolph Gehrmann of P&S was "all right" for bacteriology. Get a high-class man in hygiene, Welch advised, without mentioning names. In pure bacteriology as distinct from pathology or hygiene Welch recommended James W. Jobling, an 1896 MD from Tennessee Medical College and a pathologist at Michael Reese Hospital in Chicago since 1909. Welch also suggested Arthur I. Kendall, a PhD, not an MD, who was an instructor of preventive medicine and hygiene at Harvard.[25]

As for physiological chemistry, Welch thought that there was a type of man who was equally suited for physiological chemistry, pharmacology, or physiology. He recommended Carl Voegtlin, who was a pupil of John J. Abel, professor of pharmacology at Johns Hopkins; P. G. Hopkins at Cambridge, England, easily the best man in the subject; and Otto Folin at Harvard, a Swedish-born research chemist, formerly at McLean Hospital, Waverly, Massachusetts. In physiology Welch mentioned only George P. Dreyer of P&S, described as a first-class man.

On the matter of a dean for the junior years, Welch favored Edward F. Wells, if available, or Bardeen or Whipple, especially Bardeen. The organization of the clinical work, Welch said, was more important and more difficult than that of the laboratory years. At the head of each clinical department should be a man who gave his time exclusively to the college and the hospital, with assistants who were in private practice. It would be wise to proceed cautiously in the organization of the clinical years. There was no use, said Welch, in employing clinicians who gave most of their time to medical education without having hospital facilities for them. Pusey observed that P&S clinicians had nothing in the way of a hospital to rely on except their service in Cook County Hospital. If P&S had a reasonable part of Cook County Hospital at their service, Welch commented, it would be better than a private hospital.[26]

As in all of his faculty appointments, James wanted only the best of those recommended. As a first step he recruited men to head the departments in the junior college. Elias P. Lyon was highly recommended for physiology. He had a PhD from the University of Chicago (1897) and had been an assistant professor of physiology at Rush Medical College (1900–1904), an assistant professor of physiology and assistant dean at the University of Chicago (1901 to 1904), and professor of physiology from 1904 and dean of the St. Louis University Medical School from 1907. James B. Herrick of Rush said that Lyon, "a fine physiologist, an advanced educator and remarkably sane," was the man James wanted.[27]

James asked William H. Howell of Johns Hopkins and Jacques Loeb of the Rockefeller Institute for Medical Research for their opinions on Lyon's scientific qualifications, his general character, and his fitness for the position of junior dean. Howell wrote that Lyon was spoken of favorably by practically all who knew him and would no doubt make an excellent dean. With Lyon, Loeb said, James could not make a better selection. He was "faithful, absolutely honest and a man of excellent judgment." Scientifically he was "one of the best men in the country." He was a research man to the core and an excellent teacher. Loeb had tried to win Lyon for the Rockefeller Institute.[28]

James asked Loeb to compare Lyon with other prominent physiologists in the country. Loeb put Howell of Johns Hopkins, Lafayette B. Mendel of Yale, and possibly Anton J. Carlson of the University of Chicago first, with Lyon very closely following. Loeb rated Lyon ahead of Walter B. Cannon, the George Higginson Professor of Physiology at Harvard; Frederic S. Lee, the Dalton Professor of Physiology at Columbia from 1904; Joseph Erlanger, professor and head of the department of physiology at Washington University since 1910; and the physiologists of the state universities. Lyon was more modern than Howell and Mendel and was practically the only available scientific physiologist capable of building up the medical school. He knew the condition of affairs in medicine in the Midwest thoroughly on account of his experience as assistant dean at the University of Chicago and dean in St. Louis.[29]

At the same time, James was searching for an anatomist. He consulted Mall of Johns Hopkins, who seized the opening to discuss the medical situation in the nation. Mall congratulated James on the sixty thousand dollars appropriation and urged him to take the coming winter to assemble his staff. James had a great opportunity to develop medicine in Chicago, wrote Mall, and it would not be bad policy for him to compete at once with Washington University, Harvard, Columbia, and Johns Hopkins. It was logical that the university should ultimately control the hospital situation; to do this, the only safe course was to develop the scientific side first and to fill it with eminent men. A great prize was ahead on the clinical side. The nation was ready for it, and there was no reason why Illinois should not supply a staff of eminent scientists and practitioners who devoted all of their time to the institutions if the city supplied the hospitals.

As in Europe, the state would have a monopoly of the situation. "The medical situation in Chicago could have been solved by President Harper," Mall wrote, but "he was so blinded by numbers that he just ruined his great opportunity and lost his main support. The ten millions which went into the Rockefeller Institute he might have had. Mr. Gates tried to force him but he was blind and the 'plague spot' in medical education remains. The opportunity now is yours and if your rich and enlightened state remains behind you it will not be so very difficult to make Chicago a really great medical center."[30]

Sixty thousand dollars a year for the medical school was little more than enough to start the first two years properly, James replied. In the long run the state would dominate the situation in Illinois, "but it takes sometime [sic] for corn belt states to move in the direction of scientific education." The first step had been taken in the medical matter with the appropriation. James desired to advance standards as soon as possible, but this had to be handled with care. It takes time "to permeate" this mass of about six million people with "high scientific ideals."[31]

According to Mall, James should pay considerably more than five thousand dollars for eminent men in the basic sciences of the first two years and somewhat more on the clinical side. He viewed Clarence M. Jackson of the University of Missouri, who had declined chairs at Tulane, Bellevue, and Cincinnati, as the best man for anatomy. Next was Warren H. Lewis of Johns Hopkins, and after him came Albert C. Eycleshymer of St. Louis University and F. T. Lewis at the Harvard Medical School. Better still, Mall urged, get G. Carl Huber at seven thousand dollars.[32] Huber, professor of anatomy at the University of Michigan medical school from 1887, was being recruited at the time by the Wistar Institute of Anatomy and Biology in Philadelphia.

Milton J. Greenman, director of the Wistar Institute, thought that James had one of the finest opportunities in the country to build up a great medical school in Chicago. Greenman advised James to secure a young man who would grow with the position, for example, Warren H. Lewis or Herbert M. Evans, both of Johns Hopkins, or George L. Streeter, an embryologist who became professor of anatomy at the University of Michigan in 1907, all of whom might be tempted by five thousand dollars. Older possibilities included Clarence M. Jackson of Missouri, Frederic T. Lewis of Harvard, or Harold D. Senior at Bellevue. Greenman advised James to try to get Huber or Mall by offering from seven thousand dollars to ten thousand dollars. There was no better man for anatomy than Huber, but he would not consider an appointment in Chicago for less than seventy-five hundred dollars. Unable to pay so much, James turned to Eycleshymer.[33]

Albert C. Eycleshymer, who was born in 1867, had taken a BS at the University of Michigan and a PhD from Clark University, both in 1891. Trained as a zoologist, he taught biology and botany at Michigan and at the University of Chicago, from which he earned a PhD in 1895. He taught human embryology at Rush Medical School from 1897 to 1899 and in 1903 became director of the anatomy department at St. Louis University Medical School. In 1911, the year in which he published an important book on anatomy, St. Louis University conferred on him an honorary MD.[34]

In June when Lyon visited the university, James asked him to investigate P&S, which Lyon did, accompanied by Eycleshymer. On 29 June Lyon reported on his findings. An examination of the laboratory building showed that the school had a tremendous amount of space, much of it in large amphitheaters used for largely didactic instruction. The old building was "a hodgepodge and maze. Earthquake and lightning might properly be invoked upon it." The quarters allotted to gross anatomy were bad. "The present dissecting room is a disgrace; and clean, high class work is impossible under the conditions." The morale and discipline of students could not be maintained when a large part of their work was done in such surroundings. The large assembly hall on the fourth floor should be made into a dissecting room. The plant must be very expensive to maintain, which was probably the fundamental reason "for the mediocre educational results." Lyon disagreed with the statement repeatedly made to him in Chicago that considering the amounts spent, the educational results were very commendable. True, P&S buildings were larger, better, and better kept than those of the St. Louis University Medical School, but P&S needed men more than buildings. "Six paid professors and one janitor make a better school than *one* paid professor and six janitors."[35]

The equipment for teaching purposes of the departments of anatomy, physiology, pharmacy, and bacteriology needed some additions, Lyon found, but the immediate need was to get men and let them select the equipment that met their research and teaching requirements.

As for the organization of instruction and research, Lyon recommended that the school be organized into junior and senior colleges, with the former giving instruction in the fundamental sciences and with a dean. The first two years should be a winnowing machine that passed on only properly prepared students to the clinical years. The practice of omitting final examinations should be abandoned. Full-time instructors should teach not more than twelve hours a week. The library should be built up systematically on a university basis.

For 1911–12 Lyon recommended a budget for the departments of the junior college, building changes, equipment, and the library that ranged between $60,500 and $75,700, with certain subtractions allotted perhaps $50,000. Lyon advised James to seek out men who had already made a reputation and pay enough to get them. "The past reputation of the school is so bad that only the announcement of a superior organization will be taken in scientific circles as evidence of better conditions." Moreover, the situation was bound to be difficult because the old clinical and science teachers who had lost touch with research would look with disfavor on the growing power of the research departments.[36]

Pusey liked Lyon better than any other man mentioned as junior dean, and one point in his favor was that "he is not a Johns Hopkins man" (Pusey thought that the medical department of the University of Wisconsin, directed by Charles R. Bardeen, a 1904 Johns Hopkins MD, had not gained from being Hopkinized).[37] But Pusey criticized Lyon for a report that exhibited a snap judgment. The anatomical quarters were not entitled to Lyon's strictures, for example, and Lyon tended to exaggerate the importance of the laboratory departments. Lyon's general rating of P&S was "prejudiced and unjust," opined Pusey. Its standing and quality were as good as those of St. Louis University.[38]

James mollified Pusey by saying that his criticisms of Lyon's report were in general justified,[39] while he told Lyon that he agreed "in the main" with his exposition. James asked Lyon if he would be in a position to accept the deanship of the junior college at $5,000 a year, adding that it would be necessary to proceed on a more modest basis than Lyon recommended. The budget for 1911–12 would be about $45,000 rather than $60,500, and the clinical instruction would be reorganized only slightly. Some clinical instructors would be paid, but the school was dependent on men carrying the upper years without pay, and the university was dependent on them for securing certain hospital connections. Conditions, not theories, had to be faced. James would make no promises except to do the best he could for the interests of the medical school under the given conditions. "The situation in Chicago is further complicated by what may be called medical politics of the most virulent sort. Special problems . . . we have . . . because this is a state institution, and the prejudices of a great people have to be considered." If in peace and harmony we could develop on the basis we have, James thought that "we shall be able to line up the great commonwealth of Illinois behind medical research and medical education in a way which is absolutely without parallel."[40] Lyon agreed to accept an offer if one were made. From instinct and experience, he added, he believed in "making haste slowly."[41]

James followed Lyon's advice in reorganizing the College of Medicine. In July he recommended dividing the medical school into junior and senior colleges, corresponding roughly to the scientific departments of the first two years and the clinical departments of the last two years. He intended to name Quine as dean of the senior college and to appoint a junior dean. The instructors of professorial rank were to constitute the Executive Faculty in each college. The faculties of both colleges were to discuss matters of general interest; recommendations in such matters were to be made by the combined faculties under the chairmanship of the senior dean. Admission of students to the College of Medicine was to be in charge of the registrar of the university. The junior college was to have anatomy, physiology, and pathology departments, with the other subjects of the junior college grouped around these three. An experienced scholar and teacher was to head each department. The board approved of James's recommendations.[42]

Meanwhile, James had asked eminent anatomists to evaluate Eycleshymer. They agreed that he enjoyed a high place as an anatomist. He had proved his capacity in research, mainly in comparative embryology; was about to publish an admirable atlas of human anatomy; and was liked by students. At the University of Chicago he had lacked confidence in himself because of the uncertain future of the anatomy department there, but he had developed greatly at St. Louis University. His personality was attractive although he was inclined to be retiring socially, and he was able to work with others.[43]

On 1 August the board authorized the appointment of Lyon as junior dean in the College of Medicine and senior professor of physiology at a salary of five thousand dollars and of Eycleshymer as professor of anatomy at a salary of four thousand dollars. James informed them of the offer by both telegram and letter. Two days later, having learned that Judge Creighton had sent the application for an injunction to the Supreme Court, practically holding up the appropriation for the medical school until 15 October, James withdrew both offers.[44]

It seemed almost incredible to Eycleshymer that "a certain group of medical men" should be able and willing to obstruct the progress of medical education. If James could give him information about the moves "of that fellow at the head of the medical department of Loyola [John Dill Robertson]," Eycleshymer wrote, "I shall take great pleasure in putting the data in the hands of the Provincial of the Jesuits, whom I know and whose headquarters are here [St. Louis]."[45]

Meanwhile, concern for the lease on the premises of P&S became urgent. Although the board had decided to sign a modified lease for two years from 31 August 1911, James urged the members to execute a lease for one year from 1 September 1911, explaining that if the Supreme Court did not grant the injunction the board would be free to proceed with reorganization, but if it granted the injunction a special session of the legislature would be needed to solve the tangle, and the State Homeopathic Medical Association would undoubtedly campaign against the appropriation made by the legislature. The board took no action on the matter.[46]

On 26 September the board's Committee on the College of Medicine approved the budget for the College of Medicine for 1911–12 on condition that a satisfactory lease be concluded. It also approved the list of faculty members for 1911–12 presented by James on recommendation of Quine.[47]

On 11 November 1911, with medical matters temporarily settled, James departed for Germany. He spent more than three months visiting schools and libraries, arrived back in Chicago on 26 February 1912, and immediately resumed his efforts to reform medical education. On the day he reached Chicago he attended a meeting of the Council on Medical Education of the AMA at the Congress Hotel and went to a dinner at the Chicago Club tendered by Arthur D. Bevan. He also learned about an adverse development during his absence.

On 23 February 1912 the Illinois Supreme Court had declared the appropriation for the medical department of the university unconstitutional because the conference amendments had not been printed before final passage. The homeopaths gloated over the ruling. A letter to homeopathic doctors from the Chicago

Homeopathic Medical Society said, erroneously, that the court had declared il-
legal "the appropriation of state funds for the perpetuation of a sectarian medical school" and that the "press of Chicago" had called this "the greatest step ever
taken toward putting a stop to vicious legislation in our state." The letter attrib-
uted the result to the Illinois Homeopathic Medical Association acting jointly
with the Chicago Homeopathic Medical Society, with final success due chiefly
to Edwin M. Ashcraft. In recognition of his services, on 4 March homeopathic
officials gave Ashcraft a complimentary dinner.[48]

E. Fletcher Ingals thought that the ruling of the Supreme Court had averted
a danger. He had feared that something might occur "to disturb the relations of
Rush with the University of Chicago and to draw it into the University of Illinois." Writing to President Judson, Ingals said he realized "the validity of certain
arguments that were advanced," presumably by Bevan, Billings, and others, but
believed that "such a step," presumably absorption of Rush by the University
of Illinois, would be a positive misfortune both to Rush and to the University
of Chicago, "*providing that the University of Chicago intends any time,* to have
a fully equipped medical department." Something must be done before long,
Ingals added, to preserve to the University of Chicago the advantages it might
secure by decisive action and to relieve the teaching of medical science in Chicago from the domination of politics. The well-meant but unwise efforts made
by several of his younger colleagues a few months ago, Ingals wrote, made the
danger much more acute.[49]

The failure of the appropriation bill made it evident that the university would
have difficulty in carrying out the financial obligations of the lease. Accordingly,
on 29 March 1912 the board of directors of P&S decided to terminate the lease
at its expiration on 30 June 1912 and to reopen the school as a corporation for
profit, depending on tuition fees to meet operating expenses.[50] The school continued with the same faculty as before except for a few resignations, including
those of Charles Davison, Charles S. Bacon, and Edward L. Heintz, who had
been on the faculty since graduating from P&S in 1901. After P&S reverted to
proprietary status, an old-guard faction battled a faction of seceders for control
of the Alumni Association of the college. Heintz, representing those who had
withdrawn, won the contest.[51]

On 10 April the board of trustees severed its tie with P&S. Since there did not
seem to be any physical plant in Chicago that might be available for a medical
school at any price that the university would be willing or able to pay, the board
decided to close the medical and dental work it conducted in Chicago on 30
June 1912. The buildings of the college and the equipment, including the laboratories and library, became a part of the university but were subject to obligations in the shape of loans or mortgages amounting to $245,000. These the state
had to assume. The university also asked the legislature, then in special session,
for an appropriation of $250,000 to develop the medical work being conducted

on the campus of the university in Urbana-Champaign. The greater part of the money requested was to be used to erect, furnish, and equip a building.[52]

Two interrelated developments that affected the medical situation followed. One was the board's attempt to secure an appropriation for medical education. The other was the effort of alumni of the medical school and of the university to raise funds to enable the university to continue its medical school in Chicago. It will clarify matters to discuss each of these developments in turn.

When the second special session of the Forty-seventh General Assembly opened on 26 March, Governor Deneen informed members that since the legislature had already passed on the merits of the appropriation bill for the medical department of the university, it would be necessary only to reenact it in conformity with the constitution.[53]

Charles S. Bacon, who campaigned to secure the appropriation, noted that opposition to it appeared before the legislature met and grew during the legislative session. The chief opposition came from two sources: the Loyola College of Medicine, whose president was John Dill Robertson, and the Chicago College of Medicine and Surgery (Valparaiso), whose secretary was J. Newton Roe. Both men were politically experienced, and they secured promises from a number of legislators to oppose the university bill.[54]

On 27 March Henry M. Dunlap, a Republican from Savoy, and Joseph Carter, a Republican from Champaign, introduced in the Senate and the House, respectively, bills for an appropriation of $250,000 for a new building and $100,000 for the two basic years of medical education.[55]

In mid-April James, knowing that the fate of the bills was to be settled on 23 April, sent circular letters to members of various interest groups and to legislators asking them to support the appropriation. He also sent legislators an endorsement of the request for $250,000 by the deans of Rush Medical College and Northwestern Medical College, Arthur Bevan for the Council on Medical Education of the AMA, and twenty-nine distinguished physicians of Chicago, including Ludvig Hektoen of Rush Medical College and Otto L. Schmidt, professor of medicine in the Chicago Policlinic. Strangely, the endorsers included three known opponents of state support for the university's medical school: John Dill Robertson of Loyola and both J. Newton Roe and William J. Butler of the Chicago College of Medicine and Surgery (Valparaiso). No doubt they were playing a double game, publicly endorsing while privately opposing the appropriation. With his letters James enclosed a copy of the pamphlet *Why the State of Illinois Should Appropriate $100,000 a Year for the Biennium 1911–13 for the Maintenance of the Medical School of the University of Illinois.*[56]

The bill had rough sailing in the General Assembly. A number of P&S alumni lobbied for the bill in Springfield. Steele, Bacon, Davison, Heintz, and Archie J. Graham were all active in the cause. Bacon called on Roger Sullivan, whom he had known when Sullivan was a clerk in the County Hospital and who had, by organizing the Irish, emerged as a leader of Chicago Democrats. Although Sullivan criticized President James rather severely for having a university faculty member draw up a bill that affected one of Sullivan's business projects, he promised to do what he could for the university. But Sullivan was not in Springfield when the bill came before the appropriations committee, and many of his followers opposed the bill. When Bacon called their attention to Sullivan's promise, some of them telephoned to his son, Boethius, who confirmed Bacon's statements, which caused considerable consternation in the clan.[57]

Additional opposition developed over time. Homeopaths, strong opponents of the bill, were a forceful presence in Illinois. According to Quine, 1,046 of the avowed 4,000 homeopaths in the world were registered in the state of Illinois, and more than 800 of them were located in Chicago. Moreover, one-fourth of all the homeopathic colleges were located in or near Chicago.[58] The executive committee of the Illinois Homeopathic Medical Association sent every legislator a letter explaining why the appropriation should be denied. Six high-grade medical colleges already existed in Chicago, the homeopaths alleged; neither the public nor the profession demanded a medical department of the university; the Forty-seventh General Assembly had already provided the university a total appropriation of $2 million; and the bill for $250,000 for medicine did not specify how the money would be used. "State universities have not been conspicuously successful in their conducting of medical schools," the homeopaths added, "and their contributions in the way of medical research, have been, to say the least, insignificant." After an interview on 17 April with Joseph Carter, the university's spokesman in the House, James concluded that if Carter represented the prevailing attitude, the outlook for the medical bill was "ominous."[59]

During the campaign, wrote Bacon, some members of the legislature doubted whether the property of the medical college was worth the amount of the indebtedness. A survey showed that the value of the real estate was just about equal to the indebtedness, leaving a surplus of the laboratory equipment and the library. This report satisfied the critics and Governor Edward F. Dunne, who had not been very friendly to the acquisition of the property by the university.[60]

Contemporary accounts of how the General Assembly handled the appropriations request differ. Charles S. Bacon said that the campaign ended well. The appropriations bill passed the Senate by a good majority but encountered difficulty in the House. Although the House Appropriations Committee included many opponents of the bill, the committee referred the bill to the House without recommendation. The pro–University of Illinois people knew that they had two-thirds of the House committed to passage of the bill but feared defeat by some trick. Michael Igoe, the leader of the Democratic Party in the House, and Medill McCormick, the leader of the Progressive Party, advocated the bill, and the Republicans were generally favorable. James made an impressive appearance before the House, and the decision rested on action concerning an amendment recommended by the appropriations committee. A sharp debate followed, but on the roll call the vote was 93 for and 37 against the university.[61] Or so Bacon wrote.

The official records, however, portray a disappointing outcome. On 23 April James attended a hearing on the appropriations bill held by the Senate Committee on Appropriations. After the hearing he met with the committee, which reported the bill back with amendments. According to James, the committee recommended $120,000. The Senate Journal recorded the vote on passing the bill as 20 yeas and 4 nays. Two days later, the Senate passed all the appropriation bills that were before it by reason of the Supreme Court ruling except the one for the medical school. David Shanahan, chair of the House Committee on Appropriations, opposed the bill for the medical school, and it did not pass the House.[62]

The battle over the medical school continued after the General Assembly adjourned. At its annual meeting in Chicago on 16 May, the Illinois Homeopathic Medical Society asked for an investigation of the expenditures of the two million dollars appropriated to the university by the state and especially the school's maintenance of a lobby in Springfield. A week later the House of Delegates of the Illinois State Medical Society described the failure to appropriate as a "serious blow" that compelled the university to close its medical school. The society pledged to support adequate appropriations to enable the university to develop public health, medical research, and medical education, and it appointed a standing committee consisting of one member from each county in the state under the chairmanship of Charles S. Bacon to urge the public, the legislature, and the university to make adequate provision for this great public need.[63]

The failure to secure an appropriation for medical education inspired an effort by medical school alumni and university alumni to raise funds to enable the university to continue its medical school in Chicago.[64] Edward L. Heintz now headed the P&S Alumni Association. He and the council of the association quickly issued a statement that deplored the end of the affiliation on the grounds that the "united forces" had led to raising the standard of the school and the quality of its instruction. The council asked both P&S and the university to defer final action on cutting their ties until the legislature provided for a medical department for the university.[65]

Some of this group tried to arrange for facilities that would enable the university to continue its medical education in Chicago. Davison and Bacon, for example, talked with James about resuscitating the medical school in Chicago in buildings furnished at a nominal rent by the University Hospital Association. Davison and Bacon were among the founders of University Hospital. James pursued this possibility with Abbott, Steele, and others.[66] Architects drew up plans for a building in which to teach the clinical years with provision for two hundred students (the preclinical years would be offered in Urbana). An option on land in the vicinity of the old college was secured, and money to finance this plan was pledged.

During the summer Heintz and the council of the Alumni Association decided to gather up the stock of the P&S corporation and donate it to the university, thus enabling the university to gain control of "one of the best sites for a medical school in any American city."[67] Since 7 of the 2,170 original shares had never been issued, they had to secure 2,163 shares. In 1898 when the board of directors proposed to increase the capital stock 120 percent, they learned that Bayard Holmes had sold his shares to John B. Murphy and Henry P. Newman. As of 20 April 1900, P&S faculty members owned 635 shares valued at one hundred dollars each. John B. Murphy, with 70 shares, was the largest single stockholder. Steele, Quine, Byford, and Newman each owned 27 shares, six doctors each owned 25 shares, and others owned a lesser number. A total of 1,528 shares were in other hands.[68]

Heintz informed stockholders that many P&S faculty members had agreed to have their shares, amounting to one-third of all the stock, held in a trust until all the stock was secured. If all the stock was not secured by 1 July 1913, the stock held in trust would be returned to the owners. The council of the Alumni Association appointed Heintz, Steele, and Davison to lead a campaign to obtain the stock. P&S had 3,500 alumni, with 1,200 of them in Illinois and 800 in Chicago. Steele thought it possible to obtain donations of stock on the condition that the university reopen the school.[69]

In February 1913 Heintz and other members of the Alumni Association attended the annual meeting of the Illini Club, consisting of university alumni who lived in the city of Chicago, to urge the club to back the university's request for an appropriation for the medical school. After Heintz talked to the group, the Illini Club, headed by Fred J. Postel, Class of 1899, pledged their backing of the proposition.[70]

These outpourings of support heartened the board of trustees. At its 10 September meeting James recommended that the board request from the next legislature at least one hundred thousand dollars per annum for support of the medical school. If the appropriation were obtained and alumni secured for the university an adequate plant and site in Chicago, either by presenting to the trustees the stock of P&S or by provision of an equally good site elsewhere in the city, said James, the university would reopen a medical school in Chicago. But the university ought not try to conduct a medical school on the basis of the fees of medical students alone or without legislative support. By a vote of 7 ayes to 2 nays with four members absent, the board agreed to accept the property of P&S provided all of the stock was secured and donated to the university by 1 February 1913. Mary Busey and George A. Anthony, president of the State Board of Agriculture and an ex officio trustee, both voted no. Busey favored accepting the P&S property only on the condition that an adequate appropriation for support of the medical school was obtained from the legislature. James himself shared this view.[71]

James thought that two things were needed to ensure the success of the plan to persuade the General Assembly to provide one hundred thousand dollars to operate the school of medicine and then to secure a plant and a site in Chicago. One was to get Edward F. Dunne, the governor elect, committed to the plan. If he opposed it, the proposition was doomed; if he favored it, the plan would succeed. Thus it was essential to get both alumni and people not connected with P&S to go to Dunne, urging him to endorse the request. The other need was to secure the stock of P&S by gift or purchase.[72] In September Steele reported that he had donations promised of 1,003 shares of the stock and written options on 785 shares, making 1,788 out of a total of the 2,163 shares outstanding.[73]

James always pushed himself hard in the service of the university, and he suffered recurrent health problems. In mid-December he felt miserable physically. His doctor diagnosed stomach trouble and ordered him to the hospital. On 27 December James entered Presbyterian Hospital on the West Side in Chicago. Doctors found a stomach ulcer and severely restricted his diet. While hospitalized James continued to deal with the medical school situation, receiving visitors, phoning, and dictating letters. He kept in close touch with Abbott, Steele, Davison, Bacon, and Heintz. On 22 January James returned home, weak and weighing 149 pounds. On 28 January he had his first solid food in a month, and in late February he was still on hourly feedings.[74]

Nevertheless, while ill and convalescing James had decided how to proceed with the medical school, and on 12 February he presented his views to the board at a special meeting in Urbana. Governor Dunne and eight other trustees were present, along with Steele, Davison, Heintz, and Oliver A. Harker, the university's legal counsel.

After briefly tracing the history of relations between P&S and the university, James informed the trustees that Steele had met the challenge to acquire and turn over to the university all of the stock of the P&S corporation on or before 1 February 1913. The owners had donated 1,495 of the 2,163 outstanding shares outright. Among the leading donors were Charles Davison (218 shares), William E. Quine (192 shares), Daniel A. K. Steele (159 shares), and John B. Murphy (153 shares). Steele had obtained options on the remaining 668 shares until 1 July 1913, whereupon solicitors asked alumni to subscribe funds to purchase the stock and donate it to the university. The committee purchased these shares for $27,941.88. Even if all the subscriptions were paid, the deficit would still be $11,731.68. Steele guaranteed to make up the deficit.[75] John Dill Robertson had tried to obstruct the plan by offering a P&S stockholder $1,500 for 10 shares of stock, and J. Newton Roe of the Chicago College of Medicine and Surgery (Valparaiso) had engaged in the same practice by offering Charles Bacon $3,000 for his 20 shares of stock.[76]

On 31 January 1913 Steele had delivered the complete stock issue of P&S to Abbott, the president of the board of trustees, along with the resignations of the officers of the corporation, the charter of P&S, deeds to the real estate, a bill of sale of the personal property, and some scholarship and other funds. The transfer of property was made subject to the mortgage and bonded indebtedness of $245,000 on the property.[77]

At their meeting on 12 February the trustees formally approved the details of the transfer and directed James to reopen the medical school in the plant presented to the university, to retain the existing faculty until 30 June 1913, to admit students then in P&S to the corresponding classes in the medical school of the university, and to conduct the medical school until 30 June 1913 on the basis of the budget adopted for the current year.[78]

A month later (6 March) formal ceremonies reopened the University of Illinois College of Medicine. P&S became the University of Illinois College of Medicine.

A Retrospect on P&S

P&S had an active existence for almost exactly thirty years. Under the lease of 1900 the university hoped to be able to buy the college in twenty-five years, but the hope proved to be illusory. Scientific medicine increased the expenses of medical education far beyond the yield of tuition income, and repeated efforts to secure a legislative appropriation to invigorate the college failed. In 1912 P&S reverted to the status of a proprietary medical school.

William A. Pusey, a faculty member since 1894, offered a retrospect on the college. "It represented the sort of teaching institution that is disappearing; a sort of institution that had its defects, but that gave us nearly all of medical development that this country has shown. It became a vigorous specimen of its kind, and it made an impression upon medicine in the middle west that is large and wholesome." The teaching in the institution was varied and unequal, Pusey recalled. "There was dead timber . . . for there is always dead timber; but its faculty included many good teachers, some great ones, and many men whose names are notable in medicine." The spirit of individual faculty members was largely altruistic, and after the university affiliation "the spirit of self-effacement in the faculty ultimately became such as to do one's heart good to remember. The stockholders of the corporation were invariably willing to go as far as they were asked by their representatives in sacrificing their material interests in the corporation. And, not only this, they were willing to sacrifice their personal interest; for there was never a time when many men in the faculty did not know that absolute control of the institution by the University of Illinois meant loss of their positions." The college was fortunate, Pusey added, in having throughout its career "a continuity of ambitions and of policies" through the continued presence of Steele, Quine, King, and Pusey. Steele represented the college in its material and property interests, while Quine represented the college in its educational interests. Both had the confidence of their colleagues and could count on their support.[79]

Another retrospect comes by comparing P&S with the other university-related medical colleges in Chicago. Their admissions requirements varied. In 1904 Rush required two years of college work in addition to completion of high school, for example, whereas both P&S and Northwestern required only a high school diploma or its equivalent. Years passed before Northwestern and P&S required two years of college work for admission. In 1905 tuition at Rush was $180 a year, and at Northwestern it was $175 a year. At P&S, tuition was $145 for each of the first two years, $150 for the third year, and $175 for the fourth year.

Attendance also varied. In 1909 when Flexner visited the Chicago medical colleges, Northwestern was largest, with an attendance of 522. P&S followed with an attendance of 517, while Rush had an attendance of 488. These three schools overshadowed all of the others. The Chicago College of Medicine and Surgery (Valparaiso) had an attendance of perhaps 366, while in 1909 Bennett Medical College had an attendance of 181 and Hahnemann Medical College had an attendance of 130.

In 1905 Rush had a faculty of 254, including 69 professors and 185 others. The P&S faculty numbered 198, including 42 professors and 156 others. Northwestern had a faculty of 116, including 38 professors and 78 others. Thus 32 percent of the Northwestern faculty, 27 percent of the Rush faculty, and 21 percent of the P&S faculty were at the professorial level.

In 1910 when Flexner reported, the relative positions of the three colleges in the size of the faculty remained about the same. Rush had a staff of 230, including 89 professors and 141 others. The University of Illinois had a staff of 198, including 42 professors and 156 others. Northwestern had a staff of 143, including 54 professors and 89 others. Thus professors constituted 38.7 percent of the Rush staff, 37.7 percent of the Northwestern staff, and only 21 percent of the P&S staff.

Flexner also compared the financial resources of the three medical schools. At Rush and the University of Chicago, the total cost of the divided program of instruction was $82,452 a year with the university providing $45,738 for the first two years, while the income in fees for the clinical program, which cost $36,714, was $60,485. Northwestern, except for two endowed professorships, lived on fees that amounted to $89,076 a year. P&S depended on fees estimated at $80,155, and it had a large floating debt.[80] Thus P&S was at a disadvantage in competing with the other two.

Students entered medical school with a view to graduating and entering practice. Their first hurdle was to earn a degree. Table 6 shows the number of graduates of the medical school from 1904, the year James became president, to 1913, a

Table 6. Graduates of the medical school, 1904 to 1913

Year	Male	Female	Total	Female Percentage
1904	198	17	215	7.9
1905	199	13	212	6.1
1906	196	14	210	6.6
1907	136	9	145	6.2
1908	139	12	151	7.9
1909	117	13	130	10.0
1910	121	10	131	7.6
1911	87	6	93	6.4
1912	136	8	144	5.5
1913	121	9	130	6.9

year after the university and P&S cut the tie that bound them together. The table is broken down to show the number of males and females, the total number of graduates, and the percentage of female graduates.[81]

On occasion P&S graduated more students than either Northwestern or Rush. In 1906, for example, P&S conferred MDs on 210 students, including 14 females (6.6 percent). Northwestern graduated 125 students with the MD, but all were males. Rush graduated 83 students with the MD, including 4 females (4 percent).[82]

Graduates had to pass an examination given by one of the state medical boards in order to receive a license to practice medicine. Candidates could take the examination in any state. The standards differed from state to state. Some states licensed people who had passed the examination in another state. Graduates of low-grade colleges often took their examinations in lenient states. The Illinois State Board of Health reciprocated in licensing physicians with fifteen states in 1906 and with twenty-one states in 1913.[83]

Evidence on the performance of P&S graduates on the examinations given by the state boards gives us some sense of the academic standing of the college during the James presidency through 1912. In 1906 the Council on Medical Education published a report that showed the pass and fail rates of graduates of 1905 or previous years on state board examinations in 1905. The failure rate of all three university-related medical schools in Chicago was alarmingly high. Northwestern graduates had a failure rate of 46.7 percent. P&S graduates had a failure rate of 39.1 percent. Rush graduates had a failure rate of 23.4 percent.[84]

In the examinations given by the state boards in 1906, Northwestern did best with a failure rate of 1.9 percent; Rush followed with 2.2 percent. The American Medical Missionary College was third with 4.4 percent, P&S had a failure rate of 6.6 percent, and Bennett College had a failure rate of 8.9 percent. Hering Medical College had a failure rate of 42.8 percent, while the failure rate of the College of Medicine and Surgery (Physio-Medical) was 55.5 percent.[85]

In 1908 the state boards examined 548 graduates of 12 Chicago medical schools. Graduates of Rush did best with a failure rate of 1.8 percent. Northwestern followed with a failure rate of 3.1 percent. Hering Medical College was next with a failure rate of 6.3 percent. The Chicago College of Medicine and Surgery (Valparaiso) had a failure rate of 7 percent. P&S graduates had a failure rate of 8.7 percent.[86]

As of April 1911 the Illinois State Board of Health recognized ten medical colleges in Illinois. The board fully and unconditionally recognized Rush Medical College, Northwestern Medical School, P&S, Bennett Medical College (Loyola University), Chicago College of Medicine and Surgery (Valparaiso), and Hahnemann Medical College. The board was prepared to restore full recognition to the College of Medicine and Surgery (Physio-Medical) and Hering Medical College in 1911–12 if they complied with the conditions the board had imposed on them several months earlier. If not, recognition would be entirely withdrawn. The board was ready to withdraw recognition from Jenner Medical College and Reliance Medical School at the close of the academic year unless they changed and gave instruction in the daytime rather than during the evening.[87] The standards were remarkably lenient.

In 1911 medical schools in Chicago graduated 536 students. Of this total number, 63 percent came from the following three schools: Northwestern, 158; P&S, 94; and Rush, 87. Of the total number, 6 percent came from the following seven colleges: Chicago College of Medicine and Surgery (Valparaiso), 86; Bennett (Loyola), 56; Hahnemann, 22; Reliance, 12; Jenner, 9; Hering, 7; and College of Medicine and Surgery, Physio-Medical, 5.[88]

In 1912 the Council on Medical Education of the AMA published the results of all medical graduates of 1907 through 1911 examined by state boards during 1911. The report dealt with eleven medical schools located in Chicago. The three acknowledged as best of the group led in the ratings. Of the 99 Rush Medical College graduates who took the examinations in 17 different states, 95 passed and 4 failed (4 percent failed). Of the 198 Northwestern Medical College graduates who took the examinations in 19 different states, 181 passed and 17 failed (8.5 percent failed). Of the 116 P&S graduates who took the examinations in 17 different states, 93 passed and 23 failed (19.8 percent failed). Low failure rates no doubt correlated with high admissions standards. Rush had required two years of work in a liberal arts college since 1904, and Northwestern had required a year of college work since 1908.

The council also reported on eight other Chicago medical colleges that taught various types of medicine. The report validated Flexner's charge that in medical education Chicago was "the plague spot of the country." At the College of Medicine and Surgery, Physio-Medical, 71.4 percent failed; at National Medical University, Panpathic, 66.7 percent failed; at Reliance Medical College, a regular school, 55.6 percent failed; at Jenner Medical College, regular, 50 percent failed;

at Bennett Medical College, regular, 41.8 percent failed; at Hering Medical College, homeopathic, 36.3 percent failed; at Hahnemann Medical College, homeopathic, 29.4 percent failed; and at Chicago College of Medicine and Surgery (Valparaiso), regular, 23.9 percent failed.[89]

P&S was one of the largest medical colleges in the city in number of students, and it graduated a large number of MDs. But on the examinations given by the state boards, the percentage of failures of P&S graduates was at times nearly four times that of Rush and more than twice that of Northwestern.

While the statistics on the rate of success and failure should be viewed with caution, they probably offer a rough approximation of the quality of the various medical colleges. Rush Medical College and the Northwestern University Medical School, both private enterprises, had a competitive advantage over the University of Illinois, a public institution. But to explain the Illinois situation in terms of public versus private does not suffice. More than twenty states had tax-supported medical schools in their state universities, but James, despite his persistent efforts, had been unable to secure state-provided funds for the university's medical college. The State of Illinois was not yet ready to support a medical school as a means of advancing public welfare.

CHAPTER 10

The University of Illinois College of Medicine

Formal ceremonies reopening the University of Illinois medical school were held on 6 March 1913 in the Medical Hall of the original College of Physicians and Surgeons (P&S) building at the corner of Honore and Harrison streets. On this historic occasion President Steele handed over the deed and the bill of sale, transferring to the board of trustees the tangible property of the college along with the franchise, the goodwill, and the high ideals maintained since 1882 in developing the institution. President William L. Abbott accepted the gift for the board of trustees, sensible of the obligation that the gift imposed, and declared that P&S was now the University of Illinois College of Medicine. Among other dignitaries who spoke were William E. Quine, dean of the former P&S; Winfield S. Hall for the Northwestern University Medical School; and Arthur D. Bevan, chairman of the Council on Medical Education of the American Medical Association (AMA). Dean Frank Billings of Rush Medical College who was ill and John B. Murphy of the Northwestern Medical School sent messages. James had invited a homeopath, but no representative of that sect attended.

James delivered the main address. He described the hardscrabble effort to obtain the funds necessary to operate a medical school of the first rank and deplored the fact that the state provided generous sums to promote agriculture and engineering "but not one dollar . . . for the study of human disease." Now, however, they were entering a new era in regard to public health, James declared, and state assistance was essential to offer in Chicago the best medical training the world could afford. With the funds James was requesting, the university would be able to achieve parity in admissions requirements with the medical schools of the state universities in neighboring Indiana, Michigan, Wisconsin, Minnesota, Iowa, and Missouri, and the university would undertake to provide facilities for medical study equal to those anywhere in the world "so that our youth will not be obliged to go to New York or Philadelphia or Boston or London or Paris, or Berlin or Vienna in order to prepare themselves properly for their work as servants of the public health of this great commonwealth." James closed with a

Lincolnesque flourish: "With malice toward none, with charity toward all, hold-ing out a sympathetic and co-operating hand toward all other worthy institu-tions, public and private—asking and accepting the aid and support of all schools and sects in medicine let us, in binding up the wounds of a broken and diseased society move forward to do our part in organizing all the forces in our society to safeguard, protect, and advance the health of each and every citizen!"[1] The Uni-versity of Illinois College of Medicine was poised on the threshold of a new day.

Another Bid for State Support

A campaign to secure an appropriation for the medical school had begun be-fore the College of Medicine stood on its own. On 23 December 1912 Steele, three other medical doctors, and two representatives of the Illini Club met with Edward F. Dunne, the governor-elect, for nearly two hours. Dunne expressed himself as being strongly in favor of medical research by the university, but he wanted to be sure that the state was making a good bargain before he commit-ted himself to the purchase of a medical college. "He has been well posted," Steele informed James, "by the organized opposition Roe, Robertson and the Homeos." According to Steele, James could depend on Bevan, Billings, Hektoen, and other Rush College men as well as on Murphy and other prominent doctors from Northwestern for support. On 25 December Steele urged James to get his statement "on the Medical College proposition" in the hands of governor-elect Dunne at once, since he was waiting for it.[2]

The board included one hundred thousand dollars a year for the medical school in its appropriations request for the next biennium. The one hundred thousand dollars asked for, James observed, was half of what the University of Minnesota had for its medical school, two-thirds of what the University of Michigan had, and about one-third of what Harvard and Columbia had and was a very small sum.[3]

James and College of Medicine officials mounted a campaign to win over the General Assembly. James had dossiers prepared containing biographical infor-mation on every member of the House; he had a petition to the General As-sembly printed that contained the names of prominent Illinois, American, and European physicians who endorsed the request for funds; and he composed and distributed a pamphlet, *Why the State of Illinois Should Appropriate $100,000 a Year for the Biennium 1913–1915 for the Maintenance of the College of Medicine of the University of Illinois*. The document contained a history of the College of Medicine as a prelude to a plea for funds.[4] Steele thought that the university could again count on the support of Roger Sullivan, the Democratic Party power broker in Chicago.[5] James and Charles S. Bacon of the medical faculty worked closely together to win support for the appropriation, and James addressed the General Assembly on the subject.[6]

Bacon reported that David E. Shanahan, chairman of the House Appropriations Committee, was opposed to the state engaging in medical education and that his attitude could be changed only by pressure from his constituents and from the community.[7] Bacon enlisted fourteen prominent Chicago doctors, six from Rush, six from Northwestern, one from the Post-Graduate Medical School, and George H. Simmons, general manager of the AMA and editor of the *JAMA*, to endorse a statement that called for a state-supported medical school whose entrance requirements corresponded with those of the highest class of medical schools in the country, including two years of work in a standard American college, and that provided research laboratories for the advancement of knowledge. Bacon wanted a thousand copies of the statement for his Committee of One Hundred to distribute to legislators.[8]

Fearing that the "low brows" might feel slighted, Bacon added more names to the statement. Alfred C. Cotton, a physician who signed, thought that Bacon should get the endorsement of the Chicago Medical Society, which George W. Webster Sr. of the Illinois State Board of Health headed. Some of the signatures, Bacon believed, were "good from the political standpoint," particularly those of two Roman Catholics and one homeopath.[9]

Considerable effort went into winning the support of the press. In January while still in the hospital, James reported that Heintz saw Dennis, the number two man at the *Chicago Daily News*. Dennis said that Victor F. Lawson, publisher of both the *Daily News,* the outstanding evening newspaper of the city, and the *Chicago Record-Herald,* a morning newspaper, and his newspapers all opposed a state medical school. Charles S. Williamson of the P&S faculty planned to see the *Chicago American,* while Davison and Pusey would look after Riley of the *Chicago Evening Post.* William A. Evans, formerly on the P&S faculty, former health commissioner of Chicago, and now health editor of the *Chicago Tribune,* offered to do everything he could to win over James Keeley, managing editor of the *Chicago Tribune.* Keeley was said to favor the medical school project. Bacon saw Victor Yarrow, editorial writer of the *Record-Herald,* and Andrew M. Lawrence of the *Chicago Examiner.* Lawrence was in favor of a state medical school.[10]

Victor Lawson, an influential publisher, was a special case. His attitude as to an adequate appropriation for the support of the medical school would be determined by whether or not the university proposed to conduct "a denominational medical school to the exclusive advantage of the allopathic school of medicine, or whether it will recognize the equal rights of citizens who believe in the homeopathic school of medicine, and give that school equal representation and opportunity in the medical department of the University." Lawson noted a "long story of arrogant attempted domination by the American Medical Association respecting the profession of medicine in this country."[11]

James replied that he himself was not prejudiced for or against any particular school of medicine, but based on his experience with doctors of various schools

he thought that no one should be allowed to practice medicine without a fundamental scientific training common to all schools or sects. He would be willing
to appoint a professor of homeopathic medicine and a professor of homeopathic
materia medica on a full parity with other professors of medicine and materia
medica. More than this "our homeopathic friends" ought not to ask. As far as his
influence went, James would "stand absolutely for a scientific school of medicine with due regard to all theories and all practices which may claim a scientific
basis, no matter what the name of the theory or practice may be."[12]

While mobilizing support, Bacon encountered opposition to the medical school. Dean Quine, recalling "the usual defamatory and virulent opposition," wrote that "for the first time in the history of medical education, so far
as known, the powers of a great religious organization were used to stem the
growth of medical science in a free state."[13] Bacon provided details. He viewed
Loyola University as a source of opposition and wanted to know how much of
the talk coming from Loyola was due to John Dill Robertson's policy of making
it appear that he alone represented the Loyola medical school. "If we have the
church opposition we should know it and prepare to meet it," Bacon said, but it
hardly seemed possible that the church would wish to join issue "on this question of support of a State Medical school." Someone should go directly to the
head of Loyola, Bacon suggested, and, if necessary, to James E. Quigley, archbishop of Chicago, and get the matter settled. "This working in the dark is very
disagreeable and humiliating. To let John Dill Robertson pose as the spokesman
of the Church should not be allowed."[14]

Governor Dunne was a Roman Catholic. Bacon believed that "the Catholic
opposition with the present Governor and legislature will defeat us probably
unless we can bring it into the open and then we should have a glorious fight."
He thought of asking the trustee Ellen Henrotin to go with him, first to Bishop
John L. Spalding and then, if necessary, to Archbishop Quigley. Bacon had not
discussed the matter with anyone except his political friend, Avery Brundage,
who agreed with Bacon's plan of action.[15] As an example of the Roman Catholic
opposition, Bacon reported that Senator Edward J. Glackin, a Chicago Democrat, hoped that the opposition could be called off because he would like to favor
the measure but could not go against his friends the Loyola people, whom he
understood were opposing the appropriation.[16]

In an interview with Robertson, Bacon learned that Robertson's chief ambition was to get his school recognized as in the first class of the Council on
Medical Education's ratings. Robertson blamed the AMA for Loyola's failure
to reach this rank, and he identified the university with the AMA. "The Jesuits
are in agreement with him and he could do nothing without their consent,"
Bacon wrote. "They have an understanding with the Chicago College [Roe's
school] and Hahnemann and could not take action without consulting them.
An agreement between these three institutions and Rush and Northwestern and

the American Medical Association might be made if their right to recognition could be in some way incorporated in the law."[17]

Moreover, Robertson doubted whether the transfer of the property of P&S was valid. If its indebtedness was greater than its value, as some claimed, the transfer could be annulled. The trustees made a mistake, according to Robertson, in acting without giving Governor Dunne time to investigate. The chief thing Bacon gained from the interview was the impression that Robertson relied mainly on Governor Dunne. Robertson was well connected politically. "It seems probable that John Dill Robertson may be appointed Health Commissioner [of the city of Chicago]," Steele informed James on 21 April 1915, "and if so, Mayor [William] Thompson will give his administration and scientific sanitation a black eye at the same time." When Robertson was appointed to the office, James merely expressed the hope that Robertson "may be able to do something to advance the interest of the public health."[18]

The trustee Ellen Henrotin approved of Bacon's idea of going to Roman Catholic officials but gave good reasons for not going with Bacon to visit Bishop Spalding or Archbishop Quigley. So Bacon vowed to find "some good Catholic" to go with him.[19] His efforts led him to drum up support with students in the medical school. "I met the Catholic boys today," he informed James, "and suggested lines for work for them. We have nearly one hundred, and they seem a bright and active lot of fellows."[20]

Steele was drumming up support for the appropriation in the state legislature and making converts every day. In early April he informed James that "over fifty of our Catholic students at my suggestion met in the assembly hall of St. Jarletts Church last night and formed a club to work as a unit with the Catholic members [of the legislature] to secure a Medical College appropriation." The students, who were addressed by "Father _____ and Professor Brown," manifested "great enthusiasm," wrote Steele, who thought that they would be very helpful in the campaign. Steele also reported that Michael L. Igoe, a Democratic state representative from Chicago, "had been told by the enemy that it [the appropriation for the medical school] was a stockjobbing steal," and he had opposed the medical appropriation "until he read your argument and had the real situation explained to him when he said that he had been lied to and basely deceived and that now he would vote for and work for it [the bill]."[21] The unnamed "enemy" was Robertson, Roe, and the homeopathic doctors. James's argument was no doubt the pamphlet explaining why the medical school needed one hundred thousand dollars a year.[22]

The question of whether the debt on the property of the medical college was greater than its value led Ferdinand A. Garesche to introduce in the House a resolution asking for an investigation of the matter. Garesche favored an appropriation of one hundred thousand dollars a year for the medical school but did not want the state to appropriate money for the property and then lose it by foreclosure. Others high in the state administration were of the same mind. For example, Charles Boeschenstein, a Chicago banker and member of the Democratic National Committee, and Governor Dunne inspected the former P&S property and came away believing that the obligations on the plant might exceed its legitimate value.²³ Bacon thought that Garesche, Boeschenstein, and Dunne had been deceived by the homeopaths, Roe of the Chicago College of Medicine and Surgery (Valparaiso), and Robertson, president of the Loyola medical school.²⁴ Nevertheless, Bacon found the news about Boeschenstein and Dunne disquieting. He wondered if Roger Sullivan, the Democratic Party boss, had talked with his friend Boeschenstein and was "carrying out his threats against the University for its political activity."²⁵ In early May Governor Dunne told Edmond Beall, a House member from Alton, that under no circumstances would any appropriation be made for the medical school outside of the regular appropriation. James informed a correspondent that Governor Dunne was not fully convinced that the state ought to do anything for medicine. In mid-May members of the medical school faculty showed a number of legislators around the buildings of P&S.²⁶

At the time the Chicago *Daily News,* quoting Dr. Burton Haseltine, president of the Illinois Homeopathic Medical Association, published editorials opposing the appropriation for the medical school. Appearing before the committee on appropriations of the House in Springfield, Haseltine argued that the state would have to assume indebtedness against the college, which some said equaled the value of the property; that there were enough doctors in Illinois; that there was no need to train more at public expense; that the state should not compete with existing medical schools; and that the state should engage in medical research rather than in teaching medical students. In a letter to the editor, Charles Bacon, on behalf of the Illinois State Medical Society, which included fifty-five hundred members and endorsed the establishment of a state university medical school, effectively answered the arguments of Haseltine and the *Daily News.* He called the opposition of the *Daily News* unfortunate and unjustified.²⁷

As the vote on the bill neared, Bacon's count revealed that a majority in both houses of the General Assembly promised to vote for the bill. David Kinley, vice president of the university, was in Springfield looking after details. Late on 11 June in response to a telegram from Kinley, James rushed over to Springfield. Two days later a bill appropriating the entire proceeds of the mill tax in a lump sum ($4.5 million for the biennium) to the board of trustees for the support and development of the university, handily passed the lower House and went to Governor Dunne, who signed it on 24 June. In the House an amendment to the university appropriation bill providing that no part of the appropriation should be expended in aid of the medical school was advanced to a third reading, but a motion to table the amendment was adopted by a vote of 94 to 37. The board allotted $100,000 a year out of the proceeds to the medical school for 1913–15.

This was truly a historic occasion. It was the first time that state-provided funds were available to support the medical school in the University of Illinois. Even then, the legislature itself did not assign the funds to medical education.[28]

In October 1913 after reading in a newspaper that the Rockefeller-funded General Education Board had announced a gift of $1.5 million to Johns Hopkins University in aid of medical education and research by putting clinical professors on the same basis as laboratory professors (that is, on full-time salaries), James requested that the University of Illinois medical school be put in a position to follow the lead of Johns Hopkins in this matter. If the General Education Board would be willing to assist in this enterprise, James avowed, he could persuade the people of Illinois to follow their leadership. No place in the country offered a better opportunity for doing this work just now than in the city of Chicago under the leadership of the University of Illinois.[29]

Frederick T. Gates, who advised John D. Rockefeller, replied that Hopkins furnished an ideal that would be followed by the best medical schools as they got the funds and that it was encouraging to think that James's medical school was ripe for such a venture. He presented James's request to the board, which did not find it practicable to undertake the work suggested.[30]

Reorganizing the College of Medicine

James wanted the university to take a leading role in making Chicago a great center of medical research and education. To realize his goal he acted along two lines simultaneously. One was to reorganize the University of Illinois medical school and to elevate its quality by the appointment of new deans and faculty members and by upgrading the curriculum. The other was to persuade the leading medical schools in the city to unite in offering the work of the clinical years.

As soon as the College of Medicine was under the control of the university and money was available for the purpose, James began the task of reorganization. Since it was necessary to devote thirty-five thousand of the one hundred thousand dollars allotted for medical education to the dental department, James had only sixty-five thousand for the initial outlay for the medical school. He invited Nathan P. Colwell, secretary of the Council on Medical Education of the AMA, to inspect the school. Colwell did not comment on the marked improvements already initiated but only on the improvements most needed. On the whole, he reported, the entrance requirements had been carefully administered, but the medical school still did not have an ample corps of expert full-time professors, the laboratory departments were undermanned, the teaching departments were too extensively subdivided, in some departments there was poor discipline over students, an exceedingly small amount of research was conducted, the clinical portion of the school needed attention, the college did not have a teaching hospital, and in the clinical portion of the school too little attention was given to individual work on the part of the student. As compared with other medical schools, the histories prepared in the dispensary were not in as good a condition as they might be. The medical library was in excellent condition. Concluding, Colwell noted that a few full-time professors of unquestioned ability had recently been added to the faculty, and a decided trend toward general improvement was noticeable.[31]

Reorganization was of prime importance. In April 1913 shortly after the College of Medicine began its new career, William E. Quine retired and became professor emeritus at the age of sixty-six. Colleagues paid tribute to his self-consuming industry, fidelity to duty, faithfulness to ideals, and justice tempered by generosity and friendliness, all of which had made him the controlling personality of the faculty and the guiding spirit of the institution for years.[32] In the autumn of 1913 as the result of a grave surgical operation, Quine was unable to perform any of his duties. Doubtful as to when he would be able to resume active work, he asked Steele to assume his duties as senior dean.[33]

James accepted the existing organization of the medical school with its division into junior and senior colleges and a dean for each college. He was content to accept the clinical program pretty much as it was for the time being, but he wished to reorganize certain departments in the junior college, namely anatomy, pathology, and physiology, without delay, appointing an experienced person to head each and then creating, as soon as possible, full professorships for physiological chemistry, bacteriology, hygiene, and materia medica and therapeutics.

Steele, the acting senior dean, was critical of the existing organizational structure. In April 1914 he called the attention of James to the "somewhat chaotic condition" that existed in the college by reason of Quine's illness and the divided responsibility between the junior and senior colleges. Conditions would be greatly improved, Steele observed, when James made up his mind about the appointment of permanent college officers. Steele added that faculty members felt considerable anxiety regarding their future relations to the college in case the College of Medicine affiliated with Rush Medical College.[34]

In June 1914 a year after the College of Medicine became a part of the university, the faculty of the college showed their esteem for Daniel A. K. Steele by presenting to the university a portrait bust of him by Leonard Crunelle, a pupil of Lorado Taft and a sculptor prominent in Chicago since 1901. The faculty praised Steele, one of the founders with whom they had been associated as teacher, colleague, and friend, for his loyalty and support of the college through tumultuous years. His was the "compass hand" that had pointed the way to "this happy ending." James, accepting the gift for the university, declared that Steele more than any other one man deserved the credit for what the college had accomplished up to the present.[35]

For whatever reason, James did not reorganize the College of Medicine. Steele harbored strong views on the subject and, trusting that James would not think him meddlesome, later returned to the matter. "I do not think the present organization of the College of Medicine is at all satisfactory. I realize that we are in a transitional stage and that the present plan of organization is merely temporary. It has no cohesion, it has little opportunity for taking the initiative or making positive recommendation to the President."[36] The college had no recognized head who possessed the authority to direct and govern the affairs of the college under the orders of the president, Steele said. True, the college had a senior dean and a junior dean, but their duties and responsibilities and the coordination of their work had never been defined.

The two faculties acted independently, Steele noted, and yet their activities were so interlocked that the best work could be realized only by united effort. The president of the university appointed and dismissed faculty members without consultation with the organized faculties. True, he consulted individual faculty members and heads of departments, but at times James might misinterpret faculty and personal views. Steele wrote,

> I do not wish to criticise [*sic*] your methods, for no one could have acted more wisely than you have through this trying period of re-organization, and more or less disorganization, but I wish you to consider, if you have the time and strength, if the time is not at hand when we should have a complete Faculty Organization with a responsible Head to direct all the complex problems of a Medical department of the University. I well know that the ultimate authority rests in the hands of the President and Board of Trustees, but I think better team work would be realized if this authority was definitely delegated to the Senior Dean, the Junior Dean, and the Heads of departments and so on down the line and each one held responsible to the next higher authority until it reaches the President and Trustees, and that when suggestions or requests are made, they should come through the organization in an official way and not by individuals. In other words, Faculty action should be communicated by the Dean or Secretary of the Faculty and not by an individual member or someone who might send his individual views and have them accepted as the official report of Faculty action.[37]

James agreed substantially with Steele, he replied, and hoped that "we" could get the final organization into a shape where everything will be coming along.[38] His reply was little better than nothing. Despite Steele's urging, James did not reorganize the college. A micromanager who paid close attention to details, he may have viewed other issues as more pressing.

Next in importance to reorganization was the selection of a senior dean. Steele, as noted earlier, became acting senior dean in the autumn of 1913. Apparently he had been criticized during a board meeting the previous July, after which William L. Abbott, president of the board, felt it necessary to defend Steele. Describing the great work that Steele had done for the medical college and for the university, Abbott said that "if he [Steele] were to be humiliated in the hour of his triumph without a casual complimentary recognition of the work he has done, it might truly be said that universities are ungrateful." If it were impossible to continue Steele in his position (presumably as a professor of surgery), Abbott recommended Charles Davison as a man who was not allied with either faction of the old medical faculty but who would command the respect and support of both.[39]

John T. Montgomery, a medical doctor and trustee, was critical of Steele. Convinced that the course in surgery was largely on paper and not much more than a joke, Montgomery urged radical change in the surgical department. The senior men, he observed, turned over to junior men the clinics they were scheduled to give, and most of the junior men were not competent. Montgomery suggested a complete reorganization of the teaching faculty in the clinical years. Appointments should be given only to those who really worked, not those who held a professorship to secure the title.[40]

On 4 August James told Steele that certain trustees were opposed to his continuing as head of the surgery department. On that same day the board's Committee on Medical Education had a stormy session during which trustees John Montgomery and Ellen Henrotin opposed Steele's continuation as head of the surgery department. The committee finally approved James's list of nominations for the clinical faculty, including that of Steele as professor of surgery and head of that department.[41]

Steele became acting dean in the autumn of 1913, and on 31 August 1914 James appointed him as senior dean beginning on 1 September 1914 and continuing until further notice or until 31 August 1915. Steele protested being asked "to serve without salary." He wanted the senior dean of the College of Medicine to be paid the same as every other dean of equal rank in the university. James refused to concede the point.[42]

Relations between Steele and James were often strained. Steele complained, for example, that James failed to keep the faculty informed about his effort to unite Rush Medical College with the University of Illinois, that the work of the junior and senior years of the College of Medicine had not received the recognition and support given to every other department of the university, that the budget of the junior college faculty was more generous than that of the senior college faculty, and that although James had induced the trustees to authorize the erection of a clinical building, so far it had been talk, talk, talk and no decision about the building.[43]

James faulted Steele for various shortcomings, including the appointment of clinical assistants or instructors who lacked two years of college work, and for his appointments in the junior and senior years. "I am glad to notice," James once wrote, "that you have gotten a man with at least the preliminary training of our freshmen." Steele was doing the best he could, he countered; in the future it would be easier to obtain a higher grade of teachers.[44] When Steele erroneously informed a faculty member that the project for a clinical building had been abandoned, James said, "As usual in such cases, Dr. Steele didn't understand the real situation about our clinical building or he failed to convey the correct idea to you."[45]

Seeking to replace Steele, James invited William A. Pusey to become the senior dean. On 18 February 1914 Pusey agreed to accept the office for the next year if necessary, but in May Pusey asked James to consider him no further.[46] The search for a medical school dean frustrated James, who vented his feelings in his diary: "The doctors are a queer lot! Mont[gomery] will not have Steele as Dean; nor Steele Pusey; nor Pusey, Davison; nor Davison Bacon; nor Mrs. Henrotin any of them. Ochsner wants his brother; no surgeon wants a surgeon [e]xcept himself or brother; no medical man wants a medical man [e]xcept his brother &c."[47]

In June James told Charles Bacon and Steele that he would keep things at the medical school steady for another year, which meant Steele as dean of the senior college and head of the Department of Surgery. On 11 July 1914 at a meeting of the board's medical committee in Chicago, Abbott, Henrotin, and Montgomery had a long contest over the appointment of Steele as dean and head of the department. The trustees passed the buck to James.[48] Two days later James discussed the deanship with Steele and on 11 September appointed Steele as senior dean (this is the first time that official records named Steele as dean) as well as professor of surgery and head of the Department of Surgery.[49]

In 1915 James agreed to appoint Steele as senior dean on an annual basis at no salary on the understanding that his appointment might be terminated whenever necessary. Steele protested against this arrangement. The dean of the medical school should be paid a suitable salary, he wrote, as was the case in the universities of Iowa, Indiana, Michigan, Minnesota, Missouri, Ohio, and Wisconsin, where the salaries ranged from thirty-five hundred to six thousand dollars a year. Illinois was the only state that did not pay the medical dean a suitable salary, and its resources were very largely in excess of those of six neighboring states. James replied that he was not yet ready to take up the matter. The determination of the salary, he added, would have a relation to the man who might be appointed dean whether he was a practicing physician and whether he devoted himself full-time or part-time to the job.[50]

In an effort to clarify his position, Steele told James that he had viewed as temporary his appointments as acting dean and as senior dean while James reorganized the school. Steele knew that James wanted to keep the deanship open so as to be able to offer it to Frank Billings, dean of Rush Medical College. But since such an affiliation was unlikely and since the medical faculty urged him not to relinquish the deanship, Steele was willing to accept a permanent appointment as senior dean if it was tendered to him.[51]

Again in 1916 James appointed Steele as senior dean for a year at no salary. Accepting this arrangement, Steele said, "Under the circumstances, my dignity is not being sustained by the Trustees or yourself on the same plane that all other State Universities recognize the services of the Deans of their respective Medical Departments."[52]

While Steele filled the position, James was looking for the best man he could find for the job. His consultants recommended Charles P. Emerson, Richard M. Pearce Jr., and Roger S. Morris. Franklin P. Mall of Johns Hopkins prefaced his comments on Emerson, a Johns Hopkins MD, by observing that with money to work with, James could "now take the lead in medical education in Chicago, for it is high time for it to begin there." Mall described Emerson as a "man of ability and very high ideals." Mall would judge Emerson, who had recently become dean of the medical school at Indiana University, largely by the success he was making there. William H. Welch of Johns Hopkins thought that Emerson might be the best available man to aid in developing the medical school along advanced lines.[53]

Charles R. Bardeen, dean of the medical school at the University of Wisconsin, prefaced his evaluation of Emerson with advice. Since the violent opposition of the sectarians had died down, Bardeen could "see no reason why the medical department of the University of Illinois should not be the best medical school in the West if you can get its control into the hands of the right men." James's greatest difficulty would be in getting "the highest type of men to fill the chairs because of the somewhat unfortunate reputation the College of Physicians and Surgeons has had of not being first class." The fault was not so much the management as it was "utterly inadequate resources." The most important thing in building the medical school was to get the right man for dean, "since in some ways it will be more difficult to bring the College of Physicians and Surgeons up to the highest standards than it would be to start a medical school anew." Bardeen, who knew Emerson well, described him as a hard worker and very methodical. He would be an effective administrator. But he had never shown any originality, and "originality and resource" were important in bringing the medical school into the front rank. Any new dean would need "tact enough to handle the delicate situation at Chicago."[54]

H. Gideon Wells, dean of the medical courses at the University of Chicago, described Richard M. Pearce Jr., professor of research medicine at the University of Pennsylvania, as an administrator of much ability. Pearce had a fine reputation as a teacher, Wells added, and had done excellent research work.[55]

Nothing came of these possibilities. Several unlikely candidates sought the office, and in 1915 James confessed that "the five or six whom I thought most highly of one after another declined to be considered, all of them practically for the reason that it was not yet apparent what clinical facilities the University of Illinois was going to supply" and that the medical school had such a large number of untrained students that they did not feel like trying to organize a modern medical school on such a basis. With the prospect of a clinical building it might be possible to find a dean before many months, said James, and Steele under-stood that as soon as James found a dean Steele would yield the place to him.[56]

In 1916 having heard that Elias P. Lyon, dean of the University of Minnesota medical school, might be movable, James asked Eycleshymer to "feel him out." Lyon indicated that he was committed to his work in Minnesota and could not leave.[57]

In the spring of 1917 with Steele's retirement imminent, the faculty named a Committee on the Selection of a Dean for the College of Medicine. The commit-tee included Davis, Davison, Eycleshymer, Ochsner, and Steele. James requested each of them to furnish him with the names of five men qualified to fill the position. Steele suggested five names. In order of merit they were Dean Victor Vaughan of Michigan; Arthur I. Kendall, the thirty-nine-year-old acting dean of Northwestern; Oscar Klotz, professor of pathology and bacteriology at the Uni-versity of Pittsburgh; Charles C. Bass, a professor of experimental medicine and director of laboratories of clinical medicine at Tulane who had done research on the malaria parasite; and, in fifth place, either Lyon of Minnesota or Bardeen of Wisconsin.[58]

On 5 March 1917 James met with the selection committee, and in late March Eycleshymer told James that Bardeen should be considered. James met Bardeen in Chicago.[59] We know nothing about their discussion. Time passed. On 7 July Steele resigned as senior dean (effective 1 July), and James asked Eycleshymer to serve as both senior and junior dean until further notice. The new dean asked James to inform members of the selection committee why a member of the committee was selected. It was owing to the necessity of administrative action, James said.[60] Viewed at the time as an interim appointee, Eycleshymer served as senior dean of the College of Medicine until his untimely death in 1925.

Although Eycleshymer had been appointed, in the fall James conferred about the deanship with Leonard Rowntree, chairman of medicine at the University of Minnesota since 1915. James was "very favorably impressed" with Rowntree and would have been "only too glad to have him come." But during their talks James became convinced that Rowntree had no idea of accepting any offer James could make. Rowntree apparently bargained for a salary of seventy-five hundred dol-lars and then used this sum in bargaining for a raise at Minnesota. James saw no objection to offering seventy-five hundred dollars as soon as he could find a man worth that salary, and Rowntree had come as near making it worthwhile to pay him that amount as any man he had run across.[61]

The appointment of a junior dean was a by-product of James's efforts to strengthen the junior faculty. He proposed that all such appointments be for one year unless otherwise specifically provided, with no implication as to renewal. As always, James sought assistance in identifying and evaluating candidates.[62]

The logical man for anatomy, said the embryologist and anatomist Frank-lin P. Mall of Hopkins, was F. T. Lewis of Harvard, but he would command a large salary. Mall hesitated to recommend a younger man because it was important to secure for this chair a man who had been "thoroughly tried." Bardeen, also an anatomist, viewed the best of those available for anatomy as Herbert M. Evans of Johns Hopkins and George L. Streeter of the University of Michigan.[63]

James got in touch with Evans, who wrote in July from the Anatomical Institute at the University of Freiburg that he was "very much interested in whatever develops in this regard." Nothing further developed, so on August 28 James turned to Albert C. Eycleshymer, whom he had wanted to hire in 1911. Eycleshymer came as professor of anatomy and head of the department of anatomy at a salary of five thousand dollars.[64]

For pathology, Gideon Wells of the University of Chicago recommended Richard M. Pearce Jr. as his first choice and George H. Whipple, an assistant professor at Johns Hopkins, as his second choice. Whipple had shown great ability in research work, said Wells, and was a man of strong personality and would be a powerful factor in any faculty he joined. Among the younger men who might be available, Wells put first David J. Davis, pathologist of St. Luke's Hospital in Chicago, a man of "unusually stable qualities, of much force, and [one who] has done excellent research work." Ludvig Hektoen described Davis as "very well qualified." Wells reported that Eugene L. Opie, dean and professor of pathology at Washington University and one of the leading men in pathology in the country, might be induced to leave St. Louis. Bardeen recommended Wade Hampton Brown, "a splendid man in every way." Brown had earned an MD at Johns Hopkins in 1907; had taught pathology at the universities of Virginia, Wisconsin, and North Carolina; and had accepted a research position at the Rockefeller Institute.[65]

James tried to recruit Opie, who was in Quisett, Massachusetts, during the summer. Opie said that he enjoyed "unusual facilities" in his present position but was free to consider any place that offered wider opportunities. James invited him to Chicago to look over the ground, but Opie could not make the trip and did not believe that he should be considered further.[66]

Wade Hampton Brown visited Chicago on 9 August, but James considered him too young (he was thirty-five years old).[67] James hoped to hire Whipple, who visited Chicago on 8 August. James and Whipple conferred with various people at the medical school,[68] but Whipple chose to remain at Johns Hopkins. (In 1934 he won a Nobel Prize in pathology.) On 8 September James told David J. Davis that he would appoint him to the position. Davis had a BS from the University of Wisconsin (1898), an MD from Rush Medical College (1904), and a PhD from the University of Chicago (1906) and was teaching pathology at Rush. James appointed Davis as director of the Research Laboratory for Experimental Medicine at a salary of five thousand dollars and as acting professor of pathology and acting head of the department of pathology without additional salary.[69] Davis, born in 1875, was thirty-eight years old at the time of his appointment.

James received few names for physiological chemistry. Russell H. Chittenden of the Sheffield Scientific School at Yale named William C. Rose, a Yale PhD who was an instructor at the University of Pennsylvania, as his first choice.[70] Several people mentioned Donald R. Van Slyke of the Rockefeller Institute as a possibility.[71] In late August George P. Dreyer, a physiology professor on the faculty, asked William H. Welker if he would accept an assistant professorship in physiological chemistry at a salary of twenty-five hundred dollars. Welker, then an assistant professor of physiological chemistry in the medical department of Columbia University, accepted, and on 4 September 1913 his appointment was made on the terms described.[72]

On 6 September James made official the appointment of George P. Dreyer as professor of physiology and head of the department of physiology at thirty-five hundred dollars a year and named Dreyer junior dean with an additional five hundred dollars a year.[73] In haste James had strengthened the faculty in the junior college with as little damage to the sensitivities of the older faculty as possible.

Along with other moves, James insisted on curricular improvement in the college. Starting in 1913, the minimum requirement for admission to the medical school was one year of college work in addition to a high school diploma or its equivalent. Believing that the curriculum was overcrowded, in the autumn of 1913 James appointed a committee to report on how it could be reduced within reasonable limits. Charles S. Williamson (medicine and clinical medicine) was chairman of the committee, which included Bacon (obstetrics), Dreyer (physiology and physiological chemistry), Eycleshymer (anatomy), Ochsner (surgery and clinical surgery), and Pusey (dermatology). As a basis of comparison, members selected twelve of the leading medical colleges and the model curriculum of the Council on Medical Education of the AMA. Assuming that the collegiate year consisted of thirty-two weeks, the committee, which reported on 16 March 1914, recommended that all the work of the general curriculum be obligatory and that the total number of hours required should be approximately 4,000. The committee recommended the distribution of these hours among the various branches of study and also recommended that students, except for freshmen, be allowed to take 64 hours of elective work each year in no more than two departments. Thus the maximum number of hours a student could take was 4,192. Other recommendations dealt with the dispensary, a summer term, extern service, a hospital quiz class, the grading of students, and student ownership of microscopes.[74]

James sent the report to the deans of medical schools and prominent practitioners around the country, asking them if the proposed curriculum was a good one, if it was abreast of the best educational theory and practice in medical education, if it was workable, and what changes they might like to suggest.[75]

On the whole the respondents viewed the curriculum favorably, although some questioned the distribution of hours, usually wanting more time for their own specialty. George Blumer, dean of the Yale medical faculty, offered a long and excellent critique. The form of the curriculum, Blumer said, was less important than the administration of it, but he did not consider the curriculum presented workable. It provided for too much anatomy and too little physiology, far more dermatology than ophthalmology and diseases of the ear, nose, and throat. In addition, Blumer opposed quiz classes. "The function of a medical school," he insisted, "is to train first-class practitioners and not to train men to pass hospital or any other examinations."[76]

In the spring and early summer of 1914 and again in early 1915, James invited medical doctors in neighboring states, including Iowa, Indiana, Kentucky, Michigan, Minnesota, Ohio, and Wisconsin, to inspect the physical plant and the work of the College of Medicine with a view to informing him about admissions standards and possible improvements. Only a few visited the medical school, but a number of them wrote offering advice, none of which was useful.[77]

On 22 August 1914 the Council on Medical Education of the AMA published in the *Journal of the American Medical Association* a set of standards that represented the basis on which the council classified medical colleges. The standards dealt with the admission of students and clinical facilities and explained that the council rated medical colleges under ten heads. On this scheme twenty-nine schools were classified as A Plus (i.e., acceptable). In this category were the medical schools of Northwestern and Rush and the state universities of Indiana, Iowa, Michigan, Minnesota, Nebraska, Ohio, Missouri, and Wisconsin.

The council classified thirty-eight medical schools as A (i.e., acceptable, but could make certain improvements). The University of Illinois medical school was in this group. The twenty-two colleges classified as B (i.e., needing general improvements to make them acceptable) included Bennett College of Medicine (Loyola), Chicago College of Medicine and Surgery (Valparaiso), and Hahnemann Medical College and Hospital. Class C (i.e., requiring a complete reorganization to make them acceptable) included twenty Chicago schools, among them the Chicago Hospital College of Medicine, which had been organized in 1913, and Jenner Medical College, both of which were afternoon and night schools.[78]

As soon as these ratings were published, James asked Nathan P. Colwell, secretary of the Council on Medical Education, why the university's medical school had received an A grade and what improvement was needed to gain the higher rating. The University of Illinois medical school would be put on a first-class basis "deo volente," he declared, "and I presume that God is not going to be against it."[79]

Colwell explained the main reasons why the university's medical school could not be classed as A Plus. The entire school needed considerable overhauling, the school lacked a hospital with a sufficient number of patients who could be utilized for teaching purposes, and it did not appear that any definite plan of instruction had been well laid down in all the departments, chiefly those of the clinical years. Only a few years earlier the school had shown a lack of the best educational spirit, among other ways by the loose method of admitting students, the undue liberality shown in granting advanced standing for work done in low-grade colleges, and the apparently close relationship of some of its professors with a certain night medical school. Of course, Colwell admitted, these evils had been more than corrected since James had taken the school in hand.[80]

James sent Steele a copy of Colwell's letter and asked him to test the College of Medicine by the standards published in the *Journal of the American Medical Association* and to invite Colwell to visit the medical school.[81]

In mid-November Steele and five of his senior colleagues met with Colwell. Steele explained how the administration had organized the various departments under their respective heads in a systematic manner, and those present asked Colwell what more needed to be done to merit a higher classification. Colwell suggested that they invite two first-class disinterested men, a clinician and a laboratory man, to make a thorough inspection and report to the council and the university what more was needed to merit an A Plus rating.[82]

At Colwell's suggestion James invited Elias P. Lyon, dean of the University of Minnesota medical school, and George Dock, professor of medicine at the Washington University medical school since 1910, to make such an inspection. On 5 January 1915 they examined the laboratory building and the Cook County, West Side, and University hospitals, and they received a demonstration of the clinical instruction given groups of students in Michael Reese, Children's, St. Luke's, and Augustana hospitals.[83]

On 1 February Lyon and Dock submitted a joint report. They found the laboratories fairly well housed and fairly well equipped and did not discuss further this part of the school. They focused on the hospital. "The teaching and scientific work suffer from too much multiplication of buildings, too great distances between the various units, and from staffs not sufficiently complete, well-trained and coordinated."[84] Students did not come in close enough contact with patients and were not able to apply the knowledge they acquired during their first two years in their third and fourth years.

How to improve the situation was largely a practical question, and the authors refrained from making a specific recommendation. "So populous and wealthy a state, with a university so large, so well supplied, and so ably administered," they declared, should have a hospital with a total of about five hundred beds. The hospital should not be wholly a charity hospital but instead should be wholly a teaching and research hospital. Perhaps 20 percent of its maintenance might be charged to medical education. Many patients could pay all or part of the hospital charge.

This ideal, so far as buildings were concerned, could be attained within a comparatively short time, but it would be difficult, even with unlimited money, to form an adequate staff in a short time. It would be better to let the university obtain complete control of one or two existing hospital units convenient to the medical school building and have their administration carried on by a single head. It would also be better to subdivide the space and reorganize the staffs in the different lines so that each staff person would be brought up to the highest degree of efficiency as rapidly as possible. The primary interest and work of the staff should be given to this hospital. There should be numerous full-time men. Private practice, if allowed, should be limited to consultation work at hours that would not interfere with schoolwork. Whether to build from the existing staff or to bring in new blood would depend on conditions in different departments. The staff should have definite duties in connection with the hospital work, they should take part in teaching, and they should be encouraged to carry on original investigations.[85]

Lyon supplemented the joint report with his personal impressions. As for the laboratories, much improvement had been made since his visit two or three years earlier. But there was a lot of unused space in the building, and too much was spent in keeping up the physical plant. Economy in management could be effected by bringing the Chicago departments together under one roof.

Lyon praised the magnificence and the enormous clinical material of the County Hospital, but no positions between full staff men and interns were recognized there, and it would be difficult to bring about such a condition. The County Hospital would not be a first-class teaching institution until students were permitted in the wards, with full privilege of studying the cases, taking histories, etc. If the state could make some arrangement to take charge, medically, of a portion of the institution and would put in full-time men on an organized basis, the problem of clinical instruction would be met.

The West Side and University hospitals were essentially private institutions, and if they continued as such the most that could be expected was the same type of teaching in the college amphitheater that had been in vogue. Unless James could build a hospital or put through some effective plan at Cook County Hospital, the lease of either West Side Hospital or University Hospital might be the best plan of meeting his clinical needs for the next few years.

Michael Reese, largely a charity hospital, was in many respects a fine institution. The staff had a high concept of what a teaching hospital should be. The scientific spirit seemed unusually good. St. Luke's Hospital had the aspect of a great medical hotel. The management had no concept of a teaching institution. Augustana Hospital was much better.

The lack at the College of Medicine was not clinical material but properly controlled material with which intensive, scientific teaching could be done. The instruction in the clinical years had to have the same intensive university character as that in the fundamental branches, and men whose main interests were in competitive practice could not give it. The real introduction to medicine and surgery should be given to students by men whose primary occupation was teaching and research. "You cannot find ten such men in active practice in the whole city of Chicago. The full-time teacher is an absolute necessity."[86]

Therefore, Lyon advised, James should either build or lease a hospital and put it in charge of full-time teachers. Such hospital need not be very large. One hundred beds would be a fair number with which to begin. How would such a hospital be supported? The essential control must be with the university, but from educational funds proper need only come that amount essential to carry on teaching as distinguished from ordinary hospital activities. Another possibility was a division between state and county or between university and county. "You must have clinical teaching of university character," Lyon concluded. "You cannot get it under men whose primary interests are in medical practice. You cannot get it in hospitals whose organization and activities you do not fully control."[87]

James also asked the staff of the junior college to examine the AMA council's standards and report to him such suggestions as would enable him to put the medical school on a plane superior in every respect to the scheme proposed by the council. The faculty did a thorough job, and on 1 March 1915 Dean Dreyer submitted their report. The first of the ten items used by the council to rate schools was the showing of graduates before state boards and other evidences of the training received. Drawing on "State Board Statistics for 1913" published in *JAMA* in May 1914, the report showed that the percentage of failures for University of Illinois College of Medicine graduates in various years examined compared very favorably with the graduates of A Plus schools.[88] As for appointments to hospitals, Illinois placed as high a percentage of interns as did the A Plus schools.

The second item used to rate schools dealt with enforcement of a satisfactory educational requirement, granting of advanced standing, and the character of records. In allowing conditions on matriculation, Illinois was below the standard of the council, but remedial action had been taken. The third item, the curriculum, had been dealt with the previous year, and no further action was required. As for item four, the physical plant, the faculty's report said that Illinois was below the average of the A Plus colleges. On item five, laboratory facilities, the junior faculty believed that these were fair but not up to average and that the character of instruction was good but admittedly in need of further improvement. As for item six, dispensary facilities and instruction, all the A Plus schools had dispensaries either in a teaching hospital owned by the school or in private institutions having a number of teaching beds controlled by the school. Every criticism and improvement suggested by the report on these matters would be taken care of if the dispensary of the university was part of its teaching hospital.

As for item seven, hospital facilities and instruction, maternity work, autopsies, and specialties, Illinois was inferior in many respects to the council's standard, which was that a medical college should own or entirely control a hospital so that students could come into extended contact with patients under supervision of the attending staff. The hospital should be in close proximity to the college and have a daily average of not less than two hundred patients. Illinois met the council's standard in maternity work fairly well, but Illinois would not have a sufficient number of autopsies until the university had its own hospital. As for item eight, the size and quality of the faculty, Illinois was not as well situated as some of the A Plus schools. As for item nine, the College of Medicine was conducted for teaching the science of medicine rather than for the profit of the faculty.

As for item ten, the Quine Library of the University of Illinois College of Medicine more than met the standard set by the council. It was one of the largest medical school libraries in America. In the size of the collection, it would rank ninth among the A Plus medical school libraries. The library was housed in three large rooms on the second floor of the main medical building where it was convenient for both students and faculty, and the collections in the College of Medicine museum practically met the essentials of an acceptable medical college museum.[89]

James was resolutely determined to earn an A Plus rating for the College of Medicine, and he had assembled the best advice available as to how to proceed. But the road ahead was strewn with obstacles. The reform of medical education at the University of Illinois was a work in progress.

A number of developments unrelated to reorganization occurred, and a sampling of them reveals the complexity of affairs in the College of Medicine and the relation of the college to the university. Early in 1912 Carl Beck, a surgeon on the P&S faculty, visited the clinics of prominent surgeons in Europe, including those of Budapest, Vienna, Prague, Berlin, Leipzig, Jena, Munich, Strasbourg, Paris, and Brussels. In Jena Beck spent some time with Ernest Haeckel, author of *The Riddle of the Universe*, a pseudo-scientific work popular at the time. Beck compared Haeckel, whom he called a "giant among scientists," with Darwin and Huxley.[90]

Based on his visit, Beck wrote that American surgery was "not only recognized, but admired abroad." Beck's European conferees "conceded that the art of surgery had advanced to a high degree in the new country." American surgery, recognized European surgeons declared, "was in some respects ahead of Europe." The "tide of attraction was beginning to turn toward the west." When American surgeons became aware of their valuation abroad, Beck reported, they began to realize that it was not necessary for students to go abroad because they could learn everything in their postgraduate schools at home. Beck's comparison of European and American surgery underscores the theme of the present book.[91]

In the summer of 1913, however, Beck failed to secure a surgical appoint-ment in the County Hospital, where he had been holding a clinic for students of the medical school. Thus he would be without clinical material. Dean Steele thought it in the best interest of the college to retain on the faculty Carl's brother Joseph Beck, who had a County Hospital clinic in laryngology, rhinology, and otology with an abundance of material. But in view of the university's antine-potism policy that only one member of a family could serve on the faculty at a time, Joseph wished to give Carl preference in holding a chair in the department of surgery.[92]

Channing W. Barrett of the Department of Gynecology protested against the merging of gynecology with obstetrics under the leadership of Charles S. Bacon because he could not serve under Bacon.[93] Charles S. Williamson observed that pediatrics was the one department in the dispensary that had made no advance. The men there had shown themselves utterly lacking in reliability and teamwork and had done their work in a halfhearted fashion.[94]

In 1913 Dimiter G. Fournadjieff, a junior with an unusual background, won the Rea scholarship at the beginning of the academic year. James asked him for some biographical information, whereupon Fournadjieff related that he was born in 1881 in Samokav, Bulgaria, into a very poor family. His mother was illiterate, and his father was just barely able to read and write. The boy spent his time on the streets and in the woods. After his father became a Protestant, Fournadjieff came under the influence of Congregational missionaries sent out by the American Board of Commissioners for Foreign Missions. He attended their school, worked in their printing office, studied theology in their theologi-cal institute, taught in their mission school, and did some preaching. Studying the lives of medical missionaries, he desired to become one. He prayed over his plan for two years before departing for the United States. For two years he worked as a nurse in the New York Post-Graduate Hospital and for a year at the Battle Creek Sanitarium in Battle Creek, Michigan, where he also studied Latin and took a course in theoretical and practical massage, hydrotherapy, and electrotherapy. In 1911 after a year earning money as a nurse, he entered the freshman class at P&S.[95]

Fournadjieff was appalled at the deplorable practices he had witnessed in the school during his three years as a medical student, and after some doubt about whether to write, he concluded that it was his duty to inform James of the mis-deeds he had observed so that James could correct them. In the autumn of 1914 Fournadjieff wrote from the perspectives of a student, teacher, and churchman.

His main concerns were dishonesty and cheating. Dishonesty was rife because few instructors kept records of attendance at lectures, quizzes, laboratories, and clinics. They turned their roll books over to student assistants, who marked as present those who came late, left early, or did not even appear. Cheating was commonplace in quizzes and examinations. Many students had their books or notebooks open in quiz classes or during examinations. Instructors were blind to cribbing and on occasion supplied the answer to questions. Malefactors often won over students in charge of roll books, quizzes, and exams with a box of cigars.

According to Fournadjieff, the conditions described arose because the college depended largely on tuition to operate and had not dared to eliminate undesirable students, on professors who were paid little or nothing and had not devoted themselves to their work, on quiz masters and professors who were incapable and pandered to students for popularity, and on quiz masters and instructors who were themselves products of the system.

Fournadjieff's complaints were rooted in his moral vision. If men and women obtained their degrees by deceit and cheating, he declared, could you expect good of them after they have graduated? No! At least 70 percent of them would "sooner or later enter into the ranks of malpractitioners, abortionists, quacks, and the medical sharlatans [sic] of tomorrow." The pity of it was that quite a few young medical students, coming from Christian homes, were gradually "spoiled" by the practices they witnessed.[96]

Knowing that James was eager to reform the College of Medicine, Fournadjieff suggested seven steps that James should take to achieve this goal. Most of them were directed to correcting the evils he had registered. For example, no student should be allowed to handle the roll books or call the roll, and every professor should closely monitor classes during examinations. Perhaps the most important of the recommended measures was periodical inspection of the conduct of instruction by men sent by James who were not known to faculty or students and who would report their findings to James.[97]

James would have known that Fournadjieff's description of "rotten and shameful evils" was well intended and largely accurate. But he was a wily administrator and did not let himself get identified with the situation. He replied that he was obliged to Fournadjieff for his letter, which James had read with much interest. "You have had the good fortune to have had an interesting experience preparatory to your life work," he added. "I trust that everything will turn out to your wishes and that you will do the large service that you evidently anticipate."[98]

While the College of Medicine dealt with most student infractions internally, the imposition of severe penalties was a university matter.[99] In March 1914, for example, George P. Dreyer, on behalf of the Junior Faculty, recommended that two members of the sophomore class be dismissed for the remainder of the semester for dishonesty in class work and repeated misconduct in class. Thomas A. Clark, dean of men in the university at Urbana, endorsed the recommendation, whereupon the Council of Administration, which consisted of the president of the university and the deans on the Urbana campus, approved it.[100]

In June 1914 the Junior Faculty recommended that Rudolph A. Gries, a freshman, be suspended for the first semester of the following academic year for dishonesty in an exam. Clark approved of the recommendation provided that Gries had received a hearing before the Junior Faculty or a committee of the faculty. The Council of Administration then approved of the suspension. Gries apparently appealed to President James, who often involved himself in serious student misconduct. James took an interest in the case. Thus the Junior Faculty reconsidered the matter but refused to alter its original judgment.[101]

In June 1914 the Junior Faculty, after due investigation with hearings, found that Robert N. Arthurton, a student from Chicago in his third year who was on probation because of a previous case of dishonesty, had been guilty of purloining thirteen drawings from the laboratory notebooks of another student and handing them in as his own work. The faculty recommended that Arthurton, a native of the West Indies and a graduate of Fisk University, be expelled from the university. Clark concurred, after which the Council of Administration dismissed Arthurton from the university permanently.[102]

Eager to continue his medical education, Arthurton appealed to President James and sent Dreyer a letter with his interpretation of events. James requested that the Committee of the Junior Faculty reconsider the case and see if there was anything in Arthurton's statement that would alter the committee's opinion. The committee gave the matter a considerate hearing but refused to change their decision.[103]

James asked Steele to give Arthurton some consideration, and Arthurton wrote to Steele "in the spirit of submission." The Junior Faculty had refused to reconsider his case, Arthurton said, and Dreyer and Steele had advised him to try to enter some inferior-grade medical school, of which there were many in Chicago. Arthurton had gone over to the Chicago College of Medicine and Surgery (Valparaiso), where he was turned down on account of color. In any case, he desired to return to Illinois because it offered advantages "far in excess of most schools for colored students," and he was trying to get the best medical education for the people among whom he expected "to do missionary service." "Will you lighten my penalty, please? No other school will have me with such a record against me." He stated that he had spent years in the study of medicine "preparing for useful service among a people who are belittled and mistreated because God made them dark" and that "because of one supposed wrong" he had been punished with "too drastic a penalty." "Punish me," he pleaded, "but not with expulsion. Give me a chance . . . to go elsewhere . . . [or] let me come and redeem myself under your roof." He begged on behalf of himself, his parents, and "those millions of ignorant and uncared for Africans for whom few, white, or black, are willing to make any sacarifice [sic]."[104]

After receiving this "very appealing letter," Steele asked about the legality of the recommendation of the Junior Faculty to the Council of Administration. "I have no desire to champion the cause of a weak or dishonest student," Steele wrote, "unless his severe punishment has been brought about in an irregular manner." So, Steele inquired, would not the proper course have been for the Junior Faculty to lay the facts before the Senior Faculty, with a recommendation to the Senior Faculty, and let the recommendation of the Senior Faculty go to the Council of Administration? Was the action of the Council of Administration final, or could it be reconsidered "upon a new presentation of facts and in view of Arthurton's pitiful appeal for an amelioration of the sentence of expulsion so that he might be permitted to go to some other Medical school and finish his education or must he remain black-listed and blasted for life?"[105]

James thought that the Senior Faculty should have had some voice in the matter, and he vowed to look into the situation. "We ought to do everything we can to help our students," he assured Steele. "Mr. Arthurton seems, however, to have put himself in rather a bad position."[106] After hearing from Dreyer, James concluded that there was little evidence that Arthurton's case should be reopened, and after looking over Arthurton's correspondence, Steele also concluded that there was no reason to reopen the case.[107]

Arthurton obtained a medical degree from one of the night schools in Chicago. In 1916 he relocated to Los Angeles, but the California medical board did not reciprocate with the Illinois medical board, so Arthurton was forced to accept a position as a prescription clerk and "soda-water jerker" in a local drugstore. His marriage to the daughter of a wealthy Los Angeles real estate dealer on 30 January 1918, reported in the *Chicago Defender,* portrayed Arthurton in a bad light.[108]

CHAPTER 11

The Continued Quest for Excellence

While striving to reorganize the medical school and to secure a legislative appropriation for it, James resumed his efforts to consolidate the medical colleges in the city. His endeavors to do so intensified over time. When he arrived in Urbana, he had been given an opportunity to absorb a homeopathic school. Shortly before he assumed the presidency, Harvey Medical College and Hahnemann Medical College, homeopathic schools in Chicago, had requested affiliation with the university. Harvey conducted evening classes only and had a small enrollment. In June 1904 the board of trustees declined Harvey's proposal, explaining that the university's contract with the College of Physicians and Surgeons (P&S) precluded such a tie and that P&S was accomplishing all that the university might well do in the "regular or old school field of medicine."[1]

Andrew S. Draper, who left Urbana in April to take a job in New York but was still officially president of the university at the time, favored the affiliation of Hahnemann with the university. Quine strongly objected, and the board of directors endorsed his opposition.[2]

On 1 June 1904 George F. Shears, president of Hahnemann Medical College, a day school with a large attendance, formally applied for affiliation. He offered to give the university all of Hahnemann's property as a perpetual trust in return for which the college would become part of the medical school and its students would receive degrees from the university. Shears provided statistics purporting to show that enrollment in P&S had declined in recent years, whereas enrollment at Hahnemann Medical College had increased.[3]

The board of trustees desired to accept the offer, but Steele, Quine, and Pusey all insisted that the university honor its contract with P&S. The contract contained a provision that opposed the affiliation of the university with any other medical college in Chicago during the life of the lease, but it did not prohibit the introduction into the curriculum of any branch of study or method of instruction not included when the contract was signed.[4] The board sought legal advice from George W. Gere, a Champaign attorney, who advised that the university

might engage in the teaching of any branch of medical science taught in Hahnemann Medical College, and if Hahnemann became part of the university, P&S
could not by reason thereof terminate its contract with the university.[5]

James discussed these matters with the P&S faculty and sought to educate
himself on the issues by asking Charles S. Bacon of the medical faculty for
help. Homeopathic medicine was at the time popular among many upper-class
Americans, and while waiting for Bacon to report, James heard from some
prominent Chicagoans who favored this mode of healing. In mid-November
1904 L. F. Swift, president of Swift and Co., a stockyards and meat packing business, wrote James to express the familiar argument that homeopaths were justly
entitled to receive from the state the same educational encouragement offered to
the other school of medicine. In December 1904 and again in early 1905 Harlow
N. Higinbotham, a prominent Chicago businessman, informed James that he
and the Hahnemann trustees were in earnest about affiliation. The Hahnemann
trustees believed that they had rights with the State of Illinois, which should
arrange for the best and highest education of its future physicians and surgeons
in both schools of medicine. "Hahnemann [Medical College] now more than
ever represents the Homeopathic school in its best and largest sense," Higinbotham wrote, "and the sooner it is taken over by the state the better it will be
for all concerned." Edward F. Swift, chairman of Swift and Co., asked James for
information as to the advantages of an affiliation between the university and
Hahnemann Medical College.[6]

On 30 December 1904 Bacon informed James that Chicago had always had an
unusually large number of homeopathic physicians and that the homeopathic
schools of Chicago had graduated a considerable proportion of the homeopathic physicians of the country. Lately, however, the number of students in
homeopathic medical schools had markedly decreased. In 1903–4 the total attendance of all Chicago medical schools was 4,150, of which 3,358 (more than 82
percent) were regular, 345 (more than 8 percent) were homeopathic, 377 (more
than 9 percent) were eclectic, and 70 (less than 2 percent) were physio-medics.
Thus, Bacon concluded, the claims of the homeopaths for recognition were not
supported by their present numbers or prospects. James took no action on the
Hahnemann offer at this time.[7]

A decade later, however, the Chicago homeopathic community revived their
bid to join forces with the University of Illinois. Among the Chicagoans identified with homeopathy at the time were Harlow N. Higinbotham; Edward F.
Swift; William Wrigley Jr., the chewing gum magnate; Victor Lawson, a newspaper publisher; and Howard R. Chislett, president of Hahnemann College. In
1913 Higinbotham, the president of Hahnemann Hospital, asked James if he
would meet with Chislett about consolidation with the University of Illinois.
Steele, Quine, and other members of P&S, Higinbotham added, were not opposed to such a move.[8]

In 1916 Chislett sent James a plan for cooperation between Hahnemann Medical College and the University of Illinois. One part of the plan involved a six-year program for medical students. Chislett proposed that the university matriculate students with proper credentials sent by Hahnemann for a six-year combined course. The students would take two premedical years at the university, at the end of which the university would grant a BS, and four years at Hahnemann Hospital College, at the end of which Hahnemann would grant a medical degree. Chislett also proposed that the university make Hahnemann one of its departments of clinical medicine.[9] James appears to have considered the plan, but he concluded that the arrangements proposed were not feasible until the university had succeeded in putting its own work in first-class condition and on a perfectly sound basis.[10]

A Great Center of Medical Research and Education

Apart from Hahnemann, James was most eager to combine the clinical work of the university's College of Medicine with that of either Northwestern or Rush or of both. The presidents of those institutions—James, Harris, and Judson—had previously discussed a cooperative effort along this line. Now, in the autumn of 1913, word circulated that the University of Illinois would like to buy the Northwestern medical school. James and Harris agreed that this should not and would not happen, but there was, Harris suggested, "opportunity for the State University to take the lead and to inaugurate a new policy that may be novel and of great consequence." James agreed. It was "decidedly worth while," he believed, "to reorganize our resources for medical education and research in the city of Chicago in such a way as to produce the maximum of result with the minimum of expense."[11]

In 1914 consolidation of the medical colleges in the city of Chicago took a new turn when E. Fletcher Ingals of Rush Medical College offered James a plan of union. The University of Illinois should conduct the first two years of medical work in Chicago, Ingals proposed, provided that the university not take up the clinical work of the last two years and that the students of the first two years be kept by themselves. The medical plant that the university had already secured would be satisfactory for the purpose. Ingals envisioned a future when the University of Illinois would be doing the greater part of the fundamental medical teaching for all of the medical schools in the city. This plan, said Ingals, would combine all of the best medical schools in the state in favor of the University of Illinois, and the professional influence thus obtained would be a great benefit to the university in its other lines of work. Ingals would leave all of the work of clinical education to Rush.

Ingals closed with comments that James might have viewed as thinly veiled threats. Someone in the legislature might object to the amount that the university would pay to the other colleges under his plan, claiming that it was not really university work. But such an objection was not as likely as an objection to an appropriation for a single college if the medical teachers of the best schools were not harmonious in their action. "A considerable number of men in the other schools would feel piqued if Rush were to be taken over," Ingals opined, "and as they met members of the Legislature [they] would take an opportunity for criticism that might prove very detrimental to the University." If an obstacle like that should arise in the legislature, it could be overcome by the university appointing "all the members of the various *recognized faculties* as Professorial Lecturers in the University of Illinois without salary."[12]

Many of the points Ingals made were full of force, James replied, and he would carefully consider them. The difficulties Ingals mentioned were more serious than some of their friends realized. It would be wise to meet them by some rather different administrative arrangement. But the present opportunity would not come again for a generation, and James thought that they ought to work together to bring about the best scheme possible. "You are in a position to exercise a great influence in this matter, as I know that your colleagues set great store by your judgment."[13]

James informed the board of the informal inquiries he had received from Ingals with respect to the university's attitude toward a possible union with Rush, and the board authorized him to negotiate the terms of such consolidation with Rush.[14]

Ingals followed by sending James a condensed form of the suggestions he had made. The document provided that the university should conduct either at Urbana or Chicago the first two years, or laboratory years, of the medical course and should not directly engage in the instruction of the clinical years, leaving that to the affiliated medical schools and providing as liberally as possible for paying the cost of such instruction pro rata according to the number of graduates from each of these schools. James continued this game of cat and mouse by saying that Ingals's suggestions had some good features but that the practical difficulties in carrying them out would be very great.[15]

At the time, as Ingals knew, Rush was vulnerable. A joint committee of the boards of the University of Chicago and Rush Medical College was engaged in an effort to obtain funds for the establishment of clinical teaching on a solid basis in the two institutions. Some faculty members in the basic medical sciences on the South Side campus of the University of Chicago favored continuing relations with Rush on the grounds that Rush was a going concern with a tradition and assets. Others opposed the union. In addition to noting the inefficiency of geographically dividing the laboratory and clinical instruction between two locations, they emphasized the basic differences between the two schools. Rush was a high-grade technical school, the opponents contended, whereas the University of Chicago was a group of science departments devoted to research. A union would accentuate the differences between the two and increase the friction that existed ever since affiliation had begun years earlier.[16]

James viewed Rush as vulnerable because of its worsening financial situation. The college depended on tuition income, and as admissions requirements increased, enrollment decreased. At the time of affiliation, the Rush faculty and trustees had insisted that the college debt of $71,000 be erased. A number of faculty members had put up the money for this purpose.[17] The budget for the year 1899–1900 was favorable, prompting Ingals to assure Harper that the Rush past gave promise as to its future. A year later, however, Ingals estimated a deficit of $19,424 for the following year, and he feared that some at Rush might wish to connect with the University of Illinois.[18]

Conditions at Rush continued to deteriorate. By 1903 the number of students had decreased from 1,100 in 1898 to 750, necessitating rigid economy. In 1906 the deficit for the fiscal year was $13,635, and a year later a deficit was avoided by not paying teachers in the clinical departments with the rank of assistant professor and above, with two exceptions, and by faculty donations. For two successive years Frank Billings had secured donations of $10,000 from friends. In 1908 Ingals thought that it might be necessary to borrow to clear up a deficit of $7,000.[19]

In addition, faculty dissension weakened Rush. Some of the older faculty members were smug in resisting change. They opposed a proposal to confer with the principal medical schools in the city about medical education, convinced that Rush led the way and others could follow or not, as they chose.[20] Some faculty members, inspired by Arthur Bevan and Frank Billings, sought ways to improve Rush and the quality of medical education. As early as 1904 Bevan was losing interest in the college. The feeling of dissatisfaction was growing among members of the faculty, Ingals observed, and he saw no way of avoiding it.[21] Both Bevan and Billings complained about John Dodson, the dean of students. Billings not only wanted Dodson's salary cut but also thought that Rush should pay Dodson three thousand dollars to stay away. Most of the faculty disagreed, said Ingals, arguing that Dodson was a bulwark in favor of maintaining standards.[22] The Rush faculty had been disgruntled for the past few years, Steele told James in 1915, and they were looking for a new alliance.[23]

Knowing that Rush was vulnerable, at lunch on 15 October 1913 James told Bevan and Billings that Rush should be handed over to the University of Illinois. Later that day James made the same point to Ludvig Hektoen of Rush, and on 1 November James saw John B. Murphy, then at Northwestern, about turning over the Northwestern University medical school to the University of Illinois. Recording the encounter, James confided to his diary, "Murphy talked hot air."[24]

In November 1913, reminding President Judson of the University of Chicago of their previous discussions about reorganization of the clinical years in the various schools of Chicago, James reported that others had suggested to him that a union might be brought about between the Northwestern University medical school and the College of Medicine of the University of Illinois. Furthermore, if the University of Chicago organized an entirely different kind of medical school from anything then in existence in Chicago, it would no longer have any use for Rush Medical College, and in that case Rush might be consolidated with the University of Illinois medical school. James observed that he would not confer with others about consolidation without Judson's approval and that a consolidation of Rush with the College of Medicine of the University of Illinois, and possibly with absorption of Northwestern University Medical School, would result in a second medical school of high rank in the city. These two schools, one supplementing the other, "would be able to make Chicago one of the great historic centers of medical education and research."[25]

Judson said that the Rush authorities were free to take up the question that James suggested if they wished.[26] James replied that he would be greatly pleased if he, Judson, and Harris could, "in our day and generation, get the credit of organizing the medical education in the city of Chicago upon a basis which would challenge comparison with the best which the world has thus far achieved in the history of medicine."[27]

Knowing that the University of Chicago might sever its tie with Rush, James told Frank Billings, dean of the Rush Medical College faculty, that he wished to recommend him as dean of the University of Illinois College of Medicine. "I believe," James wrote, "that you are the only man who can, within a comparatively brief period, organize the work of clinical teaching in Chicago in such a way as to put it on a par with the best work done in any other center in the world." And Billings would be able to do this from the vantage point of dean of the state university medical school more quickly and completely than from any other location. James wanted this offer kept confidential for the present. Billings replied that he could not consider any proposition to leave Rush.[28]

In his bid to absorb Rush, James collaborated closely with Bevan and Billings. According to Bevan, "the strongest possible thing that could be done for medical education in the west would be the taking over by the University of Illinois of Rush Medical College as their last two years of medicine, provided it can be kept entirely out of political control." Bevan believed that he and James could convert Billings to their position. "I am enthusiastic about the possibilities," he assured James, "and believe that we can control the situation if the facts are properly presented to the men most interested." James was delighted to learn that there was some chance of adopting "the larger plan." With proper reorganization, James assured Billings, they might build up a great center of medical teaching and research on the West Side.[29]

Early in January 1914 James discussed the absorption of Rush with Bevan, Pusey of P&S, and Hektoen of Rush and in mid-February took up the topic

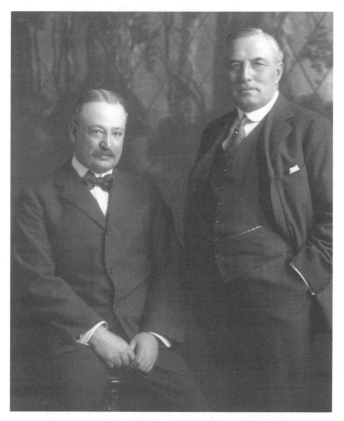

Arthur Bevan and Frank Billings. Courtesy of the Rush
University Medical Center Archives.

again with Bevan. James was indefatigable in his quest.[30] Bevan was no less vigorous in advancing the cause. He invited nine influential Rush men to dinner,
and they expressed a desire to talk over matters with James. Punctilious, James
asked Judson if it would be proper for him to proceed. Judson replied that a
considerable part of the fund to make Rush an integral part of the University of
Chicago had been raised, but if the Rush trustees desired to make another arrangement, the University of Chicago would not object.[31]

Meanwhile, Bevan had several conferences in New York and in Chicago with
Pritchett of the Carnegie Foundation. Bevan kept James informed of their talks.
According to Bevan, Pritchett had "about made arrangements to merge all the
strong medical men and institutions including the medical department of Le-
land Stanford University into one medical school to be made the department
of medicine of the University of California." This news was relevant to the local
medical situation, which Bevan had talked over further with leading lights at
Rush. He was "thoroughly convinced that we have the material at hand out of

which we can build a great medical school if it is properly utilized.... If our men could be convinced that the appointments to the medical school could be protected against political influence, I think they would be almost unanimously in favor of such a combination."[32]

Bevan sent James copies of the Rush charter, contracts, and related documents. After going over the contracts with the university's counsel, James concluded that everything could be easily handled as far as the formalities were concerned. The decision turned on whether Bevan and his colleagues were willing to seize the great opportunity. More enthusiastic than ever, James "cast all hesitation to the winds."[33]

James was probably the author of "Union between Rush Medical College and the University of Illinois." The document outlined a merger by lease of Rush for five years. Rush would be taken over by the University of Illinois in toto, which offered an opportunity to eliminate dead wood. The lease was to be made permanent if the state would develop and support the medical school. The parties to the agreement were to contract to secure four hundred thousand dollars to build a modern medical school.[34]

If the influential Rush men agreed practically unanimously on how to proceed, Bevan informed James in mid-February, they would take up the matter with the Rush trustees and then with the University of Chicago people. If the combination could be made in the right way, "it will be the best thing that can be done for medical education in this country."[35]

The collaborators tirelessly pushed forward. On 2 March Bevan called on James. Later, at dinner, James talked over the consolidation of Rush and Illinois with seven prominent members of the Rush Medical College faculty. Bevan submitted a proposed plan. On 8 March James had a two-hour interview with Hektoen "in re consolidation of Rush Medical College with the U of I." James relied on Hektoen to get Gideon Wells, dean of medical studies at the University of Chicago, into shape.[36]

These developments alarmed Ingals, the comptroller of Rush, who registered his concern to the secretary of the Board of Trustees of the University of Chicago on 4 March. Ingals wrote that

A cabal of the faculty is endeavoring to break up the affiliation of Rush Medical College with the University of Chicago and have the College taken over as the Medical Department of the University of Illinois, hoping thereby to obtain the financial assistance which we sadly need, but also, as I am informed, to make a big College with large classes which would be a misfortune.

If the University of Chicago had definitely decided that it did not want Rush Medical College as its Medical Department, it would be a good move to get into the University of Illinois, but under present conditions, the activities of the cabal appear to be untimely and unwise; and I assure you that they do not represent the judgement or desires of those who did most of the work in effecting the affiliation of the University of Chicago; or of most of those who have borne the brunt of raising the College to its present high state of efficiency in scientific work. The movement appears to be mischievous in high degree, but I do not think it can do any harm if it is not encouraged by the Trustees of the College.[37]

Ingals sent the same letter to each member of the board of trustees.

Despite Ingals, the quest for consolidation proceeded. On 17 March James saw Wells about the union of Rush and Illinois.[38] In early April Bevan and Billings presented matters at a meeting of the Rush faculty. According to Bevan, 80–90 percent of the faculty were very much in favor of Rush making a combination with the University of Illinois, "provided that the nominations to the medical department can be safe-guarded by contract in the lease for a period of at least ten years against political influence." If this could be done, Bevan informed James, the faculty would almost unanimously ask the trustees of Rush to proceed with a merger. Bevan, having met with President Abram Harris and the trustee James Patten of Northwestern University, reported that they were "willing and desirous to enter into a cooperative scheme for medical education in Chicago. We are developing a very simple and practical plan that will enable the medical departments of the University of Chicago, the University of Illinois, including Rush College if the combination is made, and Northwestern University to form separate and independent units in a big co-operative scheme."[39]

On 17 April James dined with the Council of Rush Medical College—Arthur D. Bevan, Frank Billings, John M. Dodson, Ludvig Hektoen, E. Fletcher Ingals, Oliver S. Ormsby, J. Clarence Webster, H. Gideon Wells, and William H. Wilder—at the University Club. Days later James had a long interview with Billings on consolidation with Rush. "He told me much interesting history as to Rush Medical College," James recorded. We can only speculate as to what Billings related.[40]

James was making headway. On 22 April he reported to his board that he had received informal inquiries with respect to the university's attitude toward a possible union with Rush Medical College, whereupon the trustees unanimously resolved that they looked with favor on the consolidation of Rush with the College of Medicine of the University of Illinois, "provided suitable conditions for such consolidation can be secured." The board appointed a committee to negotiate the terms of such consolidation.[41]

James immediately informed Bevan and Billings of the board's action and noted some imperatives. Do not try to make a combination with any strings attached. The board would not bind itself in any way in the matter of faculty appointments. When faculty appointments expired at the close of the academic year (31 August), it would be necessary for faculty members to resign. The university's board would then select the ablest faculty from those of Rush, the College of Medicine of the University of Illinois, and other colleges.[42]

A few days later James discussed the Rush matter with four of his deans in Urbana. Having considered the proposal to take over Rush and to make the necessary financial arrangements in the budget, David Kinley (Graduate College), Eugene Davenport (College of Agriculture), C. R. Richards (College of Engineering), and K. C. Babcock (College of Liberal Arts and Sciences) advised James to proceed. "All agreed," said James, "we ought to go ahead with the arrangement and find the necessary money in the budget."[43]

Ingals had to face realities not to his liking, so he adjusted. But he offered ambiguous counsel. All the good medical schools in Chicago should be grouped under the University of Illinois, he suggested, with each retaining its autonomy. At the same time, said Ingals, a plan for securing harmonious operation of all good colleges as *the* medical school of the university ignored human nature and was visionary. Professors were unwilling to work together with other schools unless they themselves were paramount.[44]

The faculty of Rush Medical College met on 28 April to discuss consolidation. As reported by Ingals, Bevan presented his view that within ten years great things were to happen in medical education through the University of Illinois, and he urged the faculty "to get into the band wagon at once." No one else spoke for his side, but many spoke for the other side. The sentiment of the faculty appeared to be strongly against Bevan's proposals.[45] According to Bevan, Billings reported from the faculty council on the general proposition, and the general discussion doubted the advisability of making the union. Bevan moved to appoint the faculty council to take up with the trustees of Rush Medical College the matter of union with the University of Illinois. A motion to table this lost by a vote of about 30 to 40. Bevan's motion then carried by a unanimous vote.[46]

The union was most desirable, Bevan explained, and it could be brought about if those involved could gain a little time to formulate a generally satisfactory agreement. The strong men in the Rush faculty were much in favor of union. The opposition came largely from Ingals and Dodson and some of the men who were more interested in the future of the University of Chicago than in Rush College.[47] Bevan and James had compiled a list of Rush faculty members who should be retained on the staff of the University of Illinois College of Medicine if a consolidation took place. Those on the list were Frank Billings, James B. Herrick, Bertram W. Sippy, Arthur D. Bevan, J. Clarence Webster, William H. Wilder, Ludvig Hektoen, H. Gideon Wells, Oliver S. Ormsby, and John B. Dodson. Bevan also suggested the names of men who should go over into various departments of the new college of medicine. Everyone on the prime list except Dodson was included, and also on the list were Edward C. Rosenow, Dean D. Lewis, and George E. Shambaugh.[48]

Bevan and Billings had recently met with President Abram Harris and James Patten, representing Northwestern University. Harris and Patten, Bevan reported, had obtained a million dollars from one of the Deerings, and they had about the same amount in sight for medicine from another source. They were anxious to cooperate, Bevan told James, in any way that seemed to be to the advantage of medical education in Chicago. The conferees agreed to invite three men from each university—the president, a member of the board, and a faculty member—to a dinner within the next two weeks to discuss matters. Bevan would attend as chairman of the Council on Medical Education.[49]

By mid-May Bevan and Billings realized that consolidation was going to require more time to accomplish than at first hoped. A large majority of the faculty was in favor of consolidation, Bevan attested, while Billings reported that the Rush faculty was sharply divided on the desirability of consolidation with the University of Illinois. They agreed that consolidation should be temporarily postponed. It was desirable, Billings thought, to take more time to consider the matter so as to win over opponents and secure a practically unanimous agreement. According to Bevan, Billings's hold on the faculty and trustees was such that it would be difficult to bring about the consolidation without his enthusiastic support.[50] "I presume that this disposes of the proposition for the present year at any rate," James noted, "and possibly of course indefinitely."[51]

On 29 May 1914 James conferred again with Bevan about the consolidation of Rush and the university's medical school. In mid-July Hektoen told James that he was sorry that the proposed coalition had failed. "I am holding things steady," James replied, "so that proper consolidation can be brought about any time. Let me know when you think is the time for a new attempt."[52]

As these events unfolded, James met dissension in his own ranks. As he related, the trustee John R. Trevett had voted against the resolution to consolidate Rush Medical College and the university's medical department.[53] Trevett was well known for his hostility to President James, and James sent him a powerful argument in favor of the union. The board confronted a situation, James wrote, not a theory. Owing to historical circumstances, the university had a medical school located in Chicago. The only question before the trustees was whether they were to have a first-class medical school or a mediocre school. James had organized the junior work of the College of Medicine, but the clinical work was in a "very unstable equilibrium." Not owning or having control by contract with any hospital, the university was compelled to select its clinical staff from men who had relations with private or semipublic hospitals. Ideally, the university should have a state-supported teaching hospital, but the next best thing was to take over a group of men who had actual control of hospital facilities. Such an opportunity existed in immediate proximity to the university's medical school. Billings had assembled in Rush a group of young men in medicine and surgery, and Rush had a ninety-nine-year contract with Presbyterian Hospital, a hospital of three hundred beds, whose use for medical purposes would be secured under a contract between Rush and the university to the faculty of the university's medical department. Rush also had a contract with the Central Free Dispensary, located in its own building, that had some forty thousand cases a year, and it had contracts with several hospitals, notably a hospital of infectious diseases and the Home for Destitute Crippled Children. One could not create such a group of enterprises for medical research and education as was associated around and bound up with Rush Medical College, James thought, for less than $3.5 million or $4 million. If the consolidation with Rush could be effected, James opined, it would give to the University of Illinois "one of the great medical schools of the country at the very start." And once the consolidation was effected, it would be perfectly feasible to add a chair in homeopathic medicine and to cooperate in such a way that clinical courses in homeopathic medicine could be given in Hahnemann Hospital.[54]

The trustee John T. Montgomery, a medical doctor, writing to Trevett at James's request, emphasized the fact that since the university was entirely dependent on others for clinical teaching in hospitals, the opportunity to combine with Rush should not be overlooked. Knowing that Trevett wanted the first two years of medical work done in Urbana, Montgomery explained why it was neither expedient nor advisable to do so. The opportunity presented itself to make the university's medical school "the greatest medical school in this country."[55]

Trevett replied that he lacked sufficient information about the financial and legal aspects of the Rush-Presbyterian proposition to come to a conclusion on the matter. He had been told that it was understood in Springfield that none of the university's mill tax receipts were to be spent in Chicago except for the maintenance of P&S. He would be more comfortable, Trevett added, if he felt sure that the next legislature would endorse the action by the trustees. Trevett would not oppose the proposed union but feared the attitude that the legislature was likely to take in this matter.[56]

James thought that Rush would ask the university to set aside a sum of money to support the clinical work in the medical school as a condition of turning over their property and that the trustees would probably agree to this proposition. Rush had no interest in consolidation unless the university was to put all the work on a more solid and satisfactory foundation than in the past.[57]

Montgomery saw no objection to taking in Hahnemann on the same terms as Rush. Since all of the scientific courses would be the same, it would be necessary for the university to teach only homeopathic materia medica. Montgomery understood that Hahnemann had to teach homeopathic materia medica in order to retain a large donation received years earlier.[58] James agreed that there should be no difficulty in putting in a chair for homeopathic materia medica and therapeutics so long as there was no duplicating scientific instruction in some other center in Chicago than the medical school.[59]

Montgomery was disappointed but not surprised at this turn of events. While a large majority of the best men at Rush saw that it would be to the advantage of medical education to unite with Illinois to build up the best medical college in the West, many others thought that they might not have a sufficient place in the venture or did not want to take any chances. Thus the possibility of union was not likely to come up again that year.[60] It did not, although on 13 October 1914 James interviewed Bevan again "in re Rush Medical College."[61]

Meanwhile, a number of prominent Chicago medical men were eager to improve medical education in Illinois. Franklin H. Martin took the initiative in this group. An 1880 graduate of Chicago Medical College, he specialized in diseases of the female generative organs. In addition to a private practice, he was professor of gynecology at the Post-Graduate Medical School; a founder of the journal *Surgery, Gynecology, and Obstetrics* (1905); and the prime mover in establishing the American College of Surgeons (1913).[62]

In early February 1915 Albert J. Ochsner put Martin in touch with James, whereupon Martin and James met over dinner. Shortly thereafter the presidents of the four universities along with a faculty member from each of the four medical schools and Pritchett of the Carnegie Foundation met to discuss the practicability of effecting a working agreement that would promote cooperation between the undergraduate and graduate medical schools of Chicago. The conferees appointed a committee consisting of the president and two members of the faculty of each of the four universities and the president and two members of the contemplated Graduate School of Medicine of Chicago to formulate a plan of cooperation among the five units and present the same to each of the five organizations for consideration and adoption.[63]

James did not accept membership on the committee. After hearing from Martin, James and Judson agreed that the two of them and Harris of Northwestern should meet and reach a common understanding on the subject before the committee met.[64]

Frank Billings of Rush, the chairman of the committee, doubted that it would do much good. He informed Martin that he did not desire to serve with a certain John Dill Robertson, who had been named as a representative of Loyola University. "I do not know whether President Judson knows the man," Billings wrote, "but I am sure that when he learns of his character he would act as I have in demanding the removal of the gentleman from the committee."[65] As finally constituted, the fifteen members of the Universities Committee on Medical Education included three from each of the four universities and the Graduate School of Medicine. Robertson was not on the list.[66]

In April the committee of fifteen recommended joint action by Northwestern University, the University of Chicago, Loyola University, and the University of Illinois along several lines. First, beginning in 1915–16, a standard four-year high school course or its equivalent, plus two years of college work, including one

year's study of chemistry, physics, and biology, would be a minimum requirement for admission to the medical schools of the four universities, provided that
during 1915–16 Loyola might accept one instead of two years of college work.
Second, fix a uniform standard of a four-year medical curriculum. Third, require after 1920 one year as a hospital intern in the medical course for eligibility
as a candidate for a license to practice in Illinois. Fourth, the four universities
would try to secure legislation authorizing the State Board of Health to maintain
a standard of admittance to practice in Illinois in conformity with the standards
of the named universities. The University of Chicago and Rush understood that
the associated universities would make no effort to induce the state legislature to
appropriate any money for medical education other than that furnished to the
University of Illinois. Fifth, the University of Chicago and Rush Medical College agreed to unite with Northwestern, Loyola, and the University of Illinois to
form a joint committee to formulate plans and means for the establishment of
graduate teaching in Chicago. On 27 April James presented the resolutions to
the board of trustees.[67]

The impending possibility of joint action with private universities raised a
problem for a public university. Since James was ill, on 12 April Vice President
David Kinley had sought an opinion from the attorney general of Illinois as to
the legal rights and limitations of the university in connection with a proposed
agreement with the other universities. On 17 April Attorney General Patrick J.
Lucey declared that it was not within the power of the University of Illinois as
a state institution to make an agreement with the private institutions as to the
points under discussion. James informed Martin that the University of Illinois
was not permitted by law to enter into any such agreement and told Steele that he
did not want the university represented at the meetings of the Universities Committee. Ochsner was a member of the committee in his personal capacity.[68]

Curiously, James pursued the prospect of interinstitutional cooperation on
his own. On Sunday morning, 23 May, he met with four members of the Universities Committee—William A. Evans and Martin, representatives of the Graduate School of Medicine, and Steele and Ochsner of the College of Medicine—in
what James described as a "Committee Meeting on Cooperation of Medical
Schools."[69]

The Universities Committee envisioned a graduate school of medicine, and
despite the limitations put on the University of Illinois, members of the committee continued to press for fulfillment of that goal. On 11 August Judson suggested
that it would be well for the four universities that conducted medical work in
Chicago to investigate the possibility of conducting graduate teaching in Chicago
on the basis of what was done at Harvard. Judson had appointed a committee of
five to represent the University of Chicago in such an investigation. He suggested
that if James appointed such a committee, the combined committees could report so that the authorities might consider the possibility of joint action.[70]

In September Martin, Ochsner, and Murphy proposed to James the establishment of a Universities Graduate School of Medicine of Chicago under the control of the best men in the four universities. The object of the school was to conduct a college for medical instruction of graduates of medicine. The school was to have a board of governors, an executive committee, and officers. The school was to be financially independent of the universities. Details as to the faculty were to be worked out by a committee.[71]

James met once with Martin, Ochsner, and Murphy but declined to attend additional meetings, allegedly because the board had not authorized cooperation in this enterprise.[72] The organizers of the venture adumbrated their plans more fully in a "Plan of Agreement" designed to be presented to Pritchett of the Carnegie Foundation. The plan envisioned the four universities cooperating to establish and maintain a comprehensive graduate school in Chicago under control of the universities. It laid great stress on the four universities combining to discourage the medical schools of inferior standards and to make more efficient use of the clinical facilities in the city, especially those of Cook County Hospital. The plan argued that antagonistic factors had blocked medical progress in the city for thirty years. One such factor was the inability of any one of the universities acting independently to deal with the city, county, and state situation, the first two of which controlled the city Board of Health and the great public hospitals and the last of which controlled the state university and legislation governing medical practice in the state. A second difficulty was the bitter antagonism between the two or three schools of acceptable standards and the half dozen schools of indifferent standards. The former had urged the state to furnish a high standard for license to practice medicine, and the latter had succeeded in blocking such a program. A third difficulty was the antagonism that had developed between a group of men allied with the local affairs of the American Medical Association and their following on the one hand and a self-styled "insurgents party" on the other.[73] For many years the former group had controlled the state medical society and the Chicago Medical Society, but five years earlier the insurgents had gained control. Partisans on both sides were tired of the fruitless quarrel, and those who had endeavored to remain neutral were probably a majority.

The remedy was to establish a graduate school in which the faculty would consist of all members of the faculty of the four medical schools. An executive committee of each department would nominate from the three hundred practitioners in the city who held hospital positions but were not closely allied with a university medical school, and the board of governors would elect qualified individuals to the faculty, affording them an opportunity to use the available clinical facilities.[74]

James did not endorse the plan. There was no use in attempting to do anything with the scheme until Rush Medical College was willing to join with it,

said James, who thought that the plan of utilizing the clinical facilities of Chicago for graduate work of physicians was a very good one. But he saw no reason
why the universities should back that proposition. It could manage itself. He
was interested in advanced graduate work for persons qualified to take it by
reason of their previous degrees.[75]

Instead, James focused his attention on union with Rush. "Now was the accepted time," he told Billings on 27 November 1915, "for a consolidation of Rush
Medical College and the College of Medicine of the U. of I."[76]

Billings promised to see President Judson right away and then told Judson
that it seemed impossible to secure the million dollars deemed necessary to
consummate a union between the University of Chicago and Rush Medical College, and therefore Rush prevented the University of Chicago from going forward in the development of a complete medical department at the Midway (the
area in the South Side of Chicago where the University of Chicago was located).
The situation annoyed the teachers at the University of Chicago and at Rush. It
should be changed. The state university had a policy regarding the organization
and development of a medical department in Chicago, Billings added, and the
appropriation for medicine in the university budget was now sufficient to carry
on a well-directed institution for teaching medicine in a modern way.

Judson said that the University of Chicago hoped to secure enough money to
carry on work at Rush College, but the University of Chicago would not stand in
the way if Rush might do better than continue the affiliation with Chicago. Billings asked Judson if the Rush trustees would invite James to a conference so that
James could tell them what could be done. Judson said that it would be better if
James invited the Rush trustees to meet him, so Billings advised James to write to
J. J. Glessner, president of the Rush board, and invite a conference with the Rush
trustees. Billings advised James to make a plain, straightforward statement to the
effect that the state would be able to finance medical education with Rush as the
chief part of the clinical teaching for a time with a hopeful spirit for evolution
in clinical methods elsewhere in Chicago and that the fundamental branches of
medicine would be taught in Chicago in a thorough way. It would be necessary
for the Rush trustees to transfer the property of the school to the university.[77]

On 4 December James talked with Judson about the consolidation of Rush
Medical College with the University of Illinois Medical School. Judson said
that if the University of Chicago went out of medicine it would give up the first
two years also. Judson invited James to present the matter to the governing
board of Rush.[78]

James and Glessner agreed to meet, and Glessner invited any of the Illinois
trustees to join them. The conferees gathered on 17 December in the University
of Chicago rooms in the Corn Exchange National Bank.[79] During the meeting,
James emphasized that it would be necessary to turn over the property of Rush
Medical College to the state if the desired objects were to be secured. If the

union was to be made, it had to be made under circumstances that would enable the university to obtain the necessary funds for its adequate support. The state would appropriate money only for work carried out by state agencies. Moreover, it would be necessary for the university to have a free hand in making up a faculty. The trustees of the university would appoint the clinical faculty by selecting the best men who could be obtained.[80]

Billings persuaded the Rush board to appoint a committee to confer with James in reference to the proposed union. Glessner appointed three trustees and two faculty members (Bevan and Billings) to the committee, of which he was an ex officio member. Preparing for the conference, Billings asked James to make statements on the following points in reference to the University of Illinois: first, the amount of money appropriated for the medical school for the biennium beginning 1 July 1915 and whether there was an additional sum for the purchase of ground and erection of buildings; second, the procedures in the appointment of permanent teachers in both the fundamental years and the clinical years and the methods James would follow in appointing new faculty in the clinical departments; third, the preliminary requirements of students admitted to medicine, including a statement on the status of students then in the medical department of the university; fourth, a statement as to the erection of clinical buildings in Chicago should Rush be taken over by the University of Illinois; fifth, the action necessary by the Rush board in reference to the property of the school should Rush be taken over by the university; sixth, how James would deal with the resignation of faculty members in the clinical department and how he proposed to form a new clinical faculty; and seventh, how Presbyterian Hospital, the Home for Destitute Crippled Children, and other hospitals affiliated with Rush would be connected with the University of Illinois. Billings wanted these statements as early as possible. "We should strike while the iron is hot."[81]

James acted quickly. On 6 January he sent Billings a lengthy letter that answered all the questions Billings raised except the one pertaining to the method by which a transfer of property might be made. On that same day James discussed the method of transferring Rush Medical College to the university with Oliver A. Harker, the legal counsel of the university, and Edward H. Decker, a professor in the College of Law. James hoped to meet with the committee on 11 or 12 January before leaving for New York. Billings presented James's reply to the questions to the committee and tried to arrange the meeting.[82]

On 17 January while in New York, James discussed the medical situation in Chicago with Henry S. Pritchett of the Carnegie Foundation. He "told" Pritchett to put four or five million dollars into a modern medical plant in Chicago, and he would get the money from the legislature to run it.[83] At the time James was optimistic about his prospects.

Things suddenly changed. On 24 April when James went to see Billings "in re Rush," Billings was "very non-committal." (On that same day James discussed the possibility of union with Dr. Chislett of Hahnemann Medical College.)[84] The reason for Billings being reticent is readily explained. The idea of a medical center on the University of Chicago campus, which had lain dormant since the death of President Harper in 1906, was suddenly reactivated early in 1916 when President Judson sought advice from the officers of the Rockefeller-funded General Education Board on planning for a medical school with clinical teaching on the South Side campus. The officers of the board suggested that the board might contribute as much as one million dollars for the endowment of the school. At its meeting in May, the board formally authorized its officers to continue consultation with President Judson, who promptly laid before them a plan contemplating a medical school on the campus with a hospital and an endowment. The board recommended that Judson invite Abraham Flexner, an officer of the board, to examine and report on conditions at Chicago. Flexner accepted Judson's invitation and in July presented his report.

The Flexner Report of 1916 discussed three possible directions that the University of Chicago could take in the development of medical education. One was to maintain and improve its existing medical organization, teaching the basic biological sciences on the South Side and giving the clinical years at Rush. The result would be "two half schools," separated physically from each other. A second was to concentrate the entire four years of medical training at Rush on the West Side, with the necessary teaching and research facilities being built in proximity to Presbyterian Hospital. The medical school would then be physically separated from the university. A third possibility was to develop a medical school with its own hospital on the University of Chicago campus. This option was clearly the most expensive, requiring perhaps $2.5 million in endowment alone. But only in this way could the university create a medical program in harmony with the highest modern educational ideals.

Flexner recommended that the General Education Board and the Rockefeller Foundation support the third plan and that Rush be converted to a postgraduate school as a separate enterprise. Thus there would be on the West Side, near Presbyterian Hospital and the research institutions associated with Rush, a new kind of school to which physicians could return for periodic renewal and special training.

By the end of 1916 Flexner's proposal had been accepted in principle by the General Education Board, the Rockefeller Foundation, and the Board of Trustees of the University of Chicago. The university's board appointed the Committee on the Medical School, and a campaign was initiated to raise the $5.3 million required for buildings and endowment. The General Education Board and the Rockefeller Foundation each pledged $1 million to be used for endowment, and on 11 January 1917 Frank Billings informed Judson that four donors of the Billings family, including Frank Billings himself, desired together to pledge $1 million for the hospital. By May 1917 the needed funds for the hospital, laboratory, and endowment were slightly oversubscribed, and everything seemed ready. Then the outbreak of war put a sudden stop to the plans.[85]

James had to abandon the idea of a combination with Rush but continued his campaign to reform medical education. He struck out in new directions. On 5 September 1916 writing to William B. McKinley, an Urbana traction magnate who had made a fortune and had been in the U.S. House of Representatives since 1904, James said that when the board of trustees found themselves "free from medical complications in Chicago," he had strongly advised it "to get out of the city and develop the medical school here on the campus." James was aware that the weight of the medical profession was against such a policy, but members of the medical profession, he charged, gave very little attention to real educational problems. The development of some of the small medical schools in Germany and of the medical school of the University of Michigan showed that it was perfectly possible to develop centers of worldwide interest in towns smaller than Urbana-Champaign. "In these days of express trains, interurbans, automobiles, and flying machines, it makes very little difference where a really excellent institution is located: The whole world will take advantage of its facilities." If McKinley was thinking of doing something of this kind, James urged that he could find no better place than at the University of Illinois. "Society," he added, "has no more important function than the organization of the public health service on a scientific basis,— something which no country has yet really taken up in earnest, the United States being at the very tail end of the procession among civilized people."[86]

At the same time James did not completely give up the idea of using the university to make Chicago a world center of medical research and education. On 21 February 1917 James conferred with President Thomas F. Holgate of Northwestern University and J. Rawson Pennington, a professor at Northwestern, "in re Great Clinical School in Chicago by consolidation of existing schools."[87] The reference was presumably to a union of the medical schools of Northwestern, Rush, and the University of Illinois.

While pursuing these goals, James had to deal again with dissension in his own ranks. In March 1917 when the appropriations request was before the General Assembly, James learned that "certain citizens of Champaign & Urbana" had presented to the Board of Supervisors a request to apply for an injunction to prevent the legislature from appropriating money to any department of the university not located in Champaign County. The trustee John R. Trevett, a Champaign banker well known for his hostility to James, was no doubt the instigator of the action. Joining Trevett in seeking the injunction were Matthew W. Busey, an Urbana banker, and six other local businessmen and lawyers. It would be to the economic advantage of these men to invigorate the Course Preparatory to Medicine at Urbana rather than to build up the medical school in Chicago. The Champaign County Board of Supervisors denied their request.[88]

The College of Medicine Gains Strength

The College of Medicine took on new life after becoming part of the university. In 1913 the admissions requirement rose to one year of college in addition to completion of high school, and a year later two years of college plus a high school diploma were required to matriculate. In 1913 the number of matriculants fell from 125 the previous year to 61, and in 1914 the number declined from 61 to 12.[89] And since other medical schools raised their admissions requirements, few students transferred to the medical school in their junior year. Statistics on enrollment for the medical school from 1916–17 to 1919–20 are either spotty or not available, but we know that enrollment decreased further after the nation went to war. These developments are illustrated in Table 7.

In 1918–19 the 281 students included 50 in the fourth year, 88 in the third year, 73 in the second year, 54 in the first year, 2 special students, and 14 in graduate work. In 1919–20 the 268 students included 43 in the fourth year, 51 in the third year, 71 in the second year, 100 in the first year, and 3 in graduate work. The first-year enrollment was evidence of an upward swing.[90]

In its early years the medical school that became the University of Illinois College of Medicine made little contribution to research. Only a few faculty members were investigators, and funds were not available to support their studies. But medical work required investigation because in the study of a given disease a physician needed to be trained in observation, experimentation, and induction. And although most medical schools began as commercial enterprises, they became departments of universities, and research is a distinguishing attribute of a university. In November 1913 soon after the university took over the College of Medicine, a Medical Research Club was organized. Its object was the stimulation of scientific research. Members met once a month to discuss original scientific papers. The club was a stimulus to the production of an increasing number of scientific contributions.[91]

Table 7. Enrollment and number of graduates, 1912 to 1920

Year	Enrollment				Number of Freshmen	Number of Juniors	Graduates
	M	F	Total	% Female			
1912–13	516	35	551	6.3	157	114	130
1913–14	416	34	450	7.5	72	106	113
1914–15	266	24	290	8.2	12	111	102
1915–16	210	16	226	7.0	47	48	110
1916–17	204	11	215	5.1	NA	NA	49
1917–18	252	11	263	4.2	NA	NA	30
1918–19	264	17	281	6.0	NA	NA	49
1919–20	243	25	268	9.3	NA	NA	85

The university needed to make some provision whereby students could come in contact more intimately with research methods and ideals than they did in their regular studies. Thus in the spring of 1915 the Graduate School of the university organized courses in the College of Medicine leading to the degrees of master of science and doctor of philosophy. The work was organized so late in the year that no attempt was made at the time to induce students to take this work. Only two registered for the MS degree.

In December 1915 the Junior Faculty proposed to stimulate "investigation experience" in both the teaching staff and the student body. Since the curriculum involved students so fully during the academic year, this work had to be done in a summer session. Accordingly, the Junior Faculty wanted advice and recognition from the Graduate School, and it sought permission to organize a graduate summer quarter that would include a few courses in subjects currently under direction of the Junior Faculty.[92]

Thus the College of Medicine organized a graduate summer quarter with several objects in view. One was to give medical students who had received the BS at the end of the second year of the medical course an opportunity to pursue introductory research work for three consecutive summer quarters, thereby obtaining the MS degree at the end of the summer quarter following graduation with the MD. A second object was to induce teachers from other schools to do research work in the laboratories of the College of Medicine by providing them with equipment, libraries, artists, typists, and technicians. In the first year of the program faculty members from the universities of Nebraska, Harvard, Washington University, and Kansas worked in the departments of anatomy, physiological chemistry, and physiology.

The third object of the graduate program was to bring eminent scientists from various parts of the country to the College of Medicine to report on their research and to note the problems in their particular fields. In the first phase of the program nineteen speakers came to the College of Medicine to participate. The participants were from the University of Chicago–Rush; the universities of Mississippi, Illinois, Pittsburgh, Kansas, Nebraska, Indiana, Wisconsin, Minnesota, and Kentucky; Washington University in St. Louis; Western Reserve University; Northwestern University; St. Louis University; the Rockefeller Institute; and the Mayo Foundation. Among their topics were anatomy, bacteria, biological chemistry, chemistry, histology, medicine, nephritis, parasitology, pharmacology, physiology, physiology and pharmacology, salicylates, and surgery.[93]

While student attendance and the number of graduates both declined, at the same time the performance of graduates of the College of Medicine on the examinations given by the state licensing boards improved. The record is best understood comparatively. In 1913 state boards examined graduates of seven Chicago medical schools. The failure rate of four of the colleges ranged from a high of 20 percent (Jenner) to a low of 3.68 percent (Hahnemann). All 88 Rush graduates who took the examinations passed. Of the 55 Northwestern graduates examined, 54 passed (a failure rate of 1.8 percent). Of the 126 University of Illinois graduates examined, 123 passed (a failure rate of 2.4 percent).[94]

A year later the graduates of seven Chicago medical schools took the state board examinations. For four schools, the percentage of failures ranged from a high of 40 percent (Hahnemann) to a low of 13.8 percent (Bennett). For the three university-related schools, 74 of the 76 Rush graduates who took the examinations passed (a 2.6 percent failure rate), 63 of the 66 Northwestern graduates examined passed (a 4.5 percent failure rate), and 104 of the 113 University of Illinois graduates examined passed (an 8 percent failure rate).[95]

The results of the 1915 examinations were for the most part better. Graduates of eight medical schools were examined, including those of a newcomer, Chicago Hospital College of Medicine, five of whose eight graduates passed (a 37.5 percent failure rate). Three schools had no failures. At Jenner, all nineteen graduates passed; at Northwestern, all thirty-three passed; and at Rush, all eighty-six passed. At the University of Illinois, ninety-eight of ninety-nine graduates passed (a 1 percent failure rate).[96]

The following year graduates of eight Chicago medical colleges were examined. Both the Chicago Hospital College of Medicine and Jenner had a failure rate of 33.3 percent. Loyola Medical School had a failure rate of 21.5 percent (84 passed and 23 failed). The University of Illinois led with a failure rate of 0.9 percent (110 of 111 graduates passed). Northwestern followed with a failure rate of 4.7 percent (41 of 43 passed). Rush trailed its peers with a failure rate of 2.3 percent (84 of 86 passed). The board of trustees recorded the triumph of the University of Illinois College of Medicine in its official minutes.[97]

In 1916 the College of Medicine excelled in the civil service examinations for Cook County Hospital internships. The Illinois students stood first in percentage showings, with 18 out of 37 winning places (48.6 percent) compared to 19 out of 60 Rush students (31.6 percent) and 8 out of 30 Northwestern students (26.6 percent). The Illinois students took first, third, and seventh places, the best showing the college had ever had.[98]

In the 1917 state board examinations, 145 of 146 Rush graduates passed (0.7 percent failed), 40 of 41 Northwestern graduates passed (2.4 percent failed), and 62 of 64 graduates of the University of Illinois passed (3.1 percent failed).[99]

The statistical record was at best an approximation of the quality of each of the schools.[100] Nevertheless, statistics were one measure of achievement. They suggested that the University of Illinois College of Medicine, the youngest of the three university-related medical schools in Chicago and the one most handicapped by lack of resources and by political entanglements, had reached a point of approximate parity in academic performance with Northwestern and Rush.

One way to judge the impact of the College of Medicine on the United States and abroad is to identify the places in which its graduates engaged in practice. In

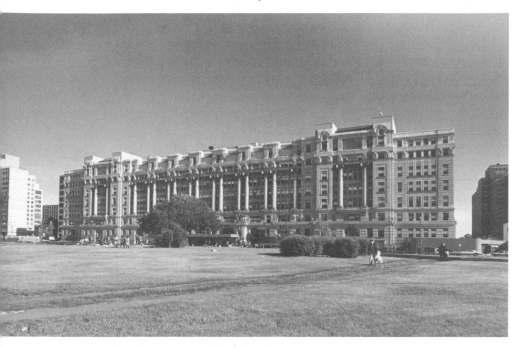

County Hospital (1916). Courtesy of the Chicago History Museum.

1910 a total of 131 individuals graduated from the medical school. At the end of the decade 125 were living. Of this number, 67 (53.6 percent) were in practice in the state of Illinois. Chicago was home to 46 (36.8 percent of the total), while 21 others (16.8 percent) were located in various places in Illinois. Another 23 graduates (18.4 percent) were scattered around in neighboring midwestern states: Wisconsin, 6; Minnesota, 5; Indiana, 3; Iowa, Michigan, and Missouri, 2 each; and Kentucky, Ohio, and Nebraska, 1 each. In the Great Plains were 9 members of the Class of 1910 (7.2 percent): Colorado, South Dakota, and Wyoming each had 2, while Kansas, North Dakota, and Montana each had 1. New York state was the residence of 2 (1 in New York City and 1 in Yonkers), while Vermont and West Virginia were the residences of 1 each. Texas and New Mexico each could boast having 2, while another 10 were in western states: Washington claimed 5 (1 of whom was in Seattle), Los Angeles claimed 3, and Idaho claimed 2. A total of 9 members of the Class of 1910 had returned to their home countries to practice their medical art and science: the Philippines, 7; Saskatchewan, Canada, 1; and Calcutta, India, 1. We can assume that these physicians and surgeons were agents of healing in their communities.[101]

CHAPTER 12

A Clinical Building and a Hospital

While striving to achieve union with Rush Medical College and the University of Chicago, James remembered that his primary obligation was to reform the university's College of Medicine. After it opened anew in 1913, James spent considerable time in examining its buildings with a view to improving them. On 21 June 1913, for example, he and Charles P. Emerson, dean of the Indiana University Medical School, inspected the physical facilities. In July and September James made additional inspections, and on 22 January 1914 he went through the entire medical school plant with Nathan P. Colwell, secretary of the Council on Medical Education of the American Medical Association. James made three more similar inspections in 1914, one in 1915, two in early 1916, and one on 6 November 1917.[1]

But his main interest was in expanding rather than improving the physical facilities and especially in acquiring a clinical building. In October 1913 Steele urged James to begin a campaign for control of Cook County Hospital in order to permanently secure its clinical advantages for the College of Medicine. Steele had discussed the subject with thirty-six of the leading surgeons of Chicago and with representatives of the leading medical schools. They all endorsed the scheme of taking the County Hospital out of the control of local politics and placing it in the hands of a commission of high-class men appointed by the governor. The commission, Steele believed, would utilize the hospital's great clinical facilities for the benefit of medical research and the development of better medical service to the taxpayers who supported the hospital. If James devoted his "great talents of organization and effort" to this practical problem, Steele predicted, it would be realized. James knew that the Cook County commissioners were not likely to surrender control over the County Hospital and that the proposed commission would involve state politics. He viewed the Cook County Hospital as hopeless as a clinic for the College of Medicine.[2]

The university needed to acquire its own clinical building. To do so required money. For the biennium 1915–17 the board asked for an appropriation of $5 million payable out of the mill tax fund. James again pleaded with alumni, editors, and prominent citizens to flood their legislators with requests to pass the appropriations bill.[3] In Springfield, legislators added to the bill a proviso that no part of the funds appropriated to the university should be used for the purchase of the buildings or grounds formerly known as the College of Physicians and Surgeons (P&S). The proviso would make it practically impossible for the trustees to conduct the medical school along sound lines, and James was instrumental in securing its removal from the bill.[4] The mill tax fund actually brought in less than $5 million, and from it the university received $4,704,242 for the biennium, none of which was specifically in the appropriations act designated for the College of Medicine.[5]

In July 1915 the board recommended that the university acquire a site for a clinical building and erect such a building as soon as possible. Steele seized the occasion to urge James to allow no delay in getting the building under way. Without it the College of Medicine could not advance. It would be good judgment, Steele advised, to postpone all building operations at Urbana for two years rather than not give the college the clinical building now. "I cannot be *constructive* if you are *obstructive*."[6]

In the fall James announced that the income from the mill tax was not adequate to the increasing demands made on the university and for a reasonable building program; the latter should include at least two million dollars for a medical plant. James wanted a site for a clinical building chosen as soon as possible. The most desirable of the several possible sites was the ballpark lying immediately south of Cook County Hospital, said James, but if that site could not be acquired, some other site should be chosen. The matter was urgent.[7]

In February 1917 the board asked for an appropriation of $6 million for operating expenses and buildings for the biennium 1917–19. The buildings request included $250,000 for a clinical building, and James declared that it ought to be erected immediately. The appropriations bill as approved included $500,000 for buildings, none of which was specified by name.[8]

Without waiting to have the funds in hand for a clinical building, James, select trustees, and some realtors devoted time and energy to looking for suitable sites for a clinical building near the medical school. They initially gave some thought to tearing down the original college building and erecting a clinical building at the corner of Harrison and Honore streets, but the site was too small, and the building could not be torn down without the consent of the bondholders.[9] James appointed a special committee of five senior medical faculty members to deal with the matter, and they unanimously recommended purchase of the Marquette School site bounded by Wood, Congress, Harrison, and Alley streets for a clinical building. It was large (289 by 126 feet) and nearby, but nothing came of the suggestion. In September James and two trustees inspected the Jenner Medical College buildings at 196 Washington Street. No doubt its location ruled it out of consideration.[10]

Far more attractive for the university's purposes was the Chicago College of Medicine and Surgery (Valparaiso) on Lincoln (later Wolcott) Street, across the street from the Cook County Hospital. J. Newton Roe, the putative owner of this property, was willing to sell the two college buildings, equipment, good-will, and contract with Frances Willard Hospital for one hundred thousand dollars. Henry S. Spalding of Loyola University was negotiating for the purchase of the property from Roe with a view to combining it with Loyola, which had only recently acquired Bennett Medical College from John Dill Robertson as its medical department. "I understand," Steele informed James, "that Roe sees the handwriting on the wall and desires to get out while the getting is good. . . . In case this deal goes through, it will simplify matters immensely as both John D. Robertson and Roe will be eliminated from the control of Medical Colleges." For anyone who wanted to conduct a university medical college, said Steele, Roe's price was a reasonable one. On 22 May 1915 Roe told Steele that his negotiations with Loyola were off because Spalding could not raise the money and that he would accept one hundred thousand dollars from any other party. James indirectly let Roe know that he was interested, and on 26 March 1916 and again on 14 May 1916 he and Roe went over the property. Nothing came of their meetings.[11] (In 1917 Loyola purchased the Chicago College of Medicine and Surgery [Valparaiso] from Roe for eighty-five thousand dollars and moved into the buildings on Lincoln [later Wolcott] Street formerly occupied by the school.)[12]

Thus James and Abbott concluded that the university had to build. The best available site was the West Side Grounds, located between Polk Street on the north, Wood Street on the east, Taylor Street on the south, and Lincoln (now Wolcott) Street on the west. Since 1894 this area had been the exclusive home of the Chicago Cubs of the National League. The ballpark, known as the West Side Grounds and located immediately south of Cook County Hospital, was in close proximity to the College of Medicine building. Abbott and James dreamed "of a grandiose expansion, of all of the Chicago departments into one great medical center surrounding the old West Side ball park. Here on an open space of ten acres, equal to two city blocks, would be a beautiful private park with recreation and athletic grounds for university students. The six adjacent blocks on the east and west would be acquired, cleared of their old two- and three-story buildings, and rebuilt with fitting structures to house the medical, dental, and pharmacy groups, including clinical hospitals and a home for the County Hospital School for Nurses."[13]

Charles W. Murphy was identified with both the West Side Grounds and the Chicago Cubs. In 1904 Murphy, a former sports writer for the *Cincinnati Times Star,* which was owned by Charles P. Taft, became publicity director for the New York Giants. A year later Murphy purchased the Chicago Cubs from James A. Hart for $105,000 advanced to him by Taft. Murphy built a five-deck stadium

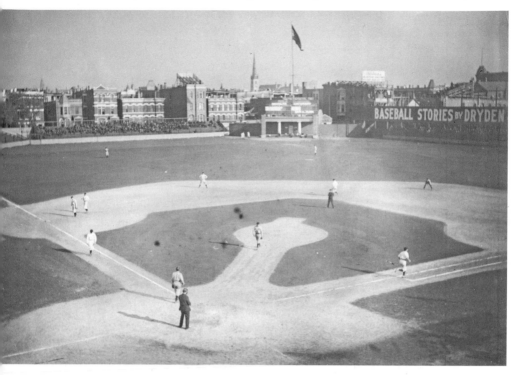

West Side Grounds, Chicago Cubs baseball players, 1907. Steeple of the St. Francis of Assisi Church. Courtesy of the Chicago History Museum.

capable of holding fifty thousand fans. For a time the Chicago Cubs were enormously successful; within a few years the club was allegedly worth more than one million dollars. But baseball magnates viewed Murphy as a bad manager of the Cubs as well as a troublemaker in organized baseball. In 1912 the president of the National League summoned him to Cincinnati to meet with Charles P. Taft and Cubs stockholders. Two years later Taft and his allies forced Murphy out of the game. Taft purchased Murphy's 53 percent of the stock, reportedly for $750,000, and in 1916 sold the franchise to a group headed by Charles H. Weeghman, a wealthy owner of Chicago lunch counters and the chief stockholder of the Whales, a baseball team in the Federal League. Weeghman and his associates, including William Wrigley Jr., the chewing gum magnate, pulled the Cubs out of the West Side Grounds. They played their last game there on 30 October 1915. In 1916 Weeghman moved the club to Weeghman Park on the North Side. By 1921 Wrigley was the sole owner of the site, and in 1926 he named it Wrigley Field.[14]

Murphy remained closely identified with the West Side Grounds. In late 1908 John R. Walsh and Albert G. Spalding, the owners, sold the property to Charles W. Murphy and Anna Sinton Taft, the wife of Charles P. Taft. The sale was closed and the title deed filed for record shortly before 29 December. "The conveyance covers the fee and the consideration is $150,000," the *Chicago Daily* reported, "but as the lease is to the Chicago National baseball club [the Cubs] the two will now be merged into one ownership." The lease, which ran from 1905 to 1 January 1922, provided for an annual rent of $7,804, payable in quarterly installments to 1912, and $10,000 a year thereafter, payable in quarterly installments. Although this affair is complicated, the available evidence indicates that probably Charles P. Taft and his wife put up most of the money for the transaction and that Murphy was their front man. Murphy was publicly identified as the owner of the West Side Grounds.[15]

James tried to interest two wealthy men in buying the site and donating it to the university for its medical center. He identified James A. Patten as one possible donor. In November 1910 when Patten, a Chicago grain commission merchant who was mayor of Evanston from 1901 to 1905, gave two hundred thousand dollars to the Northwestern University medical school to found an experimental laboratory in medical research, James congratulated him and admitted that he was enthusiastic about this subject. "If we could get Northwestern University, the University of Chicago, and the University of Illinois strongly behind medical education in the scientific sense," he wrote, "I believe we could make Chicago the center of medical education in the world, instead of being the plague spot, as somebody has described it." The following March when Patten added fifty thousand dollars to his original gift, James again congratulated him.[16]

Four years later James congratulated Patten on the great addition in "power and vigor" that had come to Northwestern University Medical School through a recent gift of James Deering to Wesley Hospital. As Patten well knew, James added, the condition of medical instruction and research in the city of Chicago had been "a reproach to the community" for the last twenty years. With the new addition made to the resources of Northwestern by Patten and Deering, with the entrance of the state into the field of medical education and research, and with the determination of the University of Chicago to take up certain specialties in that line, James strongly believed, they could organize the interests of the community in this field upon some common basis that would make Chicago "one of the great centers of medical teaching and research and practice in the world."[17]

On 11 January 1916 a professor of gynecology at Rush told James that Patten had promised Billings $250,000 for a clinical building for Rush if the medical schools of Northwestern and Rush would unite. A day later James dined with Patten and his wife in Evanston. During the evening Patten told James that he had withdrawn his offer to Billings. Thus James had reason to believe that these funds might be directed to another cause. On 13 January James and Abbott discussed the purchase of the ballpark, and James spoke with Alexander Prussing, a realtor, about buying the site for $210,000.[18]

Although James may have viewed Patten as a potential benefactor of the ball-park, he turned first to J. Ogden Armour, who had inherited the meat-packing business founded by his father, Philip Armour. On 24 January James wrote Armour proposing a meeting. In late March after they had met, James followed up on their conversation with a proposal. After describing the location and size of the property, he said that it was probably worth $257,289 for ordinary industrial purposes or $297,431 if divided up and sold for ordinary house and store purposes. James recounted the history of the leasing of the property and added that it could be acquired immediately. A day later he pleaded his case. The present condition of medical teaching and research in Chicago was a reproach to the nation, the commonwealth, and the city, James declared, and Chicago had no properly endowed and properly equipped school of medicine. If Armour were to acquire the ballpark and present it to the University of Illinois, the state would secure a well-located and ample site for a first-class medical school. With this site in possession, James was reasonably certain of obtaining gifts and legislative grants with which to erect and equip the various buildings necessary to secure a modern first-class medical school, and he could secure from the state the necessary grants to care for the buildings. Thus the whole enterprise would be provided by a combination of public and private grants. It would not be possible to carry out the proposed plan, James wrote, unless they could start it out on such a scale that people would think in large units. Other men of means in Chicago would follow Armour's example in building up a really great medical school that would be an honor to Chicago, the state, and the nation. James proposed that Armour acquire and present this site to the University of Illinois for the use of its medical school. The university would name it Armour Park. Thus Armour's connection with the University of Illinois medical school would be remembered for many generations, "and such an institution as we are planning will endure and increase as long as our civilization lasts." Two weeks later James informed Armour of the substantial sums of money that Johns Hopkins and Columbia University were devoting to their medical schools.[19]

After thinking over the suggestion James had made, Armour concluded that he did not care to purchase the ballpark and give it to the University of Illinois, "especially at this time." Any money he might wish to spend should go to meeting the needs of his own Armour Institute.[20]

Thus James quickly turned to Patten. On 13 May they had lunch at the Union League Club in Chicago, but, as James confided in his diary, "Could not get him interested in the Ball Park."[21]

Writing to Patten days later, James emphasized the development of a strong center of medical education in Chicago. He first observed that the combination of public support and private beneficence promised the largest returns in charitable and educational work. If private benefactors would put up a building, it would be possible to get public authorities to provide the funds to support and endow it. He went on to observe that the condition of medical research and teaching in Chicago was a reproach to the city, which had been called the "plague spot" of medical education in the United States a few years earlier and still stood near the bottom of the list of great cities of the world in medical instruction and research. Chicago had no properly endowed and properly equipped school of medicine, James wrote, offering as proof the situations at Rush, Northwestern, and the University of Illinois. If the ballpark could be acquired and presented to the University of Illinois, the university would secure an ample site for the development of a first-class medical school. Then, James was reasonably certain, gifts and legislative grants of from $3 million to $5 million would enable the university to erect and equip a first-class medical school. A gift of the ballpark site would inspire others in Chicago to cooperate with the University of Illinois in building up a medical school that would be an honor to the city, state, and nation. The site might be worth $260,000, James thought, although if it were divided up and sold for residential purposes it might be worth $300,000. The present owners were asking $600,000, which James called "a ridiculous price." If Patten acquired and presented the site to the university, he would give a great impulse to providing an adequate medical center for the city of Chicago whereupon James would recommend that the site be called Patten Park.[22]

Patten was not easily persuaded. "Your suggestion does not meet with my approval," he wrote, and went on to say, "You know of my opinion in regard to State Institutions, especially educational institutions. I could not give anything to any State educational institution. It would be the last thing in the world that would meet with any charitable gifts from me. I believe that a private medical institution could be run better and do better work than any State institution, and it could be run much more economically, for we see extravagance in every State and Municipal institution. I do not doubt in the least that your own institution could be run for much less money than what is now being done."[23] Patten vented his personal opinions curtly and ungraciously.

Rebuffed but resilient, James continued his effort to purchase the West Side Grounds. Some new developments made this goal more feasible. On 12 July Mrs. Taft sold her undivided half interest to Murphy for a consideration of $1. The revenue stamps affixed to the instrument were for $110, which indicated that the price paid was $110,000. James thought that the whole property might be obtained for $250,000. On 21 July the board's Committee on the College of Medicine recommended to the Executive Committee the purchase of a half interest in the ballpark, which was said to be for sale, for a clinical building on the site. The Executive Committee concurred.[24]

On 26 July James asked J. Ogden Armour if he might consider the matter again "in this new light." If the university could get this site, James observed, we could get many contributions "toward building up a center for the study of human disease which will rank among the great centers of the kind in the world." Armour replied that he could not see his way clear to changing his position with respect to the matter to which James referred.[25]

In September the board's Executive Committee directed Abbott to have the Chicago Real Estate Board appraise the West Side Grounds. Realtors appraised the land only, exclusive of improvements, at $209,533.20. James and Abbott discussed possible sites and prices of a clinical building with their agent, Alexander Prussing of McKey and Poague.[26] By this time a Chicago newspaper reported that Charles W. Murphy had put a prohibitive price on his property.[27]

In January 1917 Abbott reported on the progress he was making in the acquisition of the ballpark site, and the board authorized its Executive Committee to purchase a site for a clinical building and to proceed with the preparation of plans for such a building. A month later James proposed an appropriations bill for the 1917–19 biennium that asked for $6 million for operating and other expenses, including $250,000 for a clinical building. Abbott expected to complete the purchase of land for a site within a short time. James asked the trustee Ellen M. Henrotin to take up the matter of the appropriation for a clinical building with Chicago editors and Governor Frank O. Lowden. Henrotin talked with Lowden and learned that someone had been prejudicing him against the large amount of money spent at the university. Henrotin also talked with Mrs. Lowden who, according to Henrotin, had unlimited influence over her husband and promised to see James and to do all she could.[28]

The site for a clinical building became increasingly complicated. The Illinois Civil Administration Code of 1917 consolidated the administration of all state charitable institutions in the Department of Public Welfare, and Lowden, the newly elected governor, appointed Charles H. Thorne, a Chicago businessman, as director of the new department. Lowden had never met Thorne, who came highly recommended, but the governor persuaded the reluctant Thorne, who had resigned the presidency of Montgomery Ward and Company three years earlier, to accept a seven thousand dollars post at Springfield. An excellent choice, Thorne brought sympathy, imagination, and business skill to the task of supervising the state's twenty-three charitable and penal institutions.[29]

Thorne, like James, had a vision of the state's positive role in advancing public health. The true function of the state was advisory and supervisory, said Thorne, but the state was forced to provide custodial care for many types of people, and such care cost the state approximately one-fourth of its revenue. The state needed to insure itself against the future by premiums paid for preventive treatment. Research into the causes of diseases was essential. Since Thorne's department was administrative while research was a proper function of the university, the two agencies should coordinate their work.[30]

Thorne recommended that the state grant his department authority for the preparation of plans and the purchase of land in the city of Chicago for a central group of hospitals to be used for educational and research purposes in affiliation with universities, schools of nursing, and physicians. The group was to include the Illinois Charitable Eye and Ear Infirmary, a surgical institute for children, a psychopathic hospital, and a general hospital. The eye and ear infirmary, the one state institution that did statewide preventive work, treated only the poor, mostly children, preventing much blindness, deafness, and pauperism. The surgical institute would save children from becoming cripples and future charges on society. It was to be located in Chicago because that was the only place in the state where sufficient surgical talent was available. A psychopathic (or psychiatric) hospital was needed for the study of preventive treatment, for the training of physicians and other specialists in mental and nervous diseases, and for research work. A general hospital of about two hundred beds, needed for educational and training purposes, should be closely affiliated with the state university medical schools.[31]

On 1 August James, meeting with Thorne and others, learned that Thorne was considering the acquisition of a new site for the Illinois Charitable Eye and Ear Infirmary of Chicago, that he would consider recommending that it be located near the College of Medicine if a suitable site could be found, and that he regarded it as necessary in this development that the university should have an adequate site. So James concluded that the university should acquire, either alone or in conjunction with other state departments, all the land from Polk Street south to Twelfth Street and between Lincoln [later Wolcott] Street and Wood Street, the width corresponding to the width of the block occupied by the Cook County Hospital, and that the various state hospitals should be located on this site with an opening toward the new Twelfth Street boulevard provided in the new city plan of Chicago.[32] The area described by James was the West Side Grounds.

The situation then took a dramatic new turn. Surgeon General William C. Gorgas of the U.S. Army had selected Chicago and eighteen other big cities as sites for "reconstruction" hospitals. These institutions were to be used to enable wounded soldiers to either return to the firing line or take useful positions in civil life. The hospitals in Chicago, Boston, New York, and Washington were to be built alike. Each would contain five hundred beds with provision for enlargement to one thousand beds.[33]

Paul B. Magnuson, an orthopedic physician who was medical director of the State of Illinois Industrial Commission, had been quietly working on the plans for the reconstruction hospital with a number of well-known Chicagoans, including Edmund J. James and Samuel Insull, a utilities titan and chairman of the State Council of Defense of Illinois. On 11 August Magnuson informed James that Insull was very much interested in the hospital proposition and that with Insull and John A. Spoor of the Union Stockyards Company they could reach Governor Lowden "very forcibly."[34]

On that same day Magnuson sent James an article from the *Chicago Herald* that reported that civic leaders backed plans for a hospital to "make over" victims of war. James, Magnuson, and others had conferred relative to the state taking over, either by purchase or condemnation, the Cubs' former ballpark and erecting a hospital to hold three thousand wounded. The hospital, 600 feet long by 125 feet wide and eight stories high, would be turned over to the War Department. At the close of the war it would be given back to the University of Illinois as a teaching hospital in connection with the state medical school. Magnuson had gone to study "reconstruction hospitals" maintained by the British government in various Canadian cities, where they had been highly successful. On his return he would report to Insull, and the State Council of Defense would consider the report. The council planned to cooperate with the War Department in the matter. Some said that a special session of the legislature might be necessary to obtain an appropriation, which would probably amount to three million dollars, and that under rush orders the hospital could be completed in about four months.[35]

In early September Majors Elliott G. Brackett and Edgar King of the surgeon general's office visited Chicago to do preliminary planning for the reconstruction hospital. William L. Abbott, president of the board of trustees, met with them. What the army had in mind, Abbott learned, was some temporary buildings that would accommodate not less than one thousand and perhaps as many as three thousand wounded soldiers. Once the government was through with the buildings, it was understood, they would become the property of the state and would be turned over to the university. If this undertaking got onto the ballpark property, Abbott feared, the government would be there for four or five years, and the university would not be able to enter until the government exited.[36]

Abbott, Eycleshymer, and James M. White, the university's architect, conferred on how to advise James. The university would furnish an adequate site for building a reconstruction hospital of from five hundred to one thousand beds, they counseled, provided that the university be granted clinical instruction facilities for its students. If the hospital was to be less than one thousand beds, it could be accommodated south of the Pharmacy Buildings (that is, north of Polk Street and east of Wood Street, opposite Cook County Hospital), but if that site should not be considered adequate, the university would have to offer space on the ballpark. Eycleshymer did not favor letting the War Department on the ballpark. But, Abbott observed, the construction of this building would be of a temporary character. The government would use it for five years, the university would use it for perhaps another five years, and it could then be removed to make way for a permanent development.[37]

Writing to Major Brackett on behalf of the board of trustees, James said that the university would be glad to furnish the government with a site for a reconstruction hospital in the immediate vicinity of the Cook County Hospital. The hospital should be near the College of Medicine because there it would be in the clinical center of the Midwest, close to a number of eminent physicians and near an excellent medical library, and investigations of clinical problems could be carried on only with the aid of well-equipped laboratories.[38] James refrained from being precise as to the location.

James wrote to David E. Shanahan, Speaker of the House, and John G. Oglesby, lieutenant governor, both of whom were on a committee to report on erecting a reconstruction hospital in Chicago, urging them to line up the hospital with the state medical school.[39]

In mid-November Major King informed James that the surgeon general contemplated the establishment of one or more large hospitals somewhere in the general vicinity of the university. No details as to location could be given at the time, said King, but it was believed that it might be possible to make use to some extent, at least at a later date, of the facilities of the university. At the proper time the surgeon general would communicate further with James.

On a visit to Washington James pressed King for a description of the type of war hospital contemplated in connection with educational institutions. The War Department did not propose to build any hospital of less than five hundred beds, King explained, added to which would be buildings for administration, operating rooms, a mess hall, and the "reconstruction work." The standard was one-story frame construction, but a fireproof building of not more than eight stories would also meet the requirement.[40]

In early October while the army bureaucracy moved slowly, James, Abbott, and Eycleshymer discussed plans for the "medical outfit" with Thorne and architects Edward H. Bennett and William E. Parsons, whose practice was in comprehensive city planning. According to James, Thorne agreed to buy the block bounded by Polk, Hermitage, Taylor, and Wood streets as a location for the Illinois Charitable Eye and Ear Infirmary if the university would purchase the ballpark and if the parties could agree on a uniform scheme of architecture for the buildings to be erected.[41]

On 20 October Abbott informed the board that he had purchased two pieces of property in the Pharmacy School block with a view to obtaining a site for a clinical building. This area was across Wood Street from Cook County Hospital. One parcel was at the northeast corner of West Polk and South Wood streets; the other was several lots on South Wood Street. Both purchases included three-story and basement brick buildings, one had an apartment building, and the other had a school building. The purchase secured for the university the entire western front of South Wood Street between Flournoy and Polk streets, with the exception of a single lot twenty-five feet wide lying between the two properties. The total cost of the two purchases was $31,250, part of which had been paid and part of it represented by a mortgage.[42] This area was close to but not part of the West Side Grounds.

In December James conferred with Oliver A. Harker, the university's legal counsel, about the purchase of the baseball grounds.[43] James knew that the site for the reconstruction hospital was linked to the ballpark property. Learning from Harker that the trustees had no authority to purchase property for which it did not have the money in hand, James suggested that if someone would buy the ballpark and then sell it to the university subject to a mortgage on the property, the transaction could be handled without difficulty from a legal point of view. Charles F. Murphy, who had bought Anna Taft's interest in the ballpark property, would not sell, though the university's agent had offered him $20,000 for his contract. If Murphy would take $250,000 in cash for the property and somebody would buy it at that figure and sell it to the university for $50,000 in cash and take a mortgage on the property as security, James told Abbott, the transaction would be feasible.[44]

Abbott thought that Thorne desired to purchase the ballpark as the site for a group of state hospitals, but Thorne had done nothing and would do nothing to purchase the property until House Speaker Shanahan approved his plan. Thorne was eager to act lest the federal government beat him to it. If the government wanted it they would take it, Abbott believed, but his information indicated that the government would not want it. Abbott did not see how a partnership between the university and the federal government would benefit the university. Someone representing Thorne had virtually said that the state and the university had made a cooperative arrangement for a closer union of the medical school and the state hospitals.

Elmer Schlesinger, a lawyer, urged Abbott to say that the university would give $265,000 for the ballpark property on the assumption that his client, Charles H. Weeghman, the businessman who was president of the Chicago Federal League Baseball Club, would give $10,000 more. (Abbott had once suggested that Murphy fix his price at $275,000.) Abbott thought that the sellers might finally accept the university's offer of $250,000, and if they did he would like to say that the bank would give $200,000. Abbott wanted Harker and the attorneys for the bank to have an understanding as to what the trustees could and would do.[45]

James told Abbott that if the university could get the ballpark for $250,000, he would advise him to close the bargain immediately. If the federal government wanted the property, it would offer the university a good deal more than the university paid for it. But the university "ought to keep its hands free" of both the federal and state governments except so far as the university could cooperate with them in common enterprises. "The possession of the ball park would certainly put us in a position to begin to do things." James congratulated Abbott "upon the masterly way in which you have jewed down the Jew. Even at $250,000, it would be an extremely good bargain."[46] James's racial epithet, the only such usage in his voluminous correspondence, was a reference to Schlesinger.

James wanted the approval of Shanahan for the purchase of the ballpark before acting but thought that it would not be easy to get his wholehearted consent.

Shanahan suggested that the university take the property by condemnation. But to do so would take too long.[47]

Early in 1918 Abbott and Robert Carr, members of the executive committee of the board of trustees, concluded that it was time to crystallize the university's attitude toward the army reconstruction hospital project. Some people presupposed that the university would acquire the baseball site and would, in some unknown way, provide the larger part of the money necessary to erect the hospital.[48] Abbott and Carr, James observed, favored taking over the Home for Destitute Crippled Children as a matter of principle and buying the Cubs ballpark "if we could swing it." James told them that the university might put one hundred thousand dollars cash into it.[49]

Days later Abbott informed James that he thought he could agree on terms for the purchase of the ballpark with Schlesinger, Weeghman's attorney, that would cost the university not more than $265,000. Abbott was going to find out how much and on what terms the bank would help pay for the property. He asked James how much the university could contribute from its funds to the purchase. James thought that it would be safe for the board to put up $100,000 and in a pinch $15,000 or $20,000 more, but $75,000 would be better.[50]

Continuing the quest, in early February James interviewed Thorne "in re Reconstruction Hospital and State Hospital." According to Thorne, Major King was willing to pay rent and enough in advance to put up a million-dollar hospital if the university would furnish the ground.[51] A week later James and the board of trustees considered the blueprints for a possible clinical building to occupy the site of the ballpark or some equally available site prepared by James M. White, university architect. White's "Hospital Plan" outlined a "Typical Floor Plan" for a building of seven stories above a high basement. The plan, not site specific, was labeled "Street" at the top and "Alley" at the bottom.[52]

In mid-April James, Abbott, and Ecyleshymer discussed the terms of taking over the reconstruction hospital. Days later James sent Robert J. Dunham, vice president of Armour and Co. and Ogden Armour's agent, the plans of the proposed reconstruction hospital building. In a cover letter James said that he was delighted to know that Mr. Armour desired to help in the great work of developing medical education and research. James was especially glad that Armour was in a position to make the university the residuary legatee of the reconstruction hospital after the federal government was through with it. The university was in a position to accept the gift.[53]

James's quest to obtain a clinical building had become entangled with the proposal to erect a reconstruction hospital in Chicago. But the army moved slowly, so James proceeded independently on the matter of a hospital.

The Johns Hopkins Medical School, established in 1893, was the first to have a hospital sufficient in size and equipped well enough for research and teaching. Years passed before most medical schools had their own hospital. "It is perfectly apparent," James had told his board in 1914, "that no medical school worth the name can be conducted without a teaching hospital as one of its fundamental departments." Lacking its own hospital, the university was dependent on the goodwill of boards of directors and the medical staff of private hospitals and on such facilities as it might be able to obtain in the Cook County Hospital. The board had to provide an adequate teaching hospital, said James, or see the medical school classed among the inferior schools of the country.[54]

Students at P&S saw patients in the college dispensary and maternity clinic on Honore Street and at West Side Hospital adjacent to the college building on Harrison Street. During the period from 1 May 1912 to 30 April 1913 the West Side Dispensary treated 50,043 cases, including 16,288 adult females (32.5 percent of the total) and 10,910 female children (21.8 percent of the total). The dispensary provided 11,918 surgical treatments, 8,365 medical treatments, and 7,094 children's treatments.[55] For a short time one wing of West Side Hospital housed its outpatient department and the Post-Graduate Medical School of Chicago.[56]

University Hospital of Chicago, at the corner of Ogden Avenue and Lincoln (later Wolcott) and Congress streets, offered clinical instruction to students of P&S in its amphitheater and wards. Charles S. Bacon, Charles Davison, Lewis H. Hammers, Edward L. Heintz, and Daniel A. K. Steele of P&S had founded the hospital in 1907 to have better opportunities to treat their private patients under their own direction. The hospital, a four-story building with a capacity of 110 beds, was directly across the street from the College of Medicine. Although privately financed, the hospital was affiliated with the College of Medicine by contract with the university's board of trustees.[57]

Under certain conditions students from the university's medical school were admitted for clinical study to Cook County Hospital (the new building, completed in 1916, contained twenty-seven hundred beds and cared for about twenty thousand patients annually), and to various hospitals scattered around the city: Augustana, Baptist, Chicago, Woman's, Samaritan, Alexian Brothers', St. Mary's, and Chicago Lying-In. In addition, students could attend extramural clinical courses at the West Side Hebrew Dispensary, St. Luke's Hospital, St. Anthony's Hospital, the Illinois Charitable Eye and Ear Infirmary, and Isolation Hospital.

The students of Rush and Northwestern were more fortunate. They had access to hospitals close to their college buildings. For their clinical material, Rush students relied on Cook County Hospital; Presbyterian Hospital, with 250 beds; a college dispensary; and an obstetrical department. Northwestern students had exclusive access to Wesley Hospital, with 225 beds; Mercy Hospital, with 400 beds; Provident Hospital, with 100 beds; St. Luke's, with 200 beds; the Chicago Lying-In Hospital; and a college free dispensary. Cook County Hospital and People's Hospital were also open to them for study.[58]

In mid-March 1918 James told his board that additional provision must be made for hospital facilities. Unless improvements were made at an early date, some of the state licensing boards would strike the university from the list of ac-credited institutions on the ground that it did not possess the hospital facilities necessary to give efficient instruction.[59]

Believing that Maimonides Hospital might be bought or leased, in early April James and Eycleshymer drove out to 1519 South California Avenue to inspect it. The kosher hospital, in the heart of the Orthodox Jewish community, had opened in 1912, but for years it floundered under three governing boards and persistent financial difficulties. James and Eycleshymer talked with Morris Kurtzon about leasing or buying the property. Charles Davison of the medical school faculty, having inspected the hospital, reported that it would take at least forty-five thousand dollars to open it with one hundred beds. But Mrs. Jacob G. Grossberg, who was active in a Jewish women's hospital auxiliary, vigorously protested the sale. Thereupon Kurtzon provided the money for a new board to take over, and Maimonides Hospital was reorganized under a new name, Mount Sinai Hospital.[60]

While eyeing Maimonides, James continued to pursue other possibilities. On 4 April he interviewed "Singer and Adler" as to getting the Department of Pub-lic Welfare to build a hospital. Berthold Singer was an attorney, and Abraham K. Adler was a consulting architect and engineer in reinforced concrete. They thought that Thorne would act immediately. James met Thorne on 20 April. Eycleshymer and Abbott joined the discussion, and they all went to the office of Robert J. Dunham, "Confidential Ag[en]t of Mr. Ogden Armour," to discuss the use by the University of the "Federal Reconstruction Hospital" after the war was over. James G. Trainer, a realtor, was also present.[61]

As James knew, Ogden Armour had indicated to a syndicate of gentlemen who were considering putting up a government reconstruction hospital that he was willing to contribute to the cause, provided the structure so erected after the federal government was through with it should be of use to the cause of medical education and public health in the state of Illinois through the medium of the state university.

James responded affirmatively to Armour's offer but with certain conditions. The building proposed would not be a modern hospital building, designed with reference to the advance of medical research and training, James wrote, but it would be the shell of such a building and a valuable contribution toward the plant that the university needed to develop its medical work in the way Ar-mour conceived it. If this building was erected according to the plans suggested and on a site near the present university medical college, that is, near the Cook County Hospital, it might very well serve the purpose Armour had in mind. James wanted Armour to make it a condition of his gift that the entire property would be deeded to the university for use in the development of its medical work, it being understood that the federal government should have use of it for a reconstruction hospital during the war and for a reasonable time after the war.

The best site for such a hospital, James thought, was the old West Side Grounds, though an acceptable site not far away from the Cook County Hospital would also serve. To make the plan work, James observed, it would be necessary to secure additional legislation. The Illinois legislature did not meet until January 1919 and might not be willing to undertake the enterprise. The university would have no objection to the plan if it was sure that a man such as Charles Thorne would always be director of the Department of Public Welfare. But Thorne was special; another man in his position might easily thwart the purpose Armour had in mind, and the hospital might easily become an ordinary state hospital. Such a hospital as Armour proposed under the control of the university would become a great center of medical research and education, devoted not merely to caring for the sick but also to increasing the knowledge of diseases so as to benefit all humankind.[62]

In early May James discussed hospital arrangements with Abbott, called on Dunham to discuss plans regarding the reconstruction hospital, and briefly saw Armour, who was much interested in having the government accept his offer of half a million dollars, among other reasons because it would benefit the Armour name.[63] Young Arthur Meeker, whose father Arthur Meeker was Armour's business partner, portrayed Armour, the son and heir of a multimillionaire father, as "a simple soul, guileless and kindly. . . . He never knew what to say to you; a helpless look would steal into his handsome brown eyes as he searched in vain for the appropriate phrase. This inadequacy extended to his business life. . . . I should think," young Meeker added, "he was a classical example of the rich man's son who didn't know what to do with himself."[64] Perhaps Armour did not know what to do with James's offer.

In mid-May James had lunch at the University Club with Armour, Insull, and Shanahan.[65] Presumably they discussed the reconstruction hospital. In late June James reminded Dunham of his effort to persuade Armour to help get the ballpark as a site for the College of Medicine. Under existing conditions, Dunham replied, he thought that Armour was interested only in the government reconstruction hospital.[66]

Indefatigable in pursuing his goal, in August James called on Dunham "in re Mr. Armour's possible gift of [$]500,000 for hospital. Saw him with Mr. Armour 3 P.M. Long talk. Indifferent result." Later that day James had a "confab" with Abbott and Carr, members of the board's executive committee, "in re Red Cross Reconstruction Hospital on the Base ball Park." They agreed "to furnish a site if Armour w[oul]d put up his money to buy back the Hospital for $500,000 at the end of the War."[67]

Although Armour's gift was not forthcoming, legislative appropriations made it possible to proceed along lines adumbrated by James and Thorne. On 12 March 1919 William H. H. Miller, a state representative from Champaign, introduced in the House the appropriations bill for the university for the 1919–21 biennium. On 21 May the House approved the measure by a vote of 128 yeas to 0 nays, the Senate concurred, and on 23 June the governor signed the bill. The act appropriated five million dollars out of the funds set aside for the University of Illinois by the mill tax act plus three hundred thousand dollars for the erection of a clinical building. The General Assembly also appropriated about one million dollars to the Department of Public Welfare for the construction of a group of research and educational hospitals in the city of Chicago. The Department of Public Welfare needed the libraries, laboratories, and staff that the university possessed as well as the clinical building that the university was about to erect, while the university needed the special hospitals that the Department of Public Welfare was about to erect. Moreover, the Department of Public Welfare could provide a site for the clinical building that was much superior to that owned by the university.[68]

Arrangements between the university and the Department of Public Welfare now matured. On 12 April 1919 Thorne presented to the board of trustees the "Suggested Plan of Cooperation between the University of Illinois Medical Schools and the Department of Public Welfare." As Thorne stated, the Department of Public Welfare was about to construct a group of hospitals in Chicago, the university wished to enlarge the facilities of its medical school and to make use of the clinical facilities of the hospitals in Chicago for teaching purposes, and the Department of Public Welfare desired to avail itself of the professional staff of the university. Thorne's plan provided that the administration of the hospitals, including the Illinois Charitable Eye and Ear Infirmary, the State Psychiatric Institute, the State Surgical Institute for Children, and the University Clinical Hospital, was to be in the Department of Public Welfare. The officers of the University of Illinois medical schools were to be staff officers of the hospitals and have the use of all facilities necessary for conducting medical instruction but with no executive authority. James and Thorne were each to appoint three members of a committee to work out the details, and the report of the committee, when signed by James and Thorne, was to become a part of the agreement. The board of trustees viewed the plan as feasible and authorized James to work out the details.[69]

On 12 July 1919 the committee presented the details to the board of trustees. With few changes the agreement followed the suggested plan. The hospitals included the ones previously named plus the State Institute for Juvenile Research. The University Clinical Hospital was renamed the University Clinical Institute. The university agreed to place at the disposal of the department all funds appropriated for the erection of the University Clinical Institute, to be applied to the purpose for which they were appropriated. Things upon which doubt or dispute arose between the parties to the agreement were to be referred to a standing committee of four, with two from each party to the agreement, to facilitate cooperation. The agreement was contingent upon the General Assembly making appropriations available for the purposes described. The board approved of the agreement and recommended that the sum of three hundred thousand dollars appropriated by the legislature be used for the erection and equipment of a new clinical laboratory.[70]

The medical faculty, the board of trustees, and officials of the Department of Public Welfare held many conferences on the plan requirements for the buildings of the Illinois Research and Educational Hospitals in Chicago, which were to occupy the site of the former West Side Grounds, a ten-acre site 556 feet east and west by 800 feet north and south.[71] Edgar Martin, state architect, in association with the firm of Richard E. Schmidt, Garden, and Martin drew the plans in conformity with the advice given by medical school and Department of Public Welfare authorities. The plans were intricate, not only for the preliminary stage but also in consideration of later expansion and development. The planners aimed at creating an atmosphere of sheltered seclusion in a somewhat congested and none too attractive district of the city by choosing for the buildings of the Illinois Research and Educational Hospitals a free adaptation of English collegiate gothic architecture.

The block plan grouped the various buildings of the hospital around the perimeter of the site, turning its back on its surroundings and making its own beauty by enclosing a number of medium-sized courts and a large central quadrangle. The group of buildings included a clinical hospital for general medical purposes, an eye and ear infirmary, a psychiatric institute, and a surgical institute for crippled children. The courts and quadrangles were to receive such planting and landscape treatment as needed to make them a pleasant recreation space for convalescing patients and an attractive outlook from the wards. The construction of the buildings was to be of the most permanent and substantial character with a view to the maximum ultimate economy in maintenance costs. The walls were to be laid in a wire-cut Illinois brick, which presented sufficient variety in color and texture to approximate the charming weathered effect of old English brickwork. Bases, string courses, copings, and window trim were to be of Indiana limestone. Ornamentation was to be introduced sparingly and with discrimination, the greater reliance for effect being placed on proportion of parts and dignity of material.

The planners endeavored to make the buildings "a worthy outward expression" of the "desire of the State of Illinois to use its vast resources for the moral and physical betterment of its people." The Illinois Department of Architecture completed the drafting of the plans by the end of 1919, and construction of the Illinois Reconstruction and Educational Hospitals of Chicago on the site of the former West Side Grounds was soon under way. As contemplated, the buildings of the hospital would be costly. To make the buildings under construction operational would require a million dollars, and to complete the entire complex would bring the cost, unit by unit rather than all at once, to approximately ten million dollars.[72]

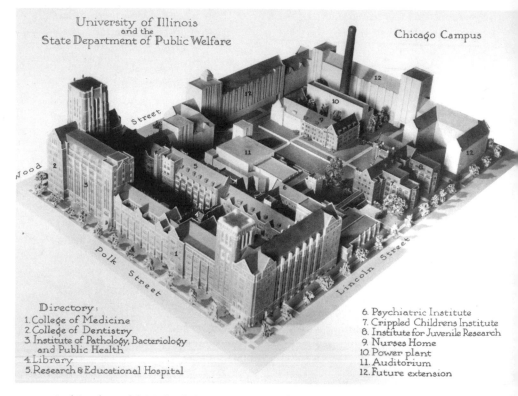

University of Illinois
and the
State Department of Public Welfare

Chicago Campus

Directory:
1. College of Medicine
2. College of Dentistry
3. Institute of Pathology, Bacteriology
   and Public Health
4. Library
5. Research & Educational Hospital

6. Psychiatric Institute
7. Crippled Childrens Institute
8. Institute for Juvenile Research
9. Nurses Home
10. Power plant
11. Auditorium
12. Future extension

Architect's model, Medical Center. Courtesy of the University of Illinois
at Urbana-Champaign Archives.

James, now sixty-four years old, had broken down under the burdens of office. On 10 June 1919 the board of trustees granted him a leave of absence with full pay from 21 June 1919 to the opening of the university in September 1920. He went to California to recuperate, but on 9 March 1920, owing to age and the condition of his health, he submitted his resignation as president. The board accepted it and elected him president emeritus beginning 1 September.[73]

Shortly after James resigned, construction of the buildings to house the College of Medicine on the West Side began.

The first unit of the Illinois Research and Educational Hospitals in Chicago was dedicated on 6 March 1924. The group of buildings completed and occupied at that time included the clinical hospital for the medical school of the University of Illinois and the orthopedic and psychopathic hospitals of the State Department of Public Welfare.

Many viewed the dedication as an epochal event in the development of the hospital and medical education facilities of Chicago and the Midwest. William E. Noble, a medical doctor and president of the university's board of trustees, pre-

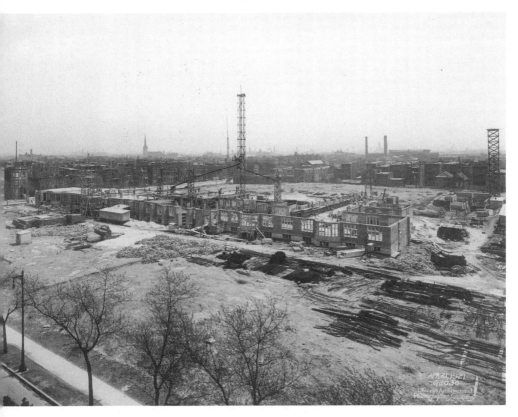

Construction of the Medical Center, 1921. Ryerson and Burham Libraries, Courtesy of the Art Institute of Chicago.

sided. The Reverend William H. Agnew, SJ, president of Loyola University, gave the invocation. Ray Lyman Wilbur, a medical doctor and president of Stanford University, gave a speech titled "The Eclipse of Magic in Medicine," while Dr. Frederick G. Banting of Toronto University gave a speech titled "Medical Research." Governor Len Small, being unable to attend, was represented by John Dill Robertson. Irony of ironies, Robertson, who had "headed the army of aliens" that opposed an appropriation for the medical school, made the address of welcome.[74]

Epilogue

A momentous transformation in medicine occurred in the transatlantic world from 1880 to 1920. In 1880 Germany was widely recognized as the world center of medical research and education, while the United States was viewed as a laggard in both areas. At the time Americans contributed relatively little to medical science. Medical education in America was largely the province of proprietary medical colleges, which depended on tuition income to cover operating expenses and return a profit. These enterprises graduated far more physicians and surgeons than needed to maintain public health, and many of them were poorly prepared. Most proprietary colleges were not affiliated with either a university or a hospital. The germ theory of disease and asepsis were only slowly making their way into medical circles.

Meanwhile, forces were at work that transformed both medicine and the intellectual and cultural life of America. Significant advances were made in the fundamental medical sciences, while at the same time the university replaced the liberal arts college as the paradigmatic form of higher education. Medical departments became an integral part of universities and acquired the attributes of universities. They emphasized research as well as education and trained students to study disease and its prevention as well as to become practitioners.

At the turn of the century the city of Chicago was home to many proprietary medical colleges. The University of Illinois College of Medicine evolved out of such an enterprise. The College of Physicians and Surgeons of Chicago (P&S), chartered in 1881, opened in 1882. For a decade thereafter internal tensions and financial hardship retarded the development of the institution. In the early 1890s new leadership reinvigorated the venture. The authorities recruited the best faculty possible within their resources, and attendance steadily increased.

Even so, it became increasingly clear that a medical college could not exist on the basis of tuition and fee income alone. Governor John P. Altgeld wanted the state university to establish a presence in Chicago in the health sciences, and some P&S officials realized that the sun was setting on proprietary medical colleges. In 1897 P&S affiliated with the University of Illinois by a lease arrangement, and in 1900 the two parties tightened their relationship by a contract that called for the university to put its share of the proceeds from tuition income into a sinking fund that would enable the university to buy the college in twenty-five years. The advent of scientific medicine, the need for large investments in laboratories and clinics, increased admissions requirements, and lower enrollments made it impossible to realize this plan.

Edmund J. James had acquired well-defined ideas about universities, scientific research, and medical education while pursuing graduate studies in Germany. His ideal university was the German university adapted to American conditions, one that emphasized the discovery of new truth and embraced a medical school. In addition, James believed that the government had an obligation to take an active role in advancing public welfare and to support medical education in order to promote the health of the people.

James had been committed to the reform of medical education since 1874, and as president of the university he made it his mission to reform American medical education, beginning with P&S. The college was, as William A. Pusey characterized it, "a vigorous specimen of its kind." During its existence it made a large and wholesome impression on medicine not only in the Midwest but also throughout the nation and in foreign countries. At various times the faculty included such luminaries as Nicholas Senn, Christian Fenger, Ludwig Hektoen, John B. Murphy, Albert J. Ochsner, and William A. Pusey. The college opened with an imposing building, and it was a pioneer among the medical colleges of the day in establishing a laboratory building. P&S moved with if not ahead of the times in introducing bacteriology into the curriculum. The four-year course of study introduced students to medicine as both an art and a science. Arrangements with the West Side Hospital and University Hospital and with Cook County Hospital provided opportunity for clinical training. The Quine Library gave faculty and students an excellent opportunity to keep abreast of the literature of medical science.

The college attracted a large and diverse student body. Many matriculants barely met the minimum admissions requirement, while others entered with considerable preparation. Despite wide differences in age and experience, medical students behaved much like American college undergraduates. Most medical students willingly submitted to hard, unremitting study, but they also enjoyed the fun and games, the rowdiness, and the fraternities that were considered a part of college life. At the same time they were serious about their commitment to medicine, and they performed well on examinations given by state boards. Most of them became practitioners in Illinois, around the country, or abroad, where they cared for the sick and injured and safeguarded public health.

P&S opened its doors to women when it affiliated with the university. While many women were in the lower faculty ranks, often in obstetrics and gynecology, Rachelle Yarros, Bertha Van Hoosen, and others held appointments as associate professor or full professor. The proportion of women in the student body was comparatively high, and several of them won academic honors.

As a body the quality of the instructional corps was high, but the faculty was pedagogically conservative. P&S was a corporation for profit, and fear of economic collapse did not encourage bold innovation. The management of the college was effective, but the college did not win a good reputation because it was handicapped by lack of resources and often by low admissions standards, weakly enforced. And yet the stockholders and alumni were fiercely loyal to the institution. They willingly sacrificed their material interests by turning over the property of P&S to the University of Illinois.

As president of the university, James made it his concern to gain control of P&S and to reform its medical education. He maintained a close watch on the operations of the school, in which effort he had the cooperation of officials at P&S. He persistently sought an appropriation from the state to advance his cause, but the General Assembly repeatedly denied his requests. James was a leader in the reform of medical education in Chicago and in the state of Illinois well before Abraham Flexner appeared on the scene.

In 1910 when Flexner reported that the city of Chicago was "in respect to medical education the plague spot of the nation," James not only agreed but also thought that Flexner had not gone far enough. He had not sufficiently criticized the medical schools of Rush-Chicago, Northwestern, and the University of Illinois. About the same time the Council on Medical Education gave the medical schools of Rush, Northwestern, and eight neighboring states of Illinois a grade A Plus, while it gave P&S a grade of only A.

James insisted that the college improve the quality of the medical education it offered, but he could not provide funds for the purpose because the legislature balked. P&S officials countered that because of a lack of resources they could not provide better laboratories and equipment and more instruction, so in 1912 they cut their tie with the university and reverted to proprietary status.

In 1913 the university reopened its College of Medicine, and the legislature finally provided funds to support it. James immediately resumed his effort to reform medical education. He reorganized the medical school into junior and senior colleges, recruited deans and faculty members, and revised and updated the curriculum.

Along with his focus on reforming medical education in the College of Medicine, James wished to consolidate the programs of the university-related medical colleges as a means of making the city of Chicago a center of medical research and education. In the early twentieth century Chicago was emerging as one of the great cities of the world. Like Boston, New York, Philadelphia, and Baltimore,

Chicago was one of the few urban areas in the United States capable of becoming a world center. In 1909 acting on a proposal by Henry S. Pritchett, president of the Carnegie Foundation for the Advancement of Teaching, to unite the medical departments of the University of Illinois, Rush Medical College–Chicago, and the Northwestern University Medical School, James and the presidents of the other two universities agreed to create a Chicago School of Medicine, which would supercede the existing schools. James actively promoted the plan, but nothing came of these efforts.

After the university opened its College of Medicine in 1913, James campaigned to unite the clinical programs of the three leading medical schools in the city. He had good reason to believe that the University of Illinois College of Medicine might be able to absorb Rush Medical College and possibly also the Northwestern University Medical School. He seemed to be close to realizing his objective when the University of Chicago received funds that enabled it to establish its own medical school, after which Rush went its own way.

At that point James devoted himself to securing a clinical building and hospital facilities for the university's College of Medicine. He was eager to acquire the West Side Grounds, former home of the Chicago Cubs baseball team, as a site for this purpose. His quest bore unanticipated fruit when the Department of Public Welfare and the university jointly agreed that the department would build research and educational hospitals on the chosen site and the faculty of the medical school would provide the staff.

The State of Illinois was late among the states in providing funds for a medical school in its state university. One reason that helps account for this tardiness is the pattern of settlement in early Illinois history. The pioneer settlers came into southern Illinois from southwestern states with no tradition of publicly supported common schools. They did not value formal education and strongly opposed taxation for public education. This habit of mind became deeply rooted and went far toward shaping a mental outlook that persisted. Thus Illinois was late among the states in enacting a law that mandated tax-supported common schools and in establishing a normal school to train teachers. The State of Illinois was the oldest and most prestigious of the commonwealths that did not found a state university before the Civil War.

A more immediate reason that helps explain the lateness of Illinois in providing public funds for a medical school was "medical politics of the most virulent sort." Chicago was home to many proprietary medical schools whose owners feared and opposed competition. John Dill Robertson, who headed one "army of aliens," spoke for the Loyola University Medical School and apparently for the Roman Catholic opposition. J. Newton Roe fought to protect his property, the Chicago College of Medicine and Surgery (Valparaiso). Homeopaths formed another block of opposition. They insisted that state funds could not be used to aid regular medicine at the expense of sectarian medicine.

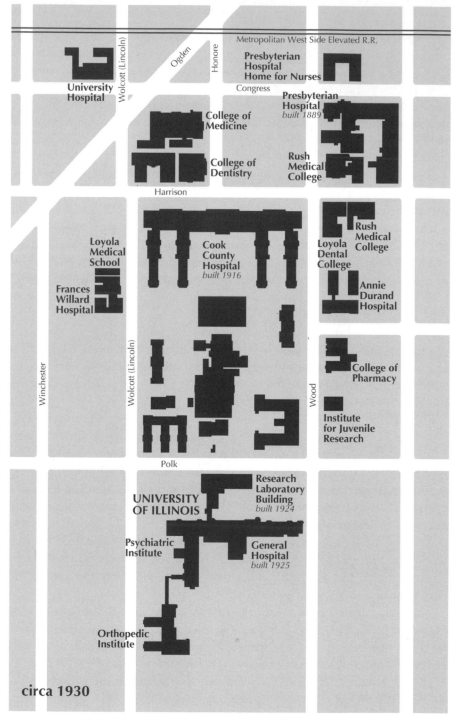

Map of the West Side Medical Center, circa 1930. Drawn by Dennis McClendon, Chicago CartoGraphic.

Despite organized resistance, James succeeded in securing state support for the College of Medicine. When he began his leave of absence in June 1919, plans were being drawn to erect the West Side Medical Center. It was undoubtedly the largest of similar enterprises in terms of more or less closely affiliated hospital and institute units concentrated in one relatively small area. By late 1919 construction was under way, and the first unit of Illinois Research and Educational Hospitals in Chicago was dedicated on 6 March 1924.

Abraham Flexner is often credited with the reform of medical education in America. To be sure, his achievement was great, but in fact the reform of medical education in America began in 1859 and then gained momentum. Edmund J. James led in the reform of medical education before and after Flexner appeared on the local scene. As president of the university, James devoted himself to the reform of medical education in the University of Illinois College of Medicine and to combining it with Rush Medical College and the Northwestern University Medical School to create a united center of clinical medical education in Chicago. James did not realize the latter objective, but he was an architect of the Illinois Medical Center on the West Side, and he deserves credit for helping to make the city of Chicago a great center of medical research and education.

NOTES

Prologue

1. Hans S. Simmer, "Principles and Problems of Medical Undergraduate Education in Germany during the Nineteenth and Early Twentieth Centuries," in C. D. O'Malley, ed., *The History of Medical Education*, UCLA Forum in Medical Sciences, No. 12 (Los Angeles: University of California Press, 1970), 173–200; Thomas N. Bonner, *American Doctors and German Universities: A Chapter in International Intellectual Relations, 1870–1914* (Lincoln: University of Nebraska Press, 1963), 89–103, 107–37; idem, *Becoming a Physician: Medical Education in Britain, France, Germany, and the United States, 1750–1945* (New York: Oxford University Press, 1995), 253–55.

2. [Charles W. Eliot], *Forty-seventh Annual Report of the President of Harvard College, 1871–72* (Cambridge: Cambridge University Press, 1873), 25–26.

3. H[orace] W[ood] Jr., "Medical Education in the United States," *Lippincott's Magazine* 16 (December 1875): 703–11.

4. William F. Norwood, "Medical Education in the United States before 1900," in O'Malley, *History of Medical Education*, 489; Bonner, *American Doctors and German Universities*, 23–39; John Field, "Medical Education in the United States: Late Nineteenth and Twentieth Centuries," in O'Malley, *History of Medical Education*, 501–5.

5. Roy Porter, *The Greatest Benefit to Mankind: A Medical History of Humanity* (New York: Norton, 1997), chaps. 11–14; idem, *Blood and Guts: A Short History of Medicine* (New York: Norton, 2002), 1–169; Richard H. Shryock, *The Development of Modern Medicine: An Interpretation of the Social and Scientific Factors Involved* (Philadelphia: University of Pennsylvania Press, 1936), 265–93; Lester S. King, *Transformations in American Medicine: From Benjamin Rush to William Osler* (Baltimore: Johns Hopkins University Press, 1991).

6. John S. Haller Jr., *Medical Protestants: The Eclectics in American Medicine, 1825–1939* (Carbondale: Southern Illinois University Press, 1994), 199–200; Victor C. Vaughan, *A Doctor's Memories* (Indianapolis: Bobbs-Merrill, 1926), 184–261.

7. Kenneth M. Ludmerer, *Learning to Heal: The Development of American Medical Education* (New York: Basic Books, 1985), 20–21, 47–63; Alan M. Chesney, *The Johns Hopkins Hospital and the Johns Hopkins University School of Medicine: A Chronicle*, Vol. 1 (Baltimore: Johns Hopkins University Press, 1943); Richard H. Shryock, *The Unique Influence of the Johns Hopkins University on American Medicine* (Copenhagen: Ejnar Munksgaard, 1953; Amsterdam: Swets & Zeitlinger, 1969).

8. Laurence R. Veysey, *The Emergence of the American University* (Chicago: University of Chicago Press, 1965), long the standard work on the subject, supplemented by John R. Thelin, *A History of American Higher Education* (Baltimore: Johns Hopkins University

Press, 2004); Roger L. Geiger, *To Advance Knowledge: The Growth of American Research Universities, 1900–1940* (New York: Oxford University Press, 1986); Winton U. Solberg, *The University of Illinois, 1867–1894: An Intellectual and Cultural History* (Urbana: University of Illinois Press, 1968); and idem, *The University of Illinois, 1894–1904: The Shaping of the University* (Urbana: University of Illinois Press, 2000).

9. On dedication to science in America in the early twentieth century and its relation to medical research and education, see J. McKeen Cattell, ed., *Science and Education,* Vol. 2, *Medical Research and Education* (New York: Science Press, 1913); Bonner, *Becoming a Physician,* 291–95.

10. Bonner, *American Doctors and German Universities,* 69–137; Rosemary Stevens, *American Medicine and the Public Interest* (New Haven, Ct.: Yale University Press, 1971), 34–171; Ronald L. Numbers, ed., *The Education of American Physicians: Historical Essays* (Berkeley: University of California Press, 1980).

Chapter 1. *The Medical Scene at the Turn of the Century*

1. H. S. Pritchett, "The Medical School and the State," *Journal of the American Medical Association* 63 (22 August 1914): 650 (hereafter *JAMA*).

2. William F. Norwood, *Medical Education in the United States before the Civil War* (Philadelphia: University of Pennsylvania Press, 1944); Joseph F. Kett, *The Formation of the American Medical Profession: The Role of Institutions, 1780–1860* (New Haven, Ct.: Yale University Press, 1968); John S. Haller Jr., *American Medicine in Transition, 1840–1910* (Urbana: University of Illinois Press, 1981); William G. Rothstein, *American Medical Schools and the Practice of Medicine: A History* (New York: Oxford University Press, 1987), 5–116.

3. Norwood, *Medical Education in the United States before the Civil War,* 32–56; William G. Rothstein, *American Physicians in the Nineteenth Century: From Sects to Science* (Baltimore: Johns Hopkins University Press, 1972), 85–87; Haller, *American Medicine in Transition,* 192–225.

4. Norwood, *Medical Education in the United States before the Civil War,* parts 3–7, describes all of these medical schools.

5. Rothstein, *American Physicians in the Nineteenth Century,* 87–100.

6. Ibid., 98.

7. George H. Simmons, "Medical Education and Preliminary Requirements," *JAMA* 42 (7 May 1904): 1205.

8. Arthur D. Bevan, "Cooperation in Medical Education and Medical Service," *JAMA* 90 (14 April 1928): 1176.

9. Rothstein, *American Physicians in the Nineteenth Century,* 45–55; Haller, *American Medicine in Transition,* 36–99; John H. Warner, *The Therapeutic Perspective: Medical Practice, Knowledge, and Identity in America, 1820–1885* (Cambridge: Harvard University Press, 1986).

10. Norman Gevitz, ed., *Other Healers: Unorthodox Medicine in America* (Baltimore: Johns Hopkins University Press, 1988), with chapters that discuss three perspectives on unorthodox medicine: alternative medical movements of the nineteenth century, divine healing in modern American Protestantism, and contemporary folk medicine.

11. John S. Haller Jr., *The People's Doctors: Samuel Thomson and the American Botanical Movement, 1790–1860* (Carbondale: Southern Illinois University Press, 2000), chaps. 1–

8; William G. Rothstein, "The Botanical Movements and Orthodox Medicine," in Gevitz, *Other Healers*, 36–37, 42–50; Rothstein, *American Physicians in the Nineteenth Century*, 125–51, 217–29; James C. Whorton, *Nature Cures: The History of Alternative Medicine in America* (New York: Oxford University Press, 2002), 25–48.

12. Haller, *Medical Protestants*, 53–55; John S. Haller Jr., *Kindly Medicine: Physio-Medicalism in America, 1836–1911* (Kent, Ohio: Kent State University Press), 139–45; John Moses and Joseph Kirkland, *History of Chicago, Illinois*, 2 vols. (Chicago: Munsell and Co., 1895), 2:292.

13. Haller, *Medical Protestants*, 66–82.

14. Ibid., 71, 76–84, 86–93.

15. Ibid., 140–52; John S. Haller Jr., *A Profile in Alternative Medicine: The Eclectic Medical College of Cincinnati, 1845–1942* (Kent, Ohio: Kent State University Press, 1999).

16. Haller, *Medical Protestants*, 167–83, 231.

17. Ibid., 231.

18. Ibid., 165, 214.

19. Martin Kaufman, "Homeopathy in America: The Rise and Fall and Persistence of a Medical Heresy," in Gevitz, *Other Healers*, 99–123; Martin Kaufman, *Homeopathy in America: The Rise and Fall of a Medical Heresy* (Baltimore: Johns Hopkins University Press, 1971); Whorton, *Nature Cures*, 49–75; Haller, *American Medicine in Transition*, 104–28. See also Harris L. Coulter, *Divided Legacy: A History of the Schism in Medical Thought*, 3 vols. (Washington, D.C.: Weehawken Book Company and McGrath, 1973–1977), a general history of medical thought and therapeutic method with special attention to homeopathy, and William Harvey King, ed., *History of Homeopathy and Its Institutions in America*, 4 vols. (New York: Lewis Publishing, 1905).

20. Haller, *American Medicine in Transition*, 165.

21. Kaufman, *Homeopathy in America*, 156–73.

22. On chiropractic, see Walter I. Wardwell, "Chiropractors: Evolution to Acceptance," in Gevitz, *Other Healers*, 157–59, and Wharton, *Nature Cures*, 165–90.

23. Norman Gevitz, *The DOs: Osteopathic Medicine in America*, 2nd ed. (Baltimore: Johns Hopkins University Press, 2004); idem, "Osteopathic Medicine: From Deviance to Difference," in Gevitz, *Other Healers*, 124–30; Whorton, *Nature Cures*, 141–63.

24. Moreau R. Brown, "Opening Address," *Plexus* 4 (October 1898): 88–89.

Chapter 2. *The Medical Situation in Chicago*

1. Bayard Holmes, "Medical History of Chicago: The Condition of Medical Thought, Medical Practice and Hospital Service after the Great Fire and before the World's Fair: 1871–1893," *Medical Life* 34 (1927): 317–35 (quotation on 332).

2. Ibid., 319.

3. Ibid., 317–25.

4. Bayard Holmes, "Medical Education in Chicago in 1882 and After: IV. The Cook County Hospital in 1884–5," *Medical Life* 28 (August 1921): 406.

5. Illinois State Board of Health, "Medical Education and Medical Colleges in the United States and Canada, 1765–1886," *Eighth Annual Report* (Springfield: n.p., 1886), 424–43. This valuable survey anticipated the 1910 Flexner Report.

6. The following discussion on the number of medical colleges in Chicago is based on Cutler, passim; Illinois State Board of Health, *Report on Medical Education and Official*

Register of Legally Qualified Physicians: 1903 (Springfield: Illinois State Register, 1903), lxi–lxxxiv, 273, 436–37; S. J. B. F., "List and Standing of Medical Schools in the United States," *Medical Notes and Queries* 3 (1907): 163–67; *Illinois Medical Directory, 1910* (Chicago: American Medical Association, [1910]), 5, 19–21; Council, 187–232; Abraham Flexner, *Medical Education in the United States and Canada,* The Carnegie Foundation for the Advancement of Teaching, Bulletin No. 4 (New York, 1910), 207–16; and Thomas N. Bonner, *Medicine in Chicago, 1850–1950: A Chapter in the Social and Scientific Development of a City,* 2nd ed. (Urbana: University of Illinois Press, 1991), 44–67. See also Illinois State Board of Health, "Medical Education and Medical Colleges in the United States and Canada, 1765–1886," *Eighth Annual Report* (1886), 377–532.

7. Arthur D. Bevan, "Cooperation in Medical Education and Medical Service," *JAMA* 90 (14 April 1928): 1173–77.

8. *Woman's Medical Journal* 15 (February 1905): 39.

9. Council, 225–28, 230–31; Leslie B. Arey, *Northwestern University Medical School, 1859–1979: A Pioneer in Educational Reform* (Evanston, Ill.: Northwestern University, 1979), 104–5; "Where Medical Science Is Taught," *Chicago Daily Tribune,* 26 February 1891, p. 3; "Celebrates Entering Its Building," *Chicago Daily Tribune,* 23 April 1893, p. 42; "For Graduate Work," *Chicago Daily Tribune,* 21 July 1893, p. 10.

10. J. H. Kellogg, "A Medical Missionary College," *Advent Review and Sabbath Herald* 72 (11 June 1895): 381–82; idem, "The American Medical Missionary College," *Medical Missionary* 5 (October 1895): 289–92; Richard W. Schwarz, *John Harvey Kellogg, M.D.* (Nashville: Southern Publishing Association, 1970), 104–7; idem, "Kellogg, John Harvey," in *American National Biography,* 24 vols., ed. John A. Garraty and Mark C. Carnes, 12:499–501 (New York: Oxford University Press, 1999); Ronald L. Numbers, *Prophetess of Health: A Study of Ellen G. White* (New York: Harper and Row, 1976), 124, 190–91; Whorton, "Patient Heal Thyself: Popular Health Reform Movements As Unorthodox Medicine," in Gevitz, *Other Healers,* 69–74; Cutler, 630–35, 636.

11. Haller, *Kindly Medicine,* 139–45; Moses and Kirkland, *History of Chicago,* 2:292; Flexner, *Medical Education in the United States and Canada,* 163n.

12. Flexner, *Medical Education in the United States and Canada,* 158, 162–63.

13. Haller, *Medical Protestants,* 213, 214, 150–51; Haller, *Kindly Medicine,* 22; J. B. McFatrich, "The Eclectic School," in Moses and Kirkland, *History of Chicago,* 2:284–92; Cutler, 235–52; Council, 211–12; Flexner, *Medical Education in the United States and Canada,* 162–63.

14. Reliable biographical information on Robertson is lacking. The most complete biographical account is "Hon. John Dill Robertson," in Edward F. Dunne, ed., *Illinois: The Heart of the Nation,* 5 vols., 5:33–34 (Chicago: Lewis Publishing Co., 1933). The biographical sketches in Dunne were by a "Special Staff of Writers." Robertson may have written his own entry. See also *Who Was Who in America,* 1:1042. The evidence on his Kansas experience is in "Beer Foils Malaria Bug?" *Chicago Daily Tribune,* 21 October 1911, p. 3.

15. *The Nineteen Hundred Sixteen Annual, Published by the Junior Medical Class of Loyola University,* 49, University Archives, Loyola University of Chicago.

16. Flexner, *Medical Education in the United States and Canada,* 210.

17. *The College Current* (of Valparaiso College), January, April, May, September, and October 1902; *Annual Announcement of the Chicago College of Medicine and Surgery, 1909–1910, Illinois Medical Directory, 1910,* 20. I thank Mr. Mel Doering, archivist of

Valparaiso University, for documentation on Valparaiso, and Mr. Kevin B. Leonard, associate archivist of Northwestern University, for information on the Northwestern University side of the transaction. Haller, *Medical Protestants,* 214, gives the number of students in 1902 as thirty-six.

18. Richard A. Matré, *Loyola University and Its Medical Center: A Century of Courage and Turmoil* ([Chicago]: Richard A. Matré, Department of Printing Services of Loyola University, 1995), 10–15. This book is not entirely reliable.

19. H. S. Spalding, SJ, "The Beginning of the Loyola University Medical School and an Account of the School during the First Ten Years," [ca. 1929]; T. H. Ahearn to J. L. Jacobs, 27 July 1934, both in William F. Kane File, B:2.5–B:6–20, B:8, B:41, University Archives, Loyola University of Chicago; *Loyola University of Chicago, 1870–1970: One Hundred Years of Knowledge in the Service of Man* (n.p., n.d.), 14–16.

20. In 1909–10, according to Flexner, there were fifteen homeopathic medical colleges in the United States. Flexner, *Medical Education in the United States and Canada,* 158–62.

21. On the early history of homeopathy in Chicago, see Reuben Ludlum, "The Homeopathic School," in Moses and Kirkland, *History of Chicago,* 2:265–84.

22. Flexner, *Medical Education in the United States and Canada,* 163. Gevitz, *The Dos,* says little about the osteopathic school in Chicago.

Chapter 3. The University-Related Medical Colleges in Chicago

1. Norwood, *Medical Education in the United States before the Civil War,* 339–44; George H. Weaver, *Beginnings of Medical Education in and Near Chicago: The Institutions and the Men* (Chicago, 1925), 19–29 [reprinted from *Proceedings of the Institute of Medicine of Chicago* 5 (1925) and *Bulletin of the Society of Medical History of Chicago* 3 (1925)].

2. Norwood, *Medical Education in the United States before the Civil War,* 344–45; Haller, *Medical Protestants,* 199.

3. Samuel J. Jones, "Northwestern University Medical School (Chicago Medical College)," in David J. Davis, ed., *History of Medical Practice in Illinois,* vol. 2, *1850–1900,* 425–31 (Chicago: Illinois State Medical Society, 1955); Arey, *Northwestern University Medical School,* 32–108.

4. Moses and Kirkland, *History of Chicago,* 2:251–52; Helga Ruud, "Woman's Medical College of Chicago," in Davis, *History of Medical Practice in Illinois,* 2:441–49.

5. "The Medical Education Situation in Illinois," *Illinois Medical Journal* 21 (May 1912): 610.

6. Frank Billings, "History of the Cook County Hospital from 1876 to the Present Time," in Council, 264–69; John G. Raffensperger and Louis G. Boshes, *The Old Lady on Harrison Street: Cook County Hospital, 1833–1995* (New York: Peter Lang, 1997), 5–102 passim. See also John Raffensperger, *Cook County Hospital, 1833–1992* (n.p., n.d.), mimeographed, 506 pp., copy in the Illinois History and Lincoln Collections, University of Illinois Library, Urbana-Champaign.

7. Cutler, 551–52; Norman Bridge and John E. Rhodes, "Rush Medical College from 1850 to 1900," in Davis, *History of Medical Practice in Illinois,* 2:424; Asa S. Bacon, "The Presbyterian Hospital of Chicago," in Dunne, *Illinois,* 3:494–96; Jim Bowman, *Good Medicine: The First 150 Years of Rush-Presbyterian-St. Luke's Medical Center* ([Chicago]: Chicago Review Press, 1987), 18–36.

8. R. French Stone, ed., *Biography of Eminent American Physicians and Surgeons* (Indianapolis: Carlon and Hollenbeck, 1894), 240; John E. Rhodes, Norman Bridge, and Stanton E. Friedberg, "Ephraim Fletcher Ingals, 1848–1918," *Proceedings of the Institute of Medicine of Chicago* 2 (1919): 173–78. See also E. Fletcher Ingals, "The Necessities of a Modern Medical College," *Bulletin of the American Academy of Medicine* 2 (August 1895): 235–46.

9. George W. Corner, *A History of the Rockefeller Institute, 1901–1953: Origins and Growth* (New York: Rockefeller Institute Press, 1964), 15–20.

10. Ingals to Harper, 18 and 26 March, 8 April, 11 May 1892, Presidents' Papers, 1889–1925, B:57, F:10, Special Collections Research Center, University of Chicago Library.

11. E. Fletcher Ingals, "Memorial Statement of President W. R. Harper," Board of Trustees, Minutes, 22 January 1906, Rush University Medical Center Archives; Thomas W. Goodspeed, *A History of the University of Chicago: The First Quarter-Century* (Chicago: University of Chicago Press, 1916), 331 (the quotation); Steven C. Wheatley, *The Politics of Philanthropy: Abraham Flexner and Medical Education* (Madison: University of Wisconsin Press, 1988), 25.

12. Ingals to Harper, 21 October, 4 November 1897, Presidents' Papers, 1889–1925, B:57, F:12 and F:10, Special Collections Research Center, University of Chicago Library; Wheatley, *The Politics of Philanthropy*, 26.

13. Corner, *History of the Rockefeller Institute*, 21–30.

14. Ibid., 581.

15. Goodspeed, *History of the University of Chicago*, 330 (the quotation); Ilza Veith and Franklin C. McLean, *The University of Chicago Clinics and Clinical Departments, 1927–1952* ([Chicago: n.p., 1952]), 3. See also Bowman, *Good Medicine*, 1–75.

16. University of Chicago Board of Trustees, Minutes, 29 December 1897; Presidents' Papers, 1889–1925, B:58, F:10, Special Collections Research Center, University of Chicago Library.

17. Ingals to Harper, 21 October 1899, Presidents' Papers, 1889–1925, B:57, F:12, Special Collections Research Center, University of Chicago Library.

18. Corner, *History of the Rockefeller Institute*, 40–41, 582 (first quotation), 582–83 (second quotation); Ingals to Harper, 24 January, 22 February 1898, Presidents' Papers, 1889–1925, B:57, F:11, Special Collections Research Center, University of Chicago Library.

19. Corner, *History of the Rockefeller Institute*, 582–83.

20. University of Chicago Board of Trustees, Minutes, 11 April 1898; Proposed articles of affiliation, 19 April 1898, Presidents' Papers, 1889–1925, B:58, F:10, Special Collections Research Center, University of Chicago Library.

21. Ingals to Harper, 6 April 1898, Presidents' Papers, 1889–1925, B:58, F:11; Copy of [affiliation] agreement, n.d., Presidents' Papers, 1889–1925, B:57, F:10, Special Collections Research Center, University of Chicago Library.

22. Corner, *History of the Rockefeller Institute*, 38, 55.

23. John D. Rockefeller Jr. and F. T. Gates to Martin A. Ryerson, 26 September 1902, Presidents' Papers, 1889–1925, B:58, F:11; Board of Trustees, Minutes, 14 November 1902, vol. 4, p. 193, Special Collections Research Center, University of Chicago Library; Goodspeed, *History of the University of Chicago*, 154, 330–33; Ernest E. Irons, *The Story of Rush Medical College* (Chicago: Board of Trustees of Rush Medical College, 1953), 32–41; Richard J. Storr, *A History of the University of Chicago: Harper's University: The Beginnings* (Chicago: University of Chicago Press, 1966), 142–46, 149, 286–91; Abraham Flexner, *An*

Autobiography, rev. ed.(1940; New York: Simon and Schuster, 1960), 167–68; Veith and McLean, *The University of Chicago Clinics and Clinical Departments,* 5.

24. Harper to Frank Billings, 7 July 1903; Harper to the Trustees of the University, 5 October 1903, Presidents' Papers, 1889–1925, B:58, F:11, Special Collections Research Center, University of Chicago Library.

25. Flexner, *An Autobiography,* 167–74; Cornelius W. Vermeulen, *For the Greatest Good to the Largest Number: A History of the Medical Center, the University of Chicago, 1927–1977* ([Chicago]: Vice President for Public Affairs, University of Chicago, 1977), 1–20.

26. James B. Herrick, "Frank Billings, 1854–1932," *Proceedings of the Institute of Medicine of Chicago* 9 (15 November 1932): 178–81; Ernest E. Irons, "Frank Billings: Physician, Teacher, Medical Statesman and Citizen," *Bulletin of the Society of Medical History of Chicago* 6 (October 1948): 1–8; Arey, *Northwestern University Medical School,* 504–10; Morris Fishbein, *A History of the American Medical Association, 1847 to 1947* (Philadelphia: W. B. Saunders, 1947), 688–91.

27. Fishbein, *History of the American Medical Association,* 741–43; Vernon C. David, "Arthur Dean Bevan, 1861–1943," *Proceedings of the Institute of Medicine of Chicago* 14 (15 November 1953): 499–501. In 1918–19 Bevan served as president of the American Medical Association.

28. John W. Farlow, "Ingals, Ephraim Fletcher," in *American Medical Biographies,* ed. Howard A. Kelly and Walter L. Burrage, 591–92 (Baltimore: Norman, Remington Co., 1920); F. M. Sperry, comp., "Ephraim Fletcher Ingals: A.M., M.D.," in *A Group of Distinguished Physicians and Surgeons of Chicago,* 107–9 (Chicago: J. H. Beers, 1904); Fishbein, *History of the American Medical Association,* 193, 220, 842, 860; Ingals to Harper, 31 January, 13 June 1900, Presidents' Papers, 1889–1925, B:57, F:13, Special Collections Research Center, University of Chicago Library.

Chapter 4. The Early Years of the College of Physicians and Surgeons

1. Charles W. Earle, "The College of Physicians and Surgeons," *Chicago Clinical Review* (October 1893): 49–56, with illustrations.

2. William E. Quine, "History of the College of Physicians and Surgeons of Chicago," *Bulletin of the Society of Medical History of Chicago* 1 (October 1911): 64–70. Also published in *Plexus,* 17 (July 1911): 255–65.

3. Carl Stephens to President David Kinley, 17 May 1922, 26/1/20, Carl Stephens Papers, B:9, F:Medicine; *Alumni Record,* vii–xxi.

4. D. A. K. Steele, "The Genesis of a Great Medical College," in *Alumni Record,* vii–xiii, reprinted in Davis, *History of Medical Practice in Illinois,* 2:431–41. Steele's article was the text of an address delivered on 20 November 1920 at the College of Medicine. See Carl Stephens to David Kinley, 17 May 1922, 26/1/20, Carl Stephens Papers, B:9, F:Medicine.

5. Many alumni of P&S criticized the history of the College of Medicine published in the *Alumni Record.* Certain faculty members, they alleged, were not given the credit they deserved. At a meeting of the Alumni Association held on 19 June 1922 in the Congress Hotel, disgruntled alumni secured the adoption of a resolution that declared that the history of the College of Medicine published in the *Alumni Record* was "inaccurate, incomplete and unjust in many particulars and therefore unworthy of the University and wholly unacceptable to the Alumni of the Medical Department." See the correspondence between Carl Stephens and William H. Browne, superintendent of P&S since 1900, in

1922 and 1942 and John M. Krasa to President David Kinley, 19 June 1922, enclosing a copy of the meeting of the Alumni Association, all in 26/1/20, Carl Stephens Papers, B:9, F:Medicine.

6. Patricia Spain Ward, "An Experiment in Medical Education: Or How the College of Physicians and Surgeons Became the University of Illinois College of Medicine," in *Medicine in Transition: The Centennial of the University of Illinois College of Medicine,* ed. Edward P. Cohen, 27–51 ([Chicago]: University of Illinois College of Medicine, 1981), draws heavily on the articles by Steele and Quine and is undocumented.

7. D. A. K. Steele, S. A. McWilliams, and A. Jackson, "To the Future Historian of Medical Colleges," 26 August 1882, 027/51/01, F:6, University Archives, University of Illinois at Chicago. A list of the contents of the lead box and a copy of the letter are also in 26/1/20, Carl Stephens Papers, B:9, F:Medicine.

8. All of these primary sources are in the University Archives, University of Illinois at Chicago.

9. Steele, "The Genesis of a Great Medical College," viii.

10. Steele, McWilliams, and Jackson, "To the Future Historian of Medical Colleges."

11. 027/01/01, F:2, 29, 30 May 1882, University Archives, University of Illinois at Chicago.

12. On this school, see Norwood, *Medical Education in the United States before the Civil War,* 94–97.

13. E[dward] P[reble], "Jackson, Abraham Reeves," in *Dictionary of American Biography,* 20 vols., ed. Allen Johnson and Dumas Malone, 9:525–26 (New York: Scribner, 1928–36); William B. Atkinson, ed., *The Physicians and Surgeons of the United States* (Philadelphia: Charles Robson, 1878), 20; Stone, *Biography of Eminent American Physicians and Surgeons,* 242; Henry T. Byford, "Jackson, Abraham Reeves," in Kelly and Burrage, *American Medical Biographies,* 596; Sperry, *A Group of Distinguished Physicians and Surgeons of Chicago,* 72–73; Leon T. Dickinson and Robert Regan, "Newspaper Letters of Another 'Innocent Abroad,' Dr. Abraham Reeves Jackson," *Mark Twain Journal* 33 (Spring 1995): 2–59.

14. William K. Beatty, "Charles Warrington Earle—Soldier, Optimist, and Hard Worker," *Proceedings of the Institute of Medicine of Chicago* 48 (October–December 1990): 124–42; Atkinson, *Physicians and Surgeons of the United States,* 356–57; Stone, *Biography of Eminent American Physicians and Surgeons,* 611–15; Council, 212; George H. Weaver, "Earle, George Washington," in Kelly and Burrage, *American Medical Biographies,* 348–49; Sperry, *A Group of Distinguished Physicians and Surgeons of Chicago,* 163–68.

15. *Catalogue of the Officers and Students of the University of Michigan, 1863,* in 027/05/01, F:3, University Archives, University of Illinois at Chicago; Samuel A. McWilliams Necrology File, Bentley Historical Library, University of Michigan, photocopies kindly furnished by Ms. Karen Wright, reference assistant; Atkinson, *Physicians and Surgeons of the United States,* 201; Davis, *History of Medical Practice in Illinois,* 2:432n. Davis gives the birth date of McWilliams as 7 February 1839.

16. Stone, *Biography of Eminent American Physicians and Surgeons,* 479–80; *Alumni Record,* 281; Council, 838; Editorial, "The Work of Dr. Daniel A. K. Steele for Medical Education," *Chicago Medical Recorder* (August 1917): 367–69. "Address by Dr. D. A. K Steele, M.D. LL.D. at Formal Opening of New Wing of Mercy Hospital, June 15, 1916," *Chicago Medical Recorder* (August 1916): 411–13, contains interesting biographical details.

17. Davis, *History of Medical Practice in Illinois,* 2:432n. I thank Ms. Carrie Schmidt, assistant in the McGill University Archives, for information about St. John. The McGill records note that St. John obtained an MRGS (the meaning of this abbreviation is unclear) from England in 1873.

18. Atkinson, *Physicians and Surgeons of the United States,* 601–2; Kelly and Burrage, *American Medical Biographies,* 147–48.

19. Stone, *Biography of Eminent American Physicians and Surgeons,* 349–50; Albert N. Marquis, *The Book of Chicagoans* (Chicago: A. N. Marquis Co., 1911), 498.

20. *The Lakeside Annual Directory of the City of Chicago, 1880* (Chicago: Chicago Directory Co., 1880), 769; *Illinois State Gazetteer and Business Directory, 1882* (Chicago: R. L. Polk and Co. and A. C. Danser, 1882), 1778.

21. Moses and Kirkland, *History of Chicago,* 2:252; Marquis, *The Book of Chicagoans,* 487.

22. Atkinson, *Physicians and Surgeons of the United States,* 473; Thomas H. Shastid, "Holtz, Ferdinand Carl," in Kelly and Burrage, *American Medical Biographies,* 547. Hotz was sometimes known as Holtz.

23. Atkinson, *Physicians and Surgeons of Chicago,* 603–4.

24. John L. Rothrock, "Stone, Alexander Johnson," in Kelly and Burrage, *American Medical Biographies,* 1109–10.

25. With the exception of the references to individuals, the following account of the founding of the college is based on 027/01/01, F:1, University Archives, University of Illinois at Chicago.

26. Ibid., 4 May meeting.

27. Ibid., 14 July meeting.

28. 027/01/01, F:2, 11 October 1881, University Archives, University of Illinois at Chicago.

29. 027/01/01, F:2, passim.

30. Steele, "The Genesis of a Great Medical College," viii–ix.

31. As quoted in Arey, *Northwestern University Medical School,* 106.

32. Earle, "The College of Physicians and Surgeons," 49.

33. Quine, "History of the College of Physicians and Surgeons of Chicago," 64.

34. The founders who purchased the lot reported that it measured ninety-seven by one hundred feet. Perhaps the building measured seventy feet by one hundred feet.

35. *First Annual Announcement of the College of Physicians and Surgeons of Chicago: Session of 1882–83* (Chicago, 1883), 12–13, University of Illinois Archives, Urbana-Champaign, and University Archives, University of Illinois at Chicago. Hereafter the Annual Announcements of P&S will be cited giving an abbreviated form of the title and the dates of the session: for example, *First Annual Announcement,* 1882–83. The place (Chicago) and year of publication were not uniformly given on the cover page, and they are omitted hereafter. Annual announcements were usually published in May or June of the year in which the session began. The Annual Announcements of P&S are available in both of the archives cited in this note.

36. "Medical Colleges," *Chicago Daily Tribune,* 27 September 1882.

37. Rush Medical College, Chicago, *Fortieth Annual Announcement, Session of 1882–1883,* RG 02300 C94-037, Rush Medical Center Archives.

38. *First Annual Announcement,* 1882–83.

39. Cutler, 575–76; *Alumni Record,* 260.

40. Cutler, 373–79.

41. Ibid., 524–27.

42. Ibid., 368–72; Stone, *Biography of Eminent American Physicians and Surgeons,* 647.

43. Cutler, 378–82.

44. Ibid., 367–68; *Alumni Record,* 268.

45. Cutler, 388, 391–92; *Alumni Record,* 245.

46. *Alumni Record,* 284; Bayard Holmes, "Medical Education in Chicago in 1882 and After. VI: An Adventure in Education," *Medical Life* 29 (January 1922): 30–31. Frank E. Waxham, "The Early History of Intubation of the Larynx in Chicago," *Bulletin of the Society of Medical History of Chicago* 1 (October 1911): 58–63, provides an account of Waxham and intubation among the poor of Chicago.

47. *First Annual Announcement,* 1882–83; Rush Medical College, *Fortieth Annual Announcement, Session of 1882–1883.*

48. *Second Annual Announcement,* 1883–84, 7.

49. *First Annual Announcement,* 1882–83. For the 1896 spring course offerings, see "Spring Course, 1896," *Plexus* 1 (March 1896): 125.

50. *Alumni Record,* ix, 1–3.

51. William A. Pusey, "The College of Physicians and Surgeons of Chicago: An Outline of Its History," in "William Edward Quine," *University of Illinois Bulletin* 20(39) (28 May 1923): 37–39; see also Bayard Holmes to T. J. Burrill, 1 April 1913, 2/5/3, F:He–Hu, 1912–13.

52. *Second Annual Announcement,* 1883–84; *Third Annual Announcement,* 1884–85.

53. Quine, "History of the College of Physicians and Surgeons of Chicago," 65.

54. 027/01/01/, F:2, 17 March 1883, University Archives, University of Illinois at Chicago.

55. "Minutes of the Annual Meeting of Trustees of Chicago Medical College," 1 April 1883, photocopy in the American College of Surgery Archives, Chicago, Illinois; 027/01/01, F:2, 12 June 1883, University Archives, University of Illinois at Chicago.

56. *Fifth Annual Announcement,* 1886–87.

57. Cutler, 96–102.

58. Ibid., 186–87; 027/01/05/02, F:21, 18 July 1893, University Archives, University of Illinois at Chicago.

59. Morris Fishbein, "Ludvig Hektoen: A Biography and an Appreciation," *Archives of Pathology* 26 (1938): 3–18 (followed by a "Bibliography of the Writings of Ludvig Hektoen," 20–31); Gert H. Brieger, "Hektoen, Ludvig," *Dictionary of Scientific Biography,* 14 vols., ed. Charles C. Gillispie, 6:232–33 (New York: Scribner, 1970–76); Paul R. Cannon, "Ludvig Hektoen, 1863–1951," in National Academy of Sciences, *Biographical Memoirs,* 28 (Washington, D.C.: National Academy of Sciences, 1954), 163–97; James B. Herrick, "Ludvig Hektoen, 1863–1951," *Proceedings of the Institute of Medicine of Chicago* 19 (15 January 1952): 3–11.

60. *Sixth Annual Announcement,* 1887–88; "Obituary," *Plexus* 4 (March 1899): 222–23 (quotation on 223).

61. *Seventh Annual Announcement,* 1888–89.

62. Quine made these remarks at a memorial service for Charles W. Earle, as reported in the *Chicago Daily,* 10 March 1894.

63. Quine, "History of the College of Physicians and Surgeons of Chicago," 65, 64.

64. 027/01/01, F:2, 24 September 1888, 277, 278, 279.

65. 027/01/01, F:3, University Archives, University of Illinois at Chicago; Quine, "History of the College of Physicians and Surgeons," 65. *Eighth Annual Announcement,* 1889–90, indicates that Earle was no longer on the board of directors or the faculty.

66. Hollis W. Field, "How Young Doctor Climbed the Ladder," *Chicago Daily Tribune*, 21 April 1907; "Downey Accepts; Dr. Evans Chosen," *Chicago Daily Tribune*, 14 April 1907 (appointed health commissioner); *Alumni Record*, 63; *The Illio 1909*, n.p.; Council, 496.

67. The data on matriculants, on graduates, and on graduates from the practitioners' course are compiled from the *First Annual Announcement*, 1882–93, through the *Eleventh Annual Announcement*, 1882–83, and from the *Alumni Record*, 1–27.

68. Rush Medical College, Medical Department of Lake Forest University, *Fiftieth Annual Announcement, 1892–1893*, Rush Medical Center Archives.

69. *Second Annual Announcement*, 1883–84, 15–17.

70. *Fifth Annual Announcement*, 1886–87, 15–18.

71. *Tenth Annual Announcement*, 1891–92, 18–20.

72. *Alumni Record*, 3–5.

73. Ibid., 12–15.

74. Ibid., 20–22.

75. Bayard Holmes, "Medical Education in Chicago in 1882 and After: VI. An Adventure in Education," *Medical Life* 29 (January 1922): 40.

76. Earle was a special lecturer in the Illinois College of Pharmacy from 1886 to 1889 while still a professor and a director at P&S. From 1891 to 1893 he was also professor of diseases of children and clinical medicine in Woman's Medical College. On this subject I thank Mr. Kevin B. Leonard of the University Archives of the Northwestern University Library.

77. *Tenth Annual Announcement*, 1891–92.

78. William A. Pusey, "Biographical Sketch," in Arthur M. Corwin, Frank Billings, William A. Pusey, Alice L. Wynekoop, William A. Harsha, and John T. Richards, "William E. Quine," *Official Bulletin of the Chicago Medical Society* (20 January 1923): 27–48 (quotation on 36).

79. Corwin, Billings, Pusey, Wynekoop, Harsha, and Richards, "William E. Quine"; David Kinley, William A. Pusey, James B. Herrick, Frank Billings, and A. C. Eycleshymer, "William Edward Quine," *University of Illinois Bulletin* 20(39) (28 May 1923): 7–55; *Eleventh Annual Announcement*, 1892–93. See also Stone, *Biography of Eminent Physicians and Surgeons of Chicago*, 414–15.

80. 027/01/01, F:3, 1 August 1891, University Archives, University of Illinois at Chicago.

81. *Eleventh Annual Announcement*, 1892–93; *Twelfth Annual Announcement*, 1893–94; *Thirteenth Annual Announcement*, 1894–95.

82. *Eleventh Annual Announcement*, 1892–93.

83. *Fourteenth Annual Announcement*, 1895–96.

84. "Bust of Dr. Jackson: Presented to the College of Physicians and Surgeons," *Chicago Daily Tribune*, 13 April 1893.

85. "Are Physicians and Surgeons," *Chicago Daily Tribune*, 14 April 1893.

86. *Twelfth Annual Announcement*, 93–94.

87. 027/01/01, F:3, 30 October 1891, University Archives, University of Illinois at Chicago.

88. Ibid., 30 October, 1 and 30 December 1891, 20 and 29 April 1892. On the stockholdings of Quine, Steele, and Murphy, see ibid., 17 April 1895.

89. *Eleventh Annual Announcement*, 1892–93.

90. William K. Beatty, "Bayard Taylor Holmes—A Forgotten Man," *Proceedings of the Institute of Medicine of Chicago* 34 (October–December 1981): 120–23. Beatty's account is based on six autobiographical sketches by Holmes published under the title "Medical

Education in Chicago in 1882 and After" in *Medical Life,* as follows: I. "Ragweed Time," 28 (January 1921): 8–12; II. "Choosing a Medical School," 28 (February 1921): 57–62; III. "The Old County Hospital," 28 (April 1921): 160–65; IV. "The Cook County Hospital in 1884–5," 28 (August 1921): 402–10; V. "Medical Libraries in Chicago," 28 (September 1921): 569–74; VI. "An Adventure in Education," 29 (January 1922): 30–41. *Medical Life* 31 (July 1924): 253–88, is a memorial to Bayard Holmes with two of his papers; *Medical Life* 37 (1930): 441–54, is a Bayard Holmes bibliography.

91. Arey, *Northwestern University Medical School,* 104.

92. The proposal to admit women to laboratory work raises a question, since the college had neither female faculty members nor female students when Holmes made his motion. Perhaps students from Woman's Medical College wanted admission to the laboratories.

93. 027/01/05/02, F:1, 8 August 1891, 2 April 1892, 17 January 1893, 21 and 28 February 1893, 1 September 1893, 13 February 1894, 11 February 1896, 12 May 1896, University Archives, University of Illinois at Chicago.

94. Holmes, "Medical Education in Chicago in 1882 and After: VI. An Adventure in Education," *Medical Life* 29 (January 1922): 33–41 (quotations on 37–38).

95. Ibid., 40.

96. Ibid., 41.

97. Crerar Ms. 95, Special Collections Research Center, University of Chicago Library. This scrapbook contains letters and documents on Holmes's background and education as well as newspaper clippings relating to his political activities. The quotation is from an unidentified, undated (mid-1890s) newspaper clipping.

98. Cutler, 382–87; Council, 436.

99. "Gehrmann, Adolph," in *American Biography: A New Cyclopedia,* 52 vols., Compiled under the Editorial Supervision of a Notable Advisory Board (New York: Published under the Direction of the American Historical Association, 1917–1932), 9:198–201.

100. Adolpho Luria, "A Few Considerations about the Murphy Button—A Critical Study," Part 1, *Plexus* 2 (October 1896): 101–6; Adolpho Luria, "A Few Considerations about the Murphy Button—A Critical Study," Part 2, *Plexus* 2 (November 1896): 124–29; "Dr. J. B. Murphy Demonstrates the Use of His Button," *Plexus* 2 (April 1896): 17.

101. Mark M. Ravitch, *A Century of Surgery: The History of the American Surgical Association,* 2 vols. (Philadelphia: Lippincott, 1981), 1:381.

102. Rush Medical College Annual Announcements, 1891–92, 1892–93, Rush Medical Center Archives. P&S catalogs list Murphy as a faculty member from 1893 through 1900; Arey, *Northwestern University Medical School, 1859–1979,* 510–18; Loyal Davis, *J. B. Murphy: Stormy Petrel of Surgery* (New York: Putnam, 1938); Stone, *Biography of Eminent American Physicians and Surgeons,* 350; J. B. Murphy, "Doctorate Address before the Graduating Class of '96," *Plexus* 2 (May 1896): 31–36 (quotation on 34).

103. Davis, *J. B. Murphy: Stormy Petrel of Surgery;* Ravitch, *A Century of Surgery,* 1:174, 227, 235, 246, 263, 288.

104. Lawrence C. Parish, "Pusey, William Allen," *American National Biography,* 17:950–51, is a brief and useful source. The most valuable treatment of Pusey is Herbert Ratner, "William Allen Pusey at Close Range," in "William Allen Pusey: An Appreciation by Friends and Co-workers," *Archives of Dermatology and Syphilology* 35 (January

1937): 1–43. These appreciations, along with a photograph of Pusey, have been separately printed as *William Allen Pusey: An Appreciation by Friends and Co-workers* (n.p., n.d.). See also Fishbein, *History of the American Medical Association,* 762–65. Pusey's *High Lights in the History of Chicago Medicine* (n.p., n.d.), reprinted from *Bulletin of the Society of Medical History of Chicago* 5 (May 1940): 159–207, was originally an address for laymen presented on 9 January 1940 at the Museum of Science and Industry in Chicago. A copy is in the University Library, University of Illinois, Urbana-Champaign.

105. William A. Pusey, *A Doctor of the 1870's and 80's* (Springfield, Ill.: Charles C. Thomas, 1931), is a charming memorial to his father as well as a valuable account of medicine as practiced before the advent of scientific medicine and university-related medical schools.

106. Ratner, "William Allen Pusey at Close Range," 9 (the quotation). The National Union Catalogue (475:627) indicates that Pusey published a book with this title in 1902 and that Pusey and Caldwell published a book with the same title in 1903 (Philadelphia: W. B. Saunders).

107. Ratner, "William Allen Pusey at Close Range," 17 (the quotations).

108. For a list of Pusey's books and articles, see "William Allen Pusey: An Appreciation by Friends and Co-workers," *Archives of Dermatology and Syphilology* 35 (January 1937): 45–49.

109. Cutler, 387–89.

110. "The P. & S. Hospital," *Plexus* 1 (February 1896): 86; "Will Start Post-Graduate School," *Chicago Daily Tribune,* 12 August 1896; "The Chicago Clinical School: Formerly West Chicago Post-Graduate School," *Plexus* 3 (September 1897): 60–61.

111. 027/01/01, F:3, 102 (1892), 10 December 1895, 4 February, 23 March 1896, University Archives, University of Illinois at Chicago; "New Corporations," *Chicago Daily Tribune,* 19 January 1896, p. 6; "Sale of a Medical School," *Chicago Daily Tribune,* 26 February 1896, p. 1; "For Y.M.C.A. Hospital," *Chicago Daily,* 20 January 1896, p. 1; D. A. K. Steele, "The West Side Hospital," *Plexus* 2 (April 1896): 8–9; "West Chicago Post-Graduate School and Polyclinic," *Plexus* 2 (September 1896): 76; Photo: "West Chicago Post-Graduate School and Polyclinic," *Plexus* 2 (December 1896): facing 160; "The Chicago Clinical School, Formerly West Chicago Post-Graduate School," *Plexus* 3 (September 1897): 60–61. On this complicated topic see also Council, 225, 227, 229–30.

112. *Alumni Record,* 27–31.

113. Bonner, *American Doctors and German Universities,* 139–56, writes about German doctors in America before 1914. The Carl Beck he mentions is not the Carl Beck of P&S.

114. William Baader and Lloyd M. Nyhus, "The Life of Carl Beck and an Important Interval with Alexis Carrel," *Surgery, Gynecology & Obstetrics* 163 (July 1986): 85–88; Joseph C. Beck, *Fifty Years in Medicine* (Chicago: McDonough & Co., 1940), 41–67; William C. Beck, "Alexis Carrel and Carl Beck: A Historical Footnote," *Perspectives in Biology and Medicine* 30 (Autumn 1986): 148–51; W. Sterling Edwards and Peter D. Edwards, *Alexis Carrel: Visionary Surgeon* (Springfield, Ill.: Charles C. Thomas, 1974), 22–37, 59.

115. Guido Kisch, *In Search of Freedom: A History of American Jews from Czechoslovakia* (London: Edward Goldston & Son, 1949), 141–42; Hyman L. Meites, ed., *History of the Jews of Chicago* (Chicago: Chicago Jewish Historical Society and Wellington Publishing, 1990), 410–11 (originally published Chicago: Jewish Historical Society of Illinois, 1924).

116. William C. Beck, *Memory Bytes: An Autobiography of a Surgeon* (Sayre, Penn.: Guthrie Foundation, 1995), 256–59.

117. Helen Clapesattle, *The Doctors Mayo,* 2nd ed. (Minneapolis: University of Minnesota Press, 1963), 236–37, 272; Clark W. Nelson, "Historical Profiles of Mayo: Dr. Carl Beck and the Mayos," *Mayo Clinical Proceedings* 66 (1991): 242 (the quotations). I am indebted to Sidney J. Blair, MD, an emeritus orthopedic surgeon at the medical school of Loyola University, for furnishing me some documents on the career of Carl Beck.

118. "Says American Schools Lead," *Chicago Daily Tribune,* 30 July 1908, p. 18.

119. *Fifteenth Annual Announcement, 1895–96,* 12–15.

120. The data on the number of matriculants are from annual college announcements; the data on the number of graduates are from *Alumni Record,* 27–49.

Chapter 5. Affiliation: The College and the University

1. *16th Report* (1892), 171–72; Altgeld to Andrew Sloan Draper, 6 March 1896, 2/5/3, B:30, F:Altgeld and Med School (the quotation); Quine, "History of the College of Physicians and Surgeons of Chicago," 66–67.

2. *17th Report* (1894), 63.

3. 027/01/01, F:3, 14 December 1894; 2 and 9 January 1895, University Archives, University of Illinois at Chicago; *18th Report* (1896), 41–42, 58, 67.

4. *Journal of the House of Representatives of the Thirty-ninth General Assembly of the State of Illinois* (Springfield, 1896), 316; [Henry M. Dunlap], "A History of the Illinois Industrial University afterward the University of Illinois 1851–1938 As Recorded in the Acts of the Illinois General Assembly," 2 vols. (1937), 1:172, 2/9/10, Legislative History, B:1.

5. Ingals to Harper, 22 April 1895, Presidents' Papers, B:57, F:10, Special Collections Research Center, University of Chicago Library.

6. 027/01/01, F:3, 26 March 1897, University Archives, University of Illinois at Chicago; *19th Report* (1898), 45.

7. Ingals to Harper, 11 March 1897, Presidents' Papers, B:57, F:10, Special Collections Research Center, University of Chicago Library.

8. 027/01/01, F:3, 23 October 1896, 13 May 1898, 26 April 1899, 28 November 1899, 20 April 1900, University Archives, University of Illinois at Chicago. On 9 March 1899, at the age of forty-one, Benson died of acute nephritis aggravated by influenza. Benson's health had not been good for more than a year; see "Obituary," *Plexus* 4 (March 1899): 222–23. Surely P&S officials could have found some way to deal with the problem other than by firing Benson.

9. *20th Report* (1901), 291–95 (quotation on 291), 125.

10. 027/01/05/02, F:1, 131 (28 April 1899), University Archives, University of Illinois at Chicago.

11. Draper to Pusey, 27 April 1899, 2/4/3, B:5, Ltrbk. 17.

12. *20th Report,* 77, 93–94.

13. 027/01/05/02, F:1, 133–34 (16 May 1899), 137–39 (29 May 1899), University Archives, University of Illinois at Chicago.

14. Quine to the Board of Trustees, 12 May 1899, 1/1/6, Board of Trustees Secretary's File, B:4, F:6/13 and 6/14/99; Draper to Quine, 13 May 1899, Draper to Mrs. Quine, 23 May 1899, Draper to Quine, 19 June 1899, 2/4/3, Andrew S. Draper, Ltrbk. B:5, Ltrbk. 17; *20th Report* (1901), 94.

15. *20th Report* (1901), 93.

16. Ibid., 94.

17. 027/01/05/02, F:2, 140–42, University Archives, University of Illinois at Chicago.

18. *20th Report* (1901), 119.

19. Ibid., 125–26. The board adopted the rules by a vote of 6 to 3. Trustee Samuel A. Bullard first voted negative but then changed his vote to affirmative so that he could move reconsideration of the matter at the next board meeting.

20. Ibid., 238, 241, 245–46, 247–53 (the contract); 027/01/01, F:3, 1 March 1900, University Archives, University of Illinois at Chicago. On the negotiations leading to the contract, see also Draper to [Trustee] Lucy Flower, 15 November, 14 December 1899, 2/4/3, Andrew S. Draper Letterbooks, B:5, Ltrbk. 19; Draper to [Trustee] Augustus F. Nightingale, 20 and 22 January 1900, 2/4/3, Andrew S. Draper Letterbooks, B:6, Ltrbk. 20; and John P. Wilson to Draper, 16 December 1899, 2/5/5, B:22, F:P & S—Early Correspondence.

21. See, for example, the *Illini,* 14 February 1900, p. 1.

22. 027/01/01, F:3, 26 June 1900–December 1903 passim, University Archives, University of Illinois at Chicago.

23. Ibid., 13 May 1898, 26 April 1899, 20 April 1900, 19 September 1900, 2 April, and 14 May 1901, 2 January 1902, 26 June 1903, 26 May 1904, and 10 May 1905.

24. *The Chicago Blue Book of Selected Names of Chicago and Suburban Towns . . . for the Year Ending 1910* (Chicago: Chicago Directory Company, [1910]), 550, 664, 692; 2/5/7, Diary entries, 3 March and 18 April 1914 (chauffeurs); W. A. Pusey, "Faculty Department," *Plexus* 2 (April 1896): 11 (the quotations).

25. *22nd Report* (1904), 20–23.

26. Council, 475; *Alumni Record,* 253; the *Illio 1912,* 436; W. L. Abbott, "How the University of Illinois Acquired Its College of Medicine," 8 June 1939, 5–7, 2/9/1, Arthur C. Willard General Correspondence, B:37, F:Medicine, College of March–August.

27. Council, 725; Allan B. Kanavel, "Albert J. Ochsner, 1858–1925," *Proceedings of the Institute of Medicine of Chicago* (1926): 47–50; Ingals to President William R. Harper, 4 January 1898, 17 January 1899, Presidents' Papers, 1889–1925, B:57, F:11, 12, Special Collections Research Center, University of Chicago Library; Ravitch, *A Century of Surgery,* 1:246; William J. Mayo and Franklin H. Martin, "Memoir—Albert J. Ochsner," *Surgery, Gynecology and Obstetrics* 41 (September 1925): 255–58; obituary in *JAMA* 85 (1 August 1925): 374 (the quotation).

28. "Bernard Fantus, M.D.," the *Illio 1909,* [145]; *Alumni Record,* 57–58; Bernard Fantus, ed., "The Therapy of the Cook County Hospital," *JAMA* 109 (10 July 1937): 128–31; Bernard Fantus, "Cook County's Blood Bank," *Modern Hospital* 50 (January 1938): 57–58; Raymond B. Allen to Carl Stephens, 12 January 1943, 26/1/20, Carl Stephens Papers, B:9, F:Medicine; Gert H. Brieger, "Hektoen, Ludvig," *Dictionary of Scientific Biography,* 6:233.

29. The *Illio 1911,* 402; *Alumni Record,* 254.

30. Charles S. Bacon, "Autobiography," 027/8/20/02, Charles S. Bacon Papers, 1895–1947, University Archives, University of Illinois at Chicago; Stone, *Biography of Eminent American Physicians and Surgeons,* 20–21.

31. Kate Campbell Hurd-Mead, *A History of Women in Medicine: From the Earliest Times to the Beginning of the Nineteenth Century* (Haddam, Conn.: Haddam, 1938); Norwood, *Medical Education in the United States before the Civil War,* 407–8.

32. Thomas N. Bonner, *To the Ends of the Earth: Women's Search for Education in Medicine* (Cambridge: Harvard University Press, 1992), 13–16; Bonner, *Becoming a Physician,* 312–15.

33. Norwood, *Medical Education in the United States before the Civil War,* 408–15; Mary Roth Walsh, *"Doctors Wanted: No Women Need Apply": Sexual Barriers in the Medical Profession, 1835–1975* (New Haven, Ct.: Yale University Press, 1977), xiv, 27–32, 61, 180; Regina M. Morantz-Sanchez, *Sympathy and Science: Women Physicians in American Medicine* (New York: Oxford University Press, 1985), 47–89, 247–48; Bonner, *To the Ends of the Earth,* 16–30; Helga Ruud, "Woman's Medical College of Chicago," in Davis, *History of Medical Practice in Illinois,* 2:441–49. See also Avis Smith et al., eds., *Woman's Medical School Northwestern University (Woman's Medical College of Chicago): The Institution and Its Founders; Class Histories, 1870–1896* (Chicago: H. G. Cutler, 1896), and Esther P. Lovejoy, *Women Doctors of the World* (New York: Macmillan, 1957), 88–94.

34. Dorothy Gies McGuigan, *A Dangerous Experiment: 100 Years of Women at the University of Michigan* (Ann Arbor: Center for Continuing Education of Women, 1970), 38 (the quotation); Walsh, "Doctors Wanted: No Women Need Apply," 176–77; Morantz-Sanchez, *Sympathy and Science,* 71; Ruth Bordin, *Women at Michigan: The "Dangerous Experiment," 1870s to the Present* (Ann Arbor: University of Michigan Press, 1999), updates McGuigan but says little about women in medicine.

35. Victor Robinson, "Elizabeth Blackwell," *Medical Life* 35 (July 1928): 327–28; Kate C. Hurd-Mead, *Medical Women of America* (New York: Froben, 1933), 25; Morantz-Sanchez, *Sympathy and Science,* 79–80. These and other secondary sources relate the episode described, but the episode cannot be substantiated from Rush Medical College records. I have not been able to locate the journal of the Illinois State Medical Society for these years.

36. Heather J. Stecklein, archivist, Rush University Medical Center Archives, to author, 30 May and 2 June 2006.

37. Ingals to Harper, undated, Presidents' Papers, 1889–1925, B:57, F:11, Special Collections Research Center, University of Chicago Library. Effa V. Davis graduated from Woman's Medical College of Chicago in 1891 (after she joined the Rush Medical College faculty). Smith et al., *Woman's Medical School Northwestern University (Woman's Medical College of Chicago),* 112.

38. *The Illinois Medical Blue Book* (Chicago: Milton E. Lowitz & Co, 1901), 157.

39. It is often difficult to identify women from names on lists of matriculants or graduates. The entry on Ora Byrd Standard in the American Medical Association's *Directory of Deceased Physicians* indicates that this person is female. I thank Heather J. Stecklein, archivist of Rush University Medical Center Archives, for help on this point.

40. Helga Ruud, "Woman's Medical College of Chicago," in Davis, *History of Medical Practice in Illinois,* 2:448; Harper to Ingals, 7 January, 1 February 1902, and Ingals to Harper, 8 and 28 January 1902, Presidents' Papers, 1880–1925, B:57, F:14, Special Collections Research Center, University of Chicago Library.

41. Council, 645; Kevin B. Leonard, Northwestern University Archives, to author, 24 and 25 May 2006.

42. *19th Report* (1898), 134; Solberg, *The University of Illinois, 1894–1904,* 252–53.

43. *Alumni Record,* 52, 53, 54. I am indebted to Ms. Susan Glover of the University Archives, University of Illinois at Chicago, and Mr. Ron Sims, Special Collections librarian,

Galter Health Sciences Library, Northwestern University, Chicago, for help in working out the details on these women students.

44. No information is available on the educational preparation of one of the seven, Sally Yingst.

45. The grades of Jenny Lind Phillips at Woman's Medical College were generally in the 80s, while Eunice B. Hamill's grades were better (a low of 78 in materia medica in the second year and a high of 98 in gynecology). I am grateful to Mr. Ron Sims, Special Collections librarian, Galter Health Sciences Library, Northwestern University, Chicago, for providing these details. On Hamill's rank in 1898, see "Roll of Honor," *Plexus* 4 (May 1898): 13.

46. *Alumni Record,* 56–63.

47. William E. Quine, "Woman's Sphere," *Plexus* 9 (January 1904): 303–4.

48. "Faculty Department," *Plexus* 4 (June 1898): 40; *The Illio 1901,* 98; "Senior Notes," *Plexus* 4 (September 1898): 79; *The Illio 1900,* 56.

49. William H. Browne (superintendent of the College of Physicians and Surgeons) to Abraham Flexner, 25 June 1909, C:23, F:University of Illinois, 1906–1907, Papers of Abraham Flexner, Manuscripts Division, Library of Congress, Washington, D.C.

50. 027/01/05/02, F:1, 116, 150–52, University Archives, University of Illinois at Chicago; Draper to Lucy L. Flower, 17 February 1899, Draper to James E. Armstrong, 17 and 21 February 1899, and Draper to Quine, 20 and 23 February 1899, 2/4/3, Andrew S. Draper Letterbooks, Ltrbks. 15, 16; *20th Report* (1901), 291.

51. University of Illinois, *Catalogue of the University of Illinois, 1897–1898,* 17. Information on faculty appointments is not entirely reliable. P&S faculty records do not always mention appointments, while catalogs and biographical dictionaries often disagree on details.

52. *Polk's Medical Register and Directory of North America, 1902,* 539; *Alumni Record,* 262.

53. *Alumni Record,* 256; Cutler, 480, 483–84; 027/01/05/01, F:1, 55, University Archives, University of Illinois at Chicago.

54. *Alumni Record,* 286 (Yarros); Council, 904 (Wynekoop), 906 (Yarros).

55. Regular medicine's stand against women physicians may have driven them to sectarian medical schools. Haller, *Medical Protestants,* 152–56. Alternative medical schools had a high proportion of women medical students. Between 1853 and 1920 a total of 118 women graduated from the Eclectic Medical Institute of Cincinnati (26 in the 1850s, 0 in the 1860s, 9 in the 1870s, 32 in the 1880s, 33 in the 1890s, 8 in the 1900s, and 10 from 1910 to 1919). Haller, *A Profile in Alternative Medicine,* 97–98, 167–69. Of 765 graduates in osteopathy up to 1900, 183 (23.9 percent) were women; see Gevits, *The DOs,* 204n42.

56. *Alumni Record,* 242.

57. *Woman's Medical College of Chicago,* 108, 109; Council, 621 (Kearsley).

58. *Woman's Medical College of Chicago,* 118 (Wynekoop, Dowiatt), 119 (Young); *Alumni Record,* 265 (Lapham), 268 (McEwen), 262 (Horton); Council, 907 (Young), 645 (Lapham). Mr. Ron Sims, Special Collections librarian, Galter Health Sciences Library, Northwestern University, Chicago, has verified and supplemented my information on women graduates of Woman's Medical College of Chicago and Northwestern University Woman's Medical School.

59. *Alumni Record,* 245, 56 (Beedy), 259, 74 (Gould).

60. Ibid., 251.

61. Ibid., 284; Cutler, 504, 507–8; Katharine W. Wright, "History of Women in Medicine, a Symposium: Nineteenth Century or Transitional Period," 19. I am indebted to Ms. Micaela Sullivan-Fowler, head of Historical Collections, Ebling Library for the Health Sciences, University of Wisconsin, for a copy of Wright's article, which lacks publications data.

62. Christopher Lasch, "Yarros, Rachelle Slobodinsky," in *Notable American Women, 1607–1950: A Biographical Dictionary,* 3 vols., ed. Edward T. James, 3:693–94 (Cambridge: Belknap Press of Harvard University Press, 1971); Marilyn E. Perry, "Yarros, Rachelle," *Dictionary of American Biography,* 24:110–11 (not entirely reliable); Alice Hamilton, *Exploring the Dangerous Trades: The Autobiography of Alice Hamilton* (Boston: Little, Brown, 1943), 43.

63. 027/01/05/02, F:1, 132, 151, 169, and 027/01/05/01, F:1, 23, 24, University Archives, University of Illinois at Chicago.

64. College of Medicine, *Annual Announcement, 1898–1899 to 1904–1905,* University Archives, University of Illinois at Chicago; Council, 906; Hamilton, *Exploring the Dangerous Trades,* 110; Morantz-Sanchez, *Sympathy and Science,* 290, 295–96; James Reed, *From Private Vice to Public Virtue: The Birth Control Movement and American Society since 1830* (New York: Basic Books, 1978), 117, 236–37.

65. University of Illinois, *Catalogue for 1902–03,* 22; Regina M. Morantz, "Van Hoosen, Bertha," in *Notable American Women: The Modern Period; A Biographical Dictionary,* ed. Barbara Sicherman and Carol Hurd Green, 706–7 (Cambridge: Belknap Press of Harvard University Press, 1980); Wright, "History of Women in Medicine, a Symposium: Nineteenth Century or Transitional Period," 20–21.

66. Bertha Van Hoosen, *Petticoat Surgeon* (Chicago: Pellegrini and Cudahy, 1947), 108 (the quotation), 135, 136–37. Mary Thompson Hospital for Women and Children was founded in 1865.

67. Ibid., 138.

68. Ibid., 139.

69. Ibid., 139–41.

70. 2/5/7, Diary entry, 18 October 1917.

71. Lovejoy, *Women Doctors of the World,* 95.

72. "Co-Education in Medical Colleges," *Woman's Medical Journal* 11 (January 1901): 13–14.

73. *Alumni Record,* 74.

Chapter 6. The Quine Library and the Students

1. "Library Notes," *Plexus* 4 (September 1898): 75.

2. Bayard Holmes, "Medical Education in Chicago in 1882 and After: V. Medical Libraries in Chicago," *Medical Life* 28 (November 1921): 574.

3. Bayard Holmes, "The Medical Library for the Medical School or the Small Community," *Bulletin of the American Academy of Medicine* 2 (August 1895): 247–301.

4. John B. Murphy often combed the medical literature in search of guidance before proceeding with a surgical operation.

5. "Library Notes," *Plexus* 3 (March 1898): 224–25; "Library Notes," *Plexus* 3 (April 1898): 244–45; "Library Notes," *Plexus* 4 (May 1898): 17; "Library Notes," *Plexus* 4 (September 1898): 75–76; "Library Notes," *Plexus* 5 (May 1899): 39–40.

6. "Library Notes," *Plexus* 4 (September 1898): 75–76.

7. 027/01/05/01, F:1, 14 December 1897, pp. 97–98, and 027/01/01, F:3, 18 January 1898, University Archives, University of Illinois at Chicago; William A. Pusey, "The Quine Library," in "William Edward Quine," *University of Illinois Bulletin* 20(39) (28 May 1923): 41–43; "Editorial," *Plexus* 4 (June 1898): 38–39; "Library Notes," *Plexus* 4 (September 1898): 75–76; "The Medical Department of the University of Illinois," [c. 1912], p. 5, 2/5/5, B:18, F:James, Edmund J. Addresses and Publications.

8. 027/01/05/02, F:1, 12 May 1896, University Archives, University of Illinois at Chicago; "Editorial," *Plexus* 2 (January 1897): 177; "Library Notes," *Plexus* 5 (November 1899): 269–72; "Library Notes," *Plexus* 5 (January 1900): 319–21; "The Quine Library," *Plexus* 9 (March 1904): 403–4.

9. *The Illio 1903*, 125; *The Illio 1908*, 147; *The Illio 1911*, 398–400.

10. Quine to James, 13 February and 17 December 1905, 2/5/5, B:22, F:P. & S.—1905 Legislative Campaign; *23rd Report* (1906), 311.

11. On 3 May 1911 Ernest Ingold, a former student at Urbana, sent James a newspaper clipping with an account of the request. 2/5/3, B:21, F:G–I 1909–11.

12. James to Wood, 26 September 1913, Wood to James, 30 September, 7 October 1913, 13 January 1914, James to Wood, 20 January 1914, 2/5/6, B:43, F:Casey A. Wood.

13. George P. Dreyer (chairman of Library Committee) to James, 31 July 1916, 2/5/3, B:81, F:Dreyer, Geo. P.; Edmund J. James, "Biennial Report of the University of Illinois," in *Thirty-first Biennial Report of the Superintendent of Public Instruction of the State of Illinois, 1914–1916* (Springfield, 1917), 436.

14. Steele to James, 3 September, 19 October 1910, 2/5/5, B:25, F:D. A. K. Steele. Steele wrote "Iowa State University." His reference should be to the State University of Iowa.

15. The data in tables 3 and 5 are from the "Summaries of Students" in the published reports of the board of trustees. See also the enrollment figures in Edmund J. James, "University of Illinois," in *Twenty-eighth Biennial Report of the Superintendent of Public Instruction of the State of Illinois, . . . 1908–1910* (Springfield, 1911), 606, for the years from 1903–4 to 1909–10, and Edmund J. James, "University of Illinois," in *Thirty-first Biennial Report of the Superintendent of Public Instruction of the State of Illinois . . . 1914–1916* (Springfield, 1911), 437, for the years from 1903–4 to 1915–16. I have ignored an occasional minor discrepancy in the totals of the different sources.

16. The data in Table 4 are from the *Alumni Record*, 50, 56, 64, 72, 81, 94, 106.

17. See n. 15.

18. Morantz-Sanchez, *Sympathy and Science*, 249.

19. *The Illio 1911*, 414.

20. "Notes from the Seniors," *Plexus* 1 (October 1895): 9; "Among the Boys," ibid., 10–11; "'98 Class Department," ibid., 12–13; "Among the Fellows," ibid., 13.

21. *The Illio 1899*, 54.

22. "The College Button," *Plexus* 1 (December 1895): 41; "Our College Button," *Plexus* 2 (December 1896): 168.

23. "Class Day and Commencement Programs," *Plexus* 2 (April 1896): 16, published the programs for both events. See also J. B. Murphy, "Doctorate Address before the Graduating Class of '96," *Plexus* 2 (May 1896): 31–36, and "Prof. Quine's Charge to the Graduating Class," *Plexus* 2 (June 1896): 54–57.

24. S. C. Garber, "Valedictory," *Plexus* 4 (May 1898): 6–11.

25. 027/01/05/02, F:1, 144, University Archives, University of Illinois at Chicago.

26. "Sophomore Notes," *Plexus* 6 (January 1901): 332–33.

27. 027/01/05/01, F:1, 113, University Archives, University of Illinois at Chicago.

28. Ibid., 116.

29. The three students were Serge Androp, William Crapple, and Charles W. Stigman. Correspondence related to this case is in 2/5/5, B:25, F:Suspended Juniors. Only Stigman graduated (*Alumni Record,* 198).

30. J. B. Murphy, "A Rare Case of Strangulated Hernia," *Plexus* 1 (October 1895): 3–5; John A. Benson, "The Value of Physiological Study," *Plexus* 1 (February 1896): 86–90; Adolph Gehrmann, "Bacteriology: A Popular Science," *Plexus* 3 (October 1897): 83–87; Carl Beck, "Our Methods of Studying Surgical Pathology," *Plexus* 4 (June 1898): 27–30; William E. Quine, "Aortic Aneurism—A Clinical Lecture," *Plexus* 4 (December 1898): 149–54; Charles S. Williamson, "Hodgkin's Disease," *Plexus* 9 (July 1903): 71–78.

31. "Prof. Quine's Charge to the Graduating Class," *Plexus* 2 (June 1896): 54–57; W. T. Eckley, "Facial Expression," *Plexus* 3 (December 1897): 129–31; Weller van Hook, "Billroth and Pean," *Plexus* 4 (June 1898): 31–36; D. A. K. Steele, "Character As an Element of Success," *Plexus* 4 (September 1898): 54–65; Andrew S. Draper, "The Personal Equation in the Medical Profession," *Plexus* 9 (June 1903): 37–42.

32. "Prof. Newman's Berlin Letter," *Plexus* 4 (January 1899): 174–76.

33. George P. Dreyer, "The College of Physicians and Surgeons: A Retrospect and a Forecast," *Plexus* 9 (October 1903): 177–92.

34. 027/01/05/02, F:1, 115–16, 146, University Archives, University of Illinois at Chicago.

35. 027/01/05/01, F:1, 136–38, 30 May 1901, University Archives, University of Illinois at Chicago.

36. Student, "To Improve Medical Colleges," *Plexus* 2 (April 1896): 20.

37. 027/01/05/02, F:1, 99–101, University Archives, University of Illinois at Chicago.

38. The *Illio 1906,* 100.

39. Patricia Spain Ward, "Old P & S in the Days of Carl Beck," *Bibliographiti: Friends of the Library of the Health Sciences* 9 and 10 (July 1984): 4.

40. Van Hoosen, *Petticoat Surgeon,* 138.

41. The *Illio 1904,* 82. On William T. Eckley, see the *Alumni Record,* 255, and the *Illio 1907,* 106.

42. Charles E. Husk, "Clinical Department, College of Physicians and Surgeons," *Plexus* 3 (June 1897): 46–47; J. S. Nagel, "Clinical Department, College of Physicians and Surgeons," *Plexus* 3 (March 1898): 222; "Clinical Department, College of Physicians and Surgeons," *Plexus* 4 (June 1898): 42; "Clinical Department, College of Physicians and Surgeons," *Plexus* 4 (November 1898): 131.

43. The *Illio 1901,* 91.

44. "Editorial," *Plexus* 9 (February 1904): 342–43.

45. A. L. Benedict, "The Life of a Medical Student," *Lippincott's Monthly Magazine* 58 (September 1896): 394; Bonner, *Becoming a Physician,* 316–18.

46. The *Illio 1902,* 113; the *Illio 1900,* 56.

47. "Sophomore Notes," *Plexus* 13 (November 1907): 469–70; James B. Herrick, *Memories of Eighty Years* (Chicago: University of Chicago Press, 1949), 45–46, describes the practice at Rush Medical College.

48. Van Hoosen, *Petticoat Surgeon,* 141–42; *The Illio 1904,* 81.

49. *20th Report* (1901), 291.

50. Winton U. Solberg, "Harmless Pranks or Brutal Practices? Hazing at the University of Illinois, 1868–1913," *Journal of the Illinois State Historical Society* 91 (Winter 1998): 233–59.

51. The *Illio 1901,* 99.

52. "Freshman Notes," *Plexus* 3 (April 1898): 250.

53. The *Illio 1907,* 113.

54. The *Illio 1913,* 479; "News," *Illinois Medical Journal,* 16 (November 1909): 627.

55. *19th Report* (1898), 235.

56. 027/01/05/02, F:1, 97, University Archives, University of Illinois at Chicago.

57. "P. & S. Shuts Rush Out and Victory Is Ours to the Tune of 8–0," *Plexus* 3 (November 1897): 117–19.

58. 027/01/05/02, F:1, 98, 101–2, 115, University Archives, University of Illinois at Chicago.

59. 027/01/05/01, F:1, 25, 34, University Archives, University of Illinois at Chicago.

60. Ibid., 64–69.

61. Ibid., 69–70.

62. The *Illio 1901,* 118.

63. The *Illio 1900,* 59; 027/01/05/02, F:1, 186, University Archives, University of Illinois at Chicago.

64. See the documents in 2/5/3, B:73, F:YMCA-Chicago.

65. Douglas F. Robbins (the executive secretary), "A Report," 1 May 1914, 2/5/3, B:57, F:YMCA-Chicago.

66. "Y.M.C.A. Notes," *Plexus* 9 (February 1904): 355.

67. 027/01/05/01, F:1, 117–18, University Archives, University of Illinois at Chicago; the *Illio 1906,* 109.

68. James to L. Wilbur Messer, 12 January 1914, William J. Parker to James, 17 January 1914, 2/5/3, B:57, F:YMCA-Chicago.

69. Jack L. Anson and Robert F. Marchesani Jr., eds., *Baird's Manual of American College Fraternities,* 20th ed. (Indianapolis: Baird's Manual Foundation, 1991), Part I:19 and Part V:34–36, 47–49, 69–70, 88–90.

70. The *Illio 1899,* 138–39; the *Illio 1904,* 92–93.

71. "Phi Rho Sigma," *Plexus* 1 (February 1896): 105; the *Illio 1902,* 118–19; the *Illio 1903,* 129; the *Illio 1904,* 96–97.

72. The *Illio 1901,* 112–13; the *Illio 1904,* 100–1; the *Illio 1911,* 416–17.

73. The *Illio 1902,* 128–29.

74. The *Illio 1904,* 104–5; the *Illio 1911,* 422–23; the *Illio 1915,* 468–69.

75. The *Illio 1907,* 126–27; the *Illio 1911,* 420–21.

76. The *Illio 1912,* 452–53.

77. The *Illio 1913,* 492–93.

78. The *Illio 1913,* 496–97.

79. The *Illio 1907,* 113.

80. The *Illio 1901,* 114–15; the *Illio 1903,* 131; the *Illio 1912,* 454–55.

81. The *Illio 1902,* 126; the *Illio 1903,* 132; the *Illio 1904,* 107–9; the *Illio 1907,* 129.

82. William W. Root, "A Brief Account of the Origin of Alpha Omega Alpha Honor Fraternity," *Pharos* (November 1952): 3–4; Ernest S. Moore to D. J. Davis, 24 March 1941, 86/01/20, B:9, F:Medicine, University Archives, University of Illinois at Chicago; *Baird's Manual of American College Fraternities,* Part VI:116–18.

83. The *Illio 1917,* 303.

84. The *Illio 1900,* 57.

Chapter 7. Early Years of the College of Medicine under President James

1. William Rainey Harper to James, 29 February 1904, 2/5/1, Edmund J. James Personal Correspondence, B:4, F:Correspondence, 1901–4.

2. Winton U. Solberg, "James, Edmund Janes," *American National Biography,* 11:813–14.

3. 2/5/7, Diary entry, 13 November 1914.

4. Howard S. Berliner, "A Larger Perspective on the Flexner Report," *International Journal of Health Services* 5 (1975): 574–75, notes a "general scientism" in American thought around 1910.

5. Edmund J. James, "The Function of the State University," in *Installation of Edmund Janes James . . . as President of the University of Illinois,* Part IV (Urbana, 1906), 131–54 (quotation on 135).

6. Edmund J. James, "The Relation of the University of Illinois to Medical Education," *Illinois Medical Journal* 19 (January 1911): 82–92. An offprint is in 52/1/812, Historical File, B:1, F:1911–13.

7. Edmund J. James, "The University of Illinois and Medical Education," *Alumni Quarterly* 6 (July 1912): 197–98.

8. Edmund J. James, "The Place of the Medical School in the American University," *Quarterly Bulletin of the Northwestern University Medical School* 4 (December 1902): 288–94.

9. Donald L. Miller, *City of the Century: The Epic of Chicago and the Making of America* (New York: Simon & Schuster, 1996); William Cronon, *Nature's Metropolis: Chicago and the Great West* (New York: Norton, 1991); Henry Harrison Lewis, "Chicago—The Evolution of a Great City," *Harper's Weekly* 49 (1905): 1558–64; Robert P. Howard, *Illinois: A History of the Prairie State* (Grand Rapids, Mich.: Eerdmans, 1972), 575.

10. Edmund J. James, "The Importance and Significance of the Northwestern University Building to the Educational Life of Chicago," *Quarterly Bulletin of the Northwestern University Medical School* 4 (December 1902): 295–97; Edmund J. James, *The Opportunity of Chicago to Become a Great City* (Chicago, 1903), reprinted from *The World Review.* See also Bonner, *Medicine in Chicago,* 19–43, 84–122.

11. James to Henry S. Pritchett, 8 November 1910, 2/5/3, B:19, F:Carnegie Foundation.

12. Stone, *Biography of Eminent American Physicians and Surgeons,* 479–80.

13. Ibid., 415; Sperry, *A Group of Distinguished Physicians and Surgeons of Chicago,* 69–72; "In Memory and Appreciation of Dr. Quine," *Illinois Alumni News* 1 (February 1923): 138–39 (quotation on 139); William K. Beatty, "William E. Quine, A Splendid Listener," *Proceedings of the Institute of Medicine* 37(2) (1984): 44–51; Council, 764.

14. Bayard Holmes, "Medical History of Chicago," 333.

15. Ibid.

16. University of Illinois, *Register for 1904–1905,* 26–33; *23rd Report* (1906), xv–xx; College of Medicine, *Annual Announcement, 1904–1905.*

17. Stone, *Biography of Eminent American Physicians and Surgeons,* 703; Sperry, *A Group of Distinguished Physicians and Surgeons of Chicago,* 203–6.

18. "Charles Spencer Williamson," *The Illio 1912,* 437; *Alumni Record,* 285–86.

19. This paragraph is based on University of Illinois catalogs and biographical information in the *Alumni Record,* 242–86, passim.

20. *23rd Report* (1906), 24 (the date was 13 December 1904); James to Quine, 19 December 1904; 17 January 1905, 2/5/4, B:1, Ltrbk. 36; Steele to James, 24 January 1905, 2/5/5, B:22, F:P. & S. 1905 Legislative Campaign Correspondence.

21. Steele to James, 28 December 1904, 2/5/5, B:22, F:P. & S. 1905 Legislative Campaign Correspondence.

22. William J. Hynes to Oscar A. King, D. A. K. Steele, and William M. Harsha, n.d. [1905], 2/5/5, B:24, F:Med School Memoranda, 1911–12.

23. James to Steele, 17 January 1905, 2/5/4, B:1, Ltrbk. 36; Oscar A. King, D. A. K. Steele, and William A. Harsha to James, 24 January 1905, 2/5/5, B:22, F:P. & S. 1905 Legislative Campaign Correspondence.

24. James to Quine, 24 January 1905, 2/5/4, B:1, Ltrbk. 36.

25. James to King, 17 January 1905, 2/5/5, B:22, F:P. & S. 1905 Legislative Campaign Correspondence. James described as his own the view of "a very influential man in Chicago." Most likely the man was Harlow N. Higinbotham (1838–1919), a prominent merchant and civic leader, president of the World's Columbian Exposition from 1892 to its close, and president of the Field Museum of Natural History from 1897 to 1909. Higinbotham cited the example of Hahnemann Medical College, whose trustees were said to be willing to donate their property, valued at one hundred thousand dollars, if the university would take over the school and permit the teaching of homeopathic medicine there.

26. *23rd Report* (1906), 38.

27. James to Kerrick, 4 February 1905, 2/5/4, B:1, Ltrbk. 37.

28. Several drafts of a bill along with what seems to be the final bill, dated 19 January 1905, are in 2/5/5, B:22, F:P. & S. Campaign—1905 Bills, Circulars, Etc. A copy of the bill introduced in Springfield is in 2/5/11, Edmund J. James Subject Scrapbooks, B:3, Vol. 11.

29. James to Steele, 20 January 1905, and James to Quine, 24 January 1905, 2/5/4, B:1, Ltrbk. 36; *23rd Report* (1906), 42–43.

30. [James] To the Stockholders of the College of Physicians and Surgeons, 28 March 1905; "Statement of Financial Relations of College of Physicians and Surgeons to the University of Illinois," [late March 1905]; James to Steele, 30 March 1905, 2/5/4, all in B:1, Ltrbk. 37.

31. James to Steele, 17 May 1905, James to Quine, 17 May 1905, 2/5/4, B:1, Ltrbk. 38.

32. [James] To the Members of the Corporation of College of Physicians and Surgeons of Chicago, 16 October 1906; 2/5/5, B:22, F:P. & S. 1905 Legislative Campaign Correspondence; James, Memorandum Concerning the College of P & S and Its Relations to the University of Illinois, 27 November 2006, 2/5/5, B:24, F:Med School Memoranda, 1911–12.

33. The medical building was appraised at $152,000 and the dental building at $61,000. The land of the medical school was appraised at $35,000; that of the dental school was appraised at $22,200. The equipment of the medical school was appraised at $98,156.50, and that of the dental school was appraised at $17,157.75. *24th Report* (1908), 45.

34. *24th Report* (1908), 45, 50. In a "Draft of a Proposed Law" James asked for an appropriation of five hundred thousand dollars (copy in 2/5/11, Edmund J. James Subject Scrapbooks, B:3, Vol. 11).

35. Steele to James, 27 December 1906, along with "Outline of Campaign," 2/5/5, B:22, F:Med School Legislative Campaign—1907.

36. A copy of the statement, dated 16 January 1907, is in 2/5/5, B:22, F:Med School Legislative Campaign—1907; also in 2/5/11, B:3, Vol. 11.

37. *Journal of the Senate of the Forty-fifth General Assembly of the State of Illinois* (Springfield, 1908), 315 (SB 120); *Journal of the House of Representatives of the Forty-fifth General Assembly of the State of Illinois* (Springfield, 1908), 150 (HB 244). A copy of the bill introduced in the Senate is in 2/5/11, B:3, Vol. 11.

38. James to Steele, 23 February 1907, and Steele to James, 25 February 1907 (two letters), 2/5/5, B:22, F:Med School Legislative Campaign—1907.

39. Copies of these documents are in 2/5/11, B:3, Vol. 11. On Busse, see Maureen A. Flanagan, "Fred A. Busse: A Silent Mayor in Turbulent Times," in *The Mayors: The Chicago Political Tradition,* 3rd ed., ed. Paul M. Green and Melvin G. Hollis, 50–60 (Carbondale: Southern Illinois University Press, 2005).

40. *Chicago Tribune,* n.d.; *Chicago American,* 16 February 1907; *Chicago Evening American,* 16 February 1907, clippings in 2/5/11, B:3, Vol. 11.

41. *Inter Ocean,* 20 February 1907, clipping in 2/5/11, B:3, Vol. 11.

42. H. S. Spalding, "The Beginning of the Loyola University Medical School and an Account of the School during the First Ten Years," p. 18, William F. Kane File, University Archives, Loyola University of Chicago. Spalding's perception was close to the truth. Roe acted as if he owned the school, and the heirs of the former president of Valparaiso University had to sue him to recover property that belonged to them. In February 1916 when members of the medical licensure boards of Pennsylvania, Ohio, and Michigan evaluated the Chicago College of Medicine and Surgery, one of them flatly stated that Roe was the owner of the college. See B. D. Harrison to John M. Baldy, 12 February 1916, 2/5/3, B:83, F:Eycleshymer, A. C.

43. Roe to Steele, 14 February 1907, 2/5/5, B:22, F:Med School Legislative Campaign—1907; *Illinois Medical Directory, 1910,* 20; Spalding, "The Beginning of the Loyola University Medical School and an Account of the School during the First Ten Years," 18, Loyola University of Chicago Archives; John Strietelmeier, *Valparaiso's First Century: A Centennial History of Valparaiso University* (Valparaiso: Published by the University, 1959), 40, 46, 53, 182; Mr. Mel Doering (archivist of Valparaiso University) to author, 6 December 2004.

44. Graham to James, 7 March 1907, 2/5/5, B:22, F:Med School Legislative Campaign—1907.

45. Shears to James, 16 February 1907, 2/5/5, B:22, F:Med School Legislative Campaign—1907.

46. William E. Quine, "The Medical Profession: The Causes of Its Division into Discordant Elements and the Reasons I Am Not a Homeopath," *JAMA* 32 (29 April 1899): 903–8; continued in *JAMA* 32 (6 May 1899), 980–85. Quine's two-part article was separately printed as a pamphlet, *The Medical Profession: The Causes of Its Division into Discordant Elements and the Reasons I Am Not a Homeopath* (Chicago: American Medical Association, 1899). The pamphlet is curiously called the "Third Edition."

47. Quine to James, 9 March 1907, 2/5/5. B:22, F:Med School Legislative Campaign—1907.

48. Steele to James, 25 February 1907, 3 March 1907, 2/5/5, B:22, F:Med School Legislative Campaign—1907.

49. "War of Pills Is Waged," *Chicago Tribune,* 7 March 1907.

50. James to Steele, 8 March 1907; Steele to James, 11, 12 March 1907; William A. Pusey to James, 12 March 1907; James to Pusey, 26 March 1907; Heinl to James, 27 March 1907; [James], "Draft of an Argument before the Illinois Legislature in Favor of the Acquisition of the Property of the College of Physicians and Surgeons by the University of Illinois," n.d., 17 pp., with a cover sheet titled "Memorandum in re College of Physicians and Surgeons." A revised and abbreviated version of fifteen pages was printed with the same title except for "Draft of." All in 2/5/5, B:22, F:Med School Legislative Campaign—1907.

51. Davison to James, 3 April 1907, 2/5/5, B:22, F:Med School Legislative Campaign— 1907.

52. *Journal of the House of Representatives of the Forty-fifth General Assembly of the State of Illinois* (Springfield, 1908), 472; *Chicago Post*, 4 April 1907, clipping in 2/5/11, B:3, Vol. 11.

53. Steele to James, 9 April 1907, 2/5/5, B:22, F:Med School Legislative Campaign— 1907.

54. James to Pusey, 5 April 1907, 2/5/5, B:22, F:Med School Legislative Campaign— 1907.

55. *Inter Ocean*, 9 May 1907; *Springfield Register*, 10 May 1907; *Chicago Post*, 10 May 1907 (the quotation), clippings in 2/5/11, B:3, Vol. 11.

56. *Chicago Examiner*, 12 May 1907, clipping in 2/5/11, B:3, Vol. 11; 2/5/7, Diary entry, 11 May 1904. The Journal of the House for 11 May runs to 213 pages but does not record the event.

57. "President J. F. Percy's Address to the House of Delegates," *Illinois Medical Journal* 12 (1907): 56–61, 71; *Chicago Tribune*, 23 May 1907, clipping in 2/5/11, B:3, Vol. 11.

58. Everett J. Brown to C. S. Bacon, n.d. [27 May 1907], 2/5/5, B:22, F:Medical School Legislative Campaign—1907.

59. *Chicago Examiner*, 28 May 1907, clipping in 2/5/11, B:3, Vol. 11; 2/5/7, Diary entry, 28 May 1907. Deneen's veto message is in the Illinois State Board of Health, *Monthly Bulletin* 3 (May–June 1907): 229, and in [Henry M. Dunlap], "A History of the Illinois Industrial University afterward the University of Illinois 1851–1938 as Recorded in the Acts of the Illinois General Assembly," 2 vols. (1937), 2:334, 2/9/10, B:1.

60. Bacon to James, 28 May 1907, 2/5/5, B:22, F:Med School Legislative Campaign— 1907. See also Everett J. Brown to Bacon, n.d., and J. Whitefield Smith to Bacon, 27 May 1907, 2/5/5, B:22, F:Medical School Legislative Campaign—1907.

61. Walter C. Jones, "Medical Education in Illinois," *Illinois Medical Journal* 19 (January 1911): 99–100.

62. James to Archie J. Graham, 19 July 1907, 52/38/20, B:1, F:unmarked.

63. *25th Report* (1911), 88–91.

64. Ibid., 158–62.

65. *Journal of the House of Representatives of the Forty-sixth General Assembly of the State of Illinois* (Springfield, 1909), 188, 861, 1205; a copy of the bill, HB 115, is in 2/5/5, B:20, F:Bills, etc. Legislative Campaign 1911 [*sic*].

66. *25th Report* (1911), 163; see the "General Summary of Appropriations for the University of Illinois," 2/5/5, B:20, F:Appropriations Memoranda, 1909–11.

67. 2/5/7, Diary entry, 29 July 1909.

68. [George P. Dreyer], "Report on the Scientific Departments in the Medical Schools of the State Universities of Minnesota, Wisconsin, Michigan, and Illinois," 50 pp. typescript, n.d., 2/6/5, Kinley Subject File, B:3, F:Medical School: Report on the Scientific

Departments in the Medical Schools of the State Universities of Minnesota, Wisconsin, Michigan, and Illinois, 1910.

69. Ibid., 46.

70. *Historical Statistics of the United States: Colonial Times to 1970* (Washington, D.C.: U.S. Department of Commerce, 1975), 27, 29, 30, 37, 243, 244, 245.

Chapter 8. Advancing the College of Medicine

1. Judson to James, 3 June 1909, 2/5/5, B:23, F:Medical Education 1910.

2. 2/5/7, Diary entry, 30 April 1909.

3. Judson to James, 14 May 1909; enclosing "A Suggested Plan for a Chicago School of Medicine," dated 13 May 1909, 2/5/5, B:23, F:Medical Education 1910.

4. James to Judson, 31 May 1909, 2/5/5, B:23, F:Medical Education 1910.

5. 2/5/7, Diary entries, 1 and 29 June 1909.

6. 2/5/7, Diary entry, 14 July 1909.

7. 2/5/7, Diary entries, 28 and 31 October, 15 and 17 November 1909.

8. 2/5/7, Diary entries, 23, 26, and 27 November, 5 December 1909.

9. *25th Report* (1911), 501–2.

10. Ibid., 502.

11. Ibid., 503.

12. Ibid., 503–4.

13. McWilliams listed "positions held with titles and dates" in a document dated 10 April 1911 in the Samuel A. McWilliams Necrology File in the Bentley Historical Library, University of Michigan. Ms. Karen Wight, reference assistant, helpfully supplied me with a photocopy.

14. 027/01/01, F:3, pp. 384–410 (these minutes, dated mainly in February 1910, are not in systematic order), University Archives, University of Illinois at Chicago.

15. *25th Report* (1911), 504.

16. 2/5/7, Diary entry, 3 February 1910.

17. *25th Report* (1911), 508.

18. 2/5/7, Diary entries, 4 and 8 February, 3, 9, and 15 March, 2 April 1910.

19. James to Judson, 15 February 1910, 2/5/5, B:23, F:Medical Education 1910.

20. Judson to James, 16 February 1910, 2/5/5, B:23, F:Medical Education 1910.

21. *25th Report* (1911), 540; James to W. L. Abbott, 18 April 1910, 2/5/3, B:18, F:Abbott, W. L.

22. *25th Report* (1911), 540–42.

23. Ibid., 541–42.

24. Ibid., 544, 557–58, 559–60; 2/5/7, Diary entry, 6 June 1910.

25. *25th Report* (1911), 602; Ward to James, 26 July 1910, 2/5/6, B:18, F:H. B. Ward.

26. James to Pritchett, 8 November 1910, Pritchett to James, 11 November 1910, 2/5/3, B:19, F:Carnegie Foundation.

27. 2/5/7, Diary entry, 6 June 1910.

28. James to Frank B. Earle, 21 February, 4 April 1905; 027/01/05/01, F:2, pp. 1–3, University Archives, University of Illinois at Chicago.

29. C. J. Ringnell to John M. Dodson, 7 April 1905; a note on Quine's action, 027/01/05/01, F:2, pp. 3–5, University Archives, University of Illinois at Chicago.

30. George T. Kemp, S. W. Parr, and S. A. Forbes, To the Faculty of the College of Science, 10 October 1905, 15/1/6, College of Science and College of Literature and Arts Minutebooks, B:1.

31. Ibid.

32. Townsend to Quine, 27 October 1905, 15/1/2, College of Science Letterbooks, B:2; Frank B. Earle to James, [n.d.], 027/01/05/01, F:2, p. 63; 4/2/1, Senate Minutes, 124–26; *23rd Report* (1906), 291–92.

33. *23rd Report* (1906), 328.

34. "Council on Medical Education of the American Medical Association, First Annual Conference," *JAMA* 44 (6 May 1905): 1470–75; Arthur D. Bevan, "Cooperation in Medical Education and Medical Service," *JAMA* 90 (14 April 1928): 1173–75; James G. Burrow, *AMA: Voice of American Medicine* (Baltimore: Johns Hopkins University Press, 1963), 21–26, 33–35; Fishbein, *History of the American Medical Association, 1891–97*.

35. Arthur D. Bevan and N. P. Colwell, "Report of the Council on Medical Education for the Year Ending June 1, 1907," 3, 2/5/5, B:23, F:Med Education, 1907–8. The other states and the number of their deficient medical schools were Missouri (fourteen), Maryland (eight), Kentucky (seven), and Tennessee (ten).

36. Bevan and Colwell, "Report of the Council on Medical Education for the Year Ending June 1, 1907," 3–5, 2/5/5, B:23, F:Med Education 1907–8; Bevan, "Cooperation in Medical Education and Medical Service," *JAMA*, 90 (14 April 1925), 1174–76.

37. Howard J. Savage, *Fruit of an Impulse: Forty-Five Years of the Carnegie Foundation, 1905–1950* (New York: Harcourt, Brace, 1953), 3–70; Ellen C. Lagemann, *Private Power for the Public Good: A History of the Carnegie Foundation for the Advancement of Teaching* (New York: College Entrance Examination Board, 1983), 59–74; Howard S. Berliner, "New Light on the Flexner Report: Notes on the AMA-Carnegie Foundation Background," *Bulletin of the History of Medicine* 51 (1977): 604–5.

38. Thomas N. Bonner, *Iconoclast: Abraham Flexner and a Life in Learning* (Baltimore: Johns Hopkins University Press, 2002), chaps. 1–6; Flexner, *An Autobiography*, 1–72; Savage, *Fruit of an Impulse*, 105–8; Abraham Flexner, *Henry S. Pritchett: A Biography* (New York: Columbia University Press, 1943), 109–10; Berliner, "New Light on the Flexner Report," 607.

39. Daniel M. Fox, "Abraham Flexner's Unpublished Report: Foundations and Medical Education, 1909–1928," *Bulletin of the History of Medicine* 54 (Winter 1980): 475–96.

40. F. Garvin Davenport, "John Henry Rauch and Public Health in Illinois, 1877–1891," *Journal of the Illinois State Historical Society* 50 (Autumn 1957): 277–93; Isaac D. Rawlings, *The Rise and Fall of Disease in Illinois*, 2 vols. (Springfield, Ill.: State Department of Public Health, 1927), 1:127–34, 137–54; Vaughan, *A Doctor's Memories*, 439 (the quotation).

41. Rawlings, *Rise and Fall of Disease in Illinois*, 1:159–74.

42. "Illinois and 'Rotten' Medical Education," *Illinois Medical Journal* 16 (December 1909): 723.

43. Carl E. Black, "Medical Education in Illinois," *Illinois Medical Journal* 17 (February 1910): 190–94; "Illinois and 'Rotten' Medical Education," *Illinois Medical Journal* 16 (December 1909): 723.

44. "Illinois and 'Rotten' Medical Education," *Illinois Medical Journal* 16 (December 1909): 723.

45. James A. Egan, "Illinois 'A Plague Spot in Medical Education, Medical Examination and Medical Licensure?'" Illinois State Board of Health, *Bulletin* 5 (December 1909): 578–87 (quotation on 579). George W. Webster Sr., president of the board, also signed this reply.

46. See "Meetings of the Councils on Medical Education and Medical Legislation in Chicago," *Illinois Medical Journal* 17 (March 1910): 333–35; James A. Egan, "Medical Education in Illinois—Dr. Egan Replies," *Illinois Medical Journal* 17 (March 1910): 338–40; Carl E. Black, "Medical Education in Illinois," *Illinois Medical Journal* 17 (March 1910): 344–48; J. F. Percy [president of the Illinois State Medical Society], "Some Facts about the Illinois State Board of Health," *Illinois Medical Journal* 17 (April 1910): 483–90; George W. Webster Sr., "Dr. Webster Comments on Our Editorial," *Illinois Medical Journal* 17 (April 1910): 490–1; and James A. Egan, "Letter from Dr. J. A. Egan," *Illinois Medical Journal* 17 (April 1910): 491–96.

47. Patricia Spain Ward, "The Other Abraham: Flexner in Illinois," *Caduceus* 2 (Spring 1986): 1–66 (quotations on 16–17).

48. Flexner to Pritchett, 19 April 1909; Pritchett to Flexner, 22 April 1909, C:19, F: Henry S. Pritchett 1909–10, Papers of Abraham Flexner, Manuscripts Division, Library of Congress, Washington, D.C.

49. Fogle to Flexner, 23 June 1909, C:22, F:State Board of Health Illinois 1906–1909, Papers of Abraham Flexner, Manuscripts Division, Library of Congress, Washington, D.C.

50. Quine to Flexner, 5 October 1909, C:23, F:University of Illinois 1906–9, Papers of Abraham Flexner, Manuscripts Division, Library of Congress, Washington, D.C.

51. A document on the budget submitted by the actuary, C:23, F:University of Illinois 1906–7, Papers of Abraham Flexner, Manuscripts Division, Library of Congress, Washington, D.C.

52. Flexner to Pritchett, 17 April 1909, C:19, F:Henry S. Pritchett 1909–10, Papers of Abraham Flexner, Manuscripts Division, Library of Congress, Washington, D.C.

53. Flexner to Pritchett, 7 February 1910, C:19, F:Henry S. Pritchett 1909–10, The Papers of Abraham Flexner, Manuscripts Division, Library of Congress, Washington, D.C.

54. 2/5/7, Diary entry, 8 February 1910.

55. Flexner to Pritchett, 8 February 1910, C:19, F:Henry S. Pritchett 1909–10, Papers of Abraham Flexner, Manuscripts Division, Library of Congress, Washington, D.C.

56. Ibid.

57. Ibid.

58. Berliner, "New Light on the Flexner Report," 608.

59. Robert P. Hudson, "Abraham Flexner in Historical Perspective," in *Beyond Flexner: Medical Education in the Twentieth Century,* ed. Barbara Barzansky and Norman Gevitz, 12–13 (New York: Greenwood, 1992).

60. Flexner, *Medical Education in the United States and Canada,* 19, 38, 39, 80–81.

61. Donald Fleming, "Welch, William Henry," *American National Biography,* 22:927.

62. Flexner, *Medical Education in the United States and Canada,* 216.

63. Ibid., 207–20; "Scores Chicago's Medical Schools," *Chicago Daily Tribune,* 6 June 1910, pp. 1, 6.

64. Flexner, *Medical Education in the United States and Canada,* 208–9, 219.

65. Flexner, *An Autobiography,* 87.

66. J. A. E[gan], "The Report of the Carnegie Foundation," Illinois State Board of Health, *Bulletin* 6 (June 1910): 63–78; idem, "Farcical Inspection of Medical Colleges," Illinois State Board of Health, *Bulletin* 7 (April 1911): 191–94; "Scores Chicago's Medical Schools," *Chicago Daily Tribune,* 6 June 1910, pp. 1, 6.

67. Spalding, "The Beginning of the Loyola University Medical School and an Account of the School during the First Ten Years," 6–7. For other reactions see "Scores Chicago's Medical Schools," *Chicago Daily Tribune,* 6 June 1910, p. 6; "Schools Protest on Criticism," *Chicago News,* 6 June 1910, clipping in 2/5/10.

68. "City's Medical Schools a Disgrace, Says E. J. James," *Chicago Examiner,* 7 June 1910; "City's Medical Schools Scored by Dr. James," *Chicago American,* 7 June 1910; "131 Are Made Physicians," *Chicago Post,* 7 June 1910; "James Pleads Guilty to Flexner Charges," *Chicago Record-Herald,* 7 June 1910; "O. K. on Medical School Roast," *Chicago Tribune,* 7 June 1910, clippings in 2/5/10.

69. James to Ira W. Allen, 10 June 1910, 2/5/5, B:23, F:Medical Education 1910.

70. "Raps School Critics," *Chicago Record-Herald,* 8 June 1910, clipping in 2/5/10.

71. "Insurgent M.D.'s to Assail Charter of Medical Body," *St. Louis Post-Dispatch,* 8 June 1910, clipping in 2/5/10.

72. This school is not listed among those in existence in 1904 by the authorities cited in chapter 2, note 6 above, and Flexner does not mention it in his report.

73. Charles McCormick to James, 7 June 1910, 2/5/5, B:23, F:Medical Education 1910.

74. Ibid.

75. Ibid.

76. Ibid.

77. James to McCormick, 9 June 1910, 2/5/5, B:23, F:Medical Education 1910.

78. Chicago city directories, 1902–1904, 1907; *The Chicago Blue Book,* 1907–1917; "Peace Ends War on Medic School," *Chicago Daily Tribune,* 3 May 1907.

79. Edmund J. James, "The Relation of the University of Illinois to Medical Education," *Illinois Medical Journal* 19 (January 1911): 82–92.

80. "Medical Education in Illinois," *Illinois Medical Journal* 19 (January 1911): 92–93.

81. Ibid., 93–95.

82. Ibid., 95–98.

83. Ibid., 98.

84. Ibid., 100–101.

Chapter 9. Medical Politics, Reorganization, and a Retrospect

1. *26th Report* (1912), 65, 76–78.

2. Ibid., 36–37.

3. James to Ingals, 25 October 1910, 2/5/3, B:21, F:G-I 1909–11.

4. Ingals to James, 27 October 1910; James to Ingals, 28 October 1910; Ingals to James, 29 October 1910, 2/5/3, B:21, F:G-I 1909–11.

5. 2/5/7, Diary entries, 1 and 9 December 1910, 6 January, 2 February 1911.

6. *Journal of the Senate of the Forty-seventh General Assembly of the State of Illinois* (Springfield, 1911), 226; *Journal of the House of Representatives of the Forty-seventh General Assembly of the State of Illinois* (Springfield, 1911), 312. For the text see a copy of the bills in 2/5/11, B:4, Vol. 15.

7. A copy of the council's resolutions is in 2/5/11, B:4, Vol. 15.

8. James to My dear Sir (physicians), 22 February 1911; James to My dear Sir (legislators and newspapers), 28 February 1911; James to My dear Sir (homeopathic physicians), 17 March 1911; William E. Quine to My Dear Doctor, n.d.; Edmund J. James, *To the Members of the General Assembly,* 29 March 1911 (the printed petition), all in 2/5/11, B:4, Vol. 15. The printed pamphlet is in 2/5/5, B:20, F:Legislature 1911, F:Bills, etc. Legislative Campaign 1911. Actually, twenty states had tax-supported medical schools: Alabama, California, Colorado, Indiana, Iowa, Kansas, Michigan, Minnesota*, Missouri*, Nebraska, North Carolina*, North Dakota*, Oklahoma*, South Dakota*, Tennessee, Texas, Utah*, Virginia, West Virginia*, and Wisconsin*. The nine states with an asterisk had a two-year program. This information is compiled from Flexner, *Medical Education in the United States and Canada.*

9. 2/5/7, Diary entry, 29 March 1911.

10. "Danger in the Bath," *Chicago Daily Tribune,* 10 December 1903, p. 1; "Beer Foils Malaria Bug," *Chicago Daily Tribune,* 21 October 1911, p. 3; "Water and Soap for City Health, Says Robertson," *Chicago Daily Tribune,* 2 May 1915, p. A3; "Hon. John Dill Robertson," in Dunne, *Illinois,* 5:34.

11. Quine to James, 2 August 1911, 2/5/5, B:25, F:William E. Quine.

12. 2/5/7, Diary entry, 2 April 1911.

13. *26th Report* (1912), 138–39.

14. James to Quine, 24 June 1911, 2/5/5, B:25, F:William E. Quine.

15. 2/5/7, Diary entries, 22, 24, 28 July 1911; James to Quine, 26 July 1911, 2/5/5, B:25, F:William E. Quine; E. M. Ashcraft to James, 27 July 1911, 2/5/5, B:25, F:Medical School Reorganization and Injunction Summer 1911; James to Abbott, 28 July 1911, 2/5/5, B:25, F:Abbott; *26th Report* (1912), 467–68.

16. James to Quine, 27 July 1911, 2/5/5, B:25, F:William E. Quine; James to Abbott, 28 July 1911, 2/5/5, B:25, F:Abbott.

17. Edwin Ashcraft to James, 27 July 1911, 2/5/5, B:23, F:Medical School Reorganization and Injunction Summer 1911.

18. Illinois State Board of Health, *Report on Medical Education and Official Register of Legally Qualified Physicians: 1903,* 218.

19. "In the Circuit Court of Sangamon County, August Term, A.D. 1911," p. 26, 2/5/5, B:23, F:Medical School Reorganization and Injunction Summer 1911.

20. "In the Circuit Court of Sangamon County, August Term, A.D. 1911," p. 26, 2/5/5, B:23, F:Medical School Reorganization and Injunction Summer 1911; *26th Report* (1912), 468.

21. 2/5/7, Diary entry, 9 June 1911; Pusey to James, 13 June 1911, 2/5/5, B:25, F:William A. Pusey.

22. Donald Fleming, "Welch, William Henry," *American National Biography,* 22:928 (the quotation).

23. Pusey to James, 19 June 1911 2/5/5, B:25, F:William A. Pusey. I have corrected spellings and provided full names as needed. Pusey listed R. D. Pierce at Pennsylvania. His reference should be to R. M. Pearce.

24. Ibid.

25. Ibid.

26. Ibid.

27. Herrick to James, 12 June 1911, 2/5/5, B:25, F:Elias P. Lyon.

28. James to Howell, 27 June 1911; James to Loeb, 29 June 1911; Howell to James, 1 July 1911; Loeb to James, 4 July 1911, 2/5/5, B:23, F:Elias P. Lyon.

29. James to Loeb, 7 July 1911; Loeb to James, 13 July, 1911, B:23, F:Elias P. Lyon.

30. Mall to James, 1 and 8 July 1911 (the quotation), 2/5/5, B:23, F:Med School Reorganization and Injunction Summer 1911.

31. James to Mall, 5 July 1911, 2/5/5, B:23, F:Med School Reorganization and Injunction Summer 1911.

32. Mall to James, 8 July 1911, 2/5/5, B:23, F:Med School Reorganization and Injunction Summer 1911.

33. Greenman to James, 18 July 1911, 2/5/5, B:23, F:Med School Reorganization and Injunction Summer 1911.

34. 2/5/15, Albert C. Eycleshymer Appointment File; Albert C. Eycleshymer and Daniel M. Shoemaker, *A Cross-Section Anatomy* (New York: D. Appleton Century, 1911).

35. E. P. Lyon, "Report on the College of Physicians and Surgeons," 29 June 1911 (quotations on 1–2, 7, and 3), 2/5/5, B:25, F:Elias P. Lyon.

36. Ibid., 13.

37. Pusey to James, 8 July 1911, 2/5/5, B:25, F:William A. Pusey.

38. Pusey to James, 13 July 1911, 2/5/5, B:25, F:William A. Pusey.

39. James to Pusey, 14 July 1911, 2/5/5, B:25, F:William A. Pusey.

40. James to Lyon, 18 July 1911 (draft), 20 July 1911, 2/5/5, B:25, F:Elias P. Lyon.

41. Lyon to James, 25 July 1911, 2/5/5, B:25, F:Elias P. Lyon.

42. *26th Report* (1912), 434–35.

43. Letters to James from R. R. Bensley (University of Chicago), Charles S. Minot (Harvard), Lewellys F. Barker (Johns Hopkins), and Henry B. Ward (University of Illinois); 2/5/15, Albert C. Eycleshymer Appointment File.

44. *26th Report* (1912), 468, 492; 2/5/7, Diary entry, 4 August 1911. Lyon later became dean of the University of Minnesota Medical School. See Owen Wangensteen, *Elias Potter Lyon: Minnesota's Leader in Medical Education* (St. Louis: W. H. Green, 1981).

45. Eycleshymer to James, 7 August 1911, 2/5/15, Albert C. Eycleshymer Appointment File.

46. *26th Report* (1912), 491–93.

47. Ibid., 495–504, 525–26.

48. Unsigned form letter to "Dear Doctor" on the letterhead of the Chicago Homeopathic Medical Society, n.d. [late February 1913], 2/5/5, B:25, F:Homeopaths.

49. Ingals to Harry Pratt Judson, 10 March 1912, Presidents' Papers, B:57, F:14, Special Collections Research Center, University of Chicago.

50. James to Arthur Meeker, 3 April 1912, 2/5/3, B:28, F:Arthur Meeker; Charles Davison, "The 1912–1914 Period," in *Alumni Record*, xiii; *26th Report* (1912), 578.

51. *Alumni Record*, 75; *The Illio 1913*, 470.

52. *26th Report* (1912), 578–81; Charles S. Bacon, "The Story of Legislation in 1912 and 1912 [*sic*: read 1913] Which Authorized the Trustees of the University to Create a Medical School," 6 pp. typescript in 26/1/20, Carl Stephens Papers, B:9, F:Medicine.

53. *Journals of the Senate and House of Representatives: Second and Third Special Sessions of the Forty-seventh General Assembly of the State of Illinois* (Springfield, 1912), 8 (Senate Journal), 9 (House Journal).

54. Bacon, "The Story of Legislation," 1–2.

55. *Journals of the Senate and House of Representatives: Second and Third Special Sessions of the Forty-seventh General Assembly of the State of Illinois,* 13 (Senate Journal), 10 (House Journal). The bills were for "An Act Making an Appropriation for the Equipment, Maintenance and Extension of the College of Medicine at the University of Illinois." The full text of the bills specified an appropriation of $60,000 per annum (2/5/11, B:4, Vol. 11). The $250,000 and $100,000 are reported in the [Champaign] *News,* 19 April 1912, clipping in 2/5/10.

56. James to My dear Sir, 12 April 1912, James to My dear Sir, 13 April 1912, James to Members of the Legislature, 15 April 1912, James to My dear Sir, 16 April 1912, "Statement Concerning Medical School of the University of Illinois," James to My dear Sir, 19 April 1912, 2/5/11, B:4, Vol. 11; Bacon, "The Story of Legislation," 2–3. See also [Champaign] *News,* 19 April 1912, clipping in 2/5/10.

57. Bacon, "The Story of Legislation," 4.

58. Quine, "The Medical Profession: The Causes of Its Division into Two Discordant Elements and the Reasons I Am Not a Homeopath," 982.

59. [Champaign] *News,* 23 April 1912, clipping in 2/5/10; Diary entry, 17 April 1912.

60. Bacon, "The Story of Legislation," 4.

61. Ibid., 4–5.

62. *Journals of the Senate and House of Representatives: Second and Third Special Sessions of the Forty-seventh General Assembly of the State of Illinois,* 31, 38, 43 (Senate Journal), 87 (House Journal); 2/5/7, Diary entry, 23 April 1912; "Legislature Takes Recess," [Champaign] *Gazette,* 26 April 1912, clipping in 2/5/10. The Senate Journal (p. 43) writes, "the question being, 'Shall this bill [making an appropriation for the College of Medicine] pass?' it was decided in the negative by the following vote: Yeas 20, nays, 4."

63. "Homeopaths Will Not Quit," [Champaign] *Gazette,* 17 May 1912, clipping in 2/5/10; *27th Report* (1914), 116–17; *Illinois Medical Journal,* 22 (July 1912), 80, 85, 86–90.

64. Davison, "The 1912–1914 Period," *Alumni Record,* xiii.

65. A. J. Graham, "Lobbying Days, 1913: Foundation of the College of Medicine and Dentistry, University of Illinois by the 48th General Assembly 1913–15," 34, 52/38/20, Archie J. Graham Papers, B:1.

66. 2/5/7, Diary entries, 23 and 24 May, 14 July, 23 and 26 August 1912.

67. Davison, "The 1912–1914 Period," *Alumni Record,* xiv; *27th Report* (1914), 98–99.

68. For a list of the P&S faculty stockholders as of 20 April 1900, see the statement accompanying Heintz to James, 7 October 1912, 2/5/3, B:33, F:Dr. Edward L. Heintz. See also Bayard Holmes to T. J. Burrill, 1 April 1913, 2/5/3, B:33, F:1912–13 He–Hu. E. Fletcher Ingals related the following story about Murphy and his stock holdings: "I find that my impressions regarding Dr. Murphy were not correct though they were given to me by one who thought he knew, some months ago. Instead of being a catholic, he is a very straight laced Presbyterian. There is a curious history connected with his property. I am told that a number of years ago he had saved, in a bank for investment some fifty or sixty thousand dollars which was about the sum of his earthly possessions. The bank failed and the doctor going to his surgical case took out a long knife and called upon the bank President. Upon entering the President's room he locked the door produced his knife and said to the President that unless he gave him deeds for sufficient property sufficient to cover the amount which he had in the bank he would forthwith carve him with that particular knife. The President is said to have stepped to his safe and taking out the deeds

made them over to him at once. The property at the time was not very valuable but has since grown to be immense." Ingals to William Rainey Harper, 7 June 1897, Presidents' Papers, B:57, F:9, Special Collections Research Center, University of Chicago Library. Murphy was a Roman Catholic. The story seems preposterous. It tells more about Ingals than about Murphy.

69. *27th Report* (1914), 98–99, 117; "Medical School May Be Obtained," [Champaign] *News*, 6 September 1912, clipping in 2/5/10; 2/5/7, Diary entry, 10 January 1913.

70. Heintz to James, 21 February 1913, 2/5/3, B:33, F:Dr. Edward L. Heintz; Davison, "The 1912–1914 Period," *Alumni Record*, xiv; *27th Report* (1914), 117.

71. *27th Report* (1914), 118; 2/5/7, Diary entry, 18 September 1912; Davison, "The 1912–1914 Period," *Alumni Record*, xiv.

72. James to Heintz, 12 and 23 December 1912, 2/5/3, B:33, F:Dr. Edward L. Heintz.

73. *27th Report* (1914), 118.

74. 2/5/7, Diary entries, 27 December 1912 to 24 February 1913.

75. For a list of the donations and subscriptions see the attachment to Heintz to James, 22 February 1913, 2/5/3, B:33, F:Dr. Edward L. Heintz.

76. Abbott to James, 4 February 1913, 2/5/6, B:28, F:Med School; Bacon to James, 10 March 1913, 2/5/3, B:30, F:C. S. Bacon, 1912–13.

77. *27th Report* (1914), 172–74; Davison, "The 1912–1914 Period," *Alumni Record*, xv.

78. *27th Report* (1914), 172–74.

79. Pusey, "The College of Physicians and Surgeons of Chicago," 53–55.

80. These figures for the early years of the century are compiled from reports of the Council on Medical Education in *JAMA* and from Flexner, *Medical Education in the United States and Canada*, 207–14.

81. The figures for 1904 are from the *22nd Report* (1904), 281–82. With one exception the other figures are from the lists of graduates of the College of Medicine published each June in the minutes of the board of trustees. The figures for 1912 are from the *Alumni Record*, 182–91.

82. "Medical Schools of the United States," *JAMA* 47, pt. 1 (25 August 1906): 615–16.

83. Illinois State Board of Health, *Bulletin* 2 (August 1906): 148; idem, *Annual Report* (1913), 133–34.

84. "Medical Schools of the United States," table D: Graduates of 1905 or Previous Examined by State Boards during 1905, *JAMA* 47 (25 August 1906): 612ff.

85. Arthur D. Bevan and N. P. Colwell, "Report of the Council on Medical Education for the Year Ending June 1, 1907," 10–13, 2/5/5, B:23, F:Med Education 1907–8.

86. "Medical Education and State Boards of Registration," *JAMA* 52, pt. 2 (22 May 1909): 1702–3. Graduates of the American Medical Missionary College and National Medical University had 0 percent failures. In both cases three candidates passed and none failed. The results are statistically insignificant.

87. Illinois State Board of Health, *Supplement to Bulletin* 7 (April 1911): 3–4.

88. Illinois State Board of Health, *Monthly Bulletin* 7 (August 1911): 430.

89. [Council on Medical Education], "State Board Statistics for 1911," *JAMA* 58, pt. 2 (25 May 1912): 1583–99. See also N. P. Colwell, "A Statement of the Entrance Requirements and the Didactic and Laboratory Positions of the Medical Courses at Colleges Requiring Studies beyond the High School Course Equivalent to One or More Years at College," reprint from the *Bulletin of the American Academy of Medicine* 10 (June 1909): 3, 5, in 2/5/5, B:23, F:Medical Education 1910.

Chapter 10. The University of Illinois College of Medicine

1. Edmund J. James, "Reopening of the Medical School," *Alumni Quarterly* 7 (April 1913): 67–77; *Addresses Delivered upon the Re-Opening of the Medical Department of the University of Illinois, March 6, 1913,* copy in 52/1/8/2, B:1, F:1911–1913. See also [Champaign] *Gazette,* 25 February and 5, 7, and 8 March 1913; and [Champaign] *News,* 7 March 1913, clippings in 2/5/10. Many letters and documents on the legal and financial aspects of the transfer of P&S to the University of Illinois from 1912 to 1913 are in 2/5/6, B:28, F: Med School.

2. Steele to James, 25 December 1912, 2/5/6, B:29, F:D. A. K. Steele.

3. James to George M. Kreider, 27 March 1913, 2/5/3, B:33, F:George M. Kreider.

4. The dossiers are in 2/5/5, B:21, F:Illinois Legislature 1913. The petition is in 2/5/5, B:21, F:Legislat [*sic*] (the third folder with the same title). The printed pamphlet is in 2/5/5, B:21, F:Legislature 1915.

5. Bacon to James, 28 January 1913, 2/5/3, B:30, F:C. S. Bacon.

6. *27th Report* (1914), 186–92; C. S. Bacon, "The Medical School of the University of Illinois," *Illinois Medical Journal* 23 (March 1913): 327–28.

7. Bacon to James, 8 February 1913, 2/5/3, B:30, F:C. S. Bacon.

8. Bacon to James, 24 February, 10 March 1913, 2/5/3, B:30, F:C. S. Bacon.

9. Bacon to James, 14 March 1913, 2/5/3, B:30, F:C. S. Bacon.

10. 2/5/7, Diary entries, 7 January to 15 January 1913.

11. Lawson to James, 5 March 1912, 2/5/3, B:34, F:Victor F. Lawson.

12. James to Lawson, 10 March 1913, 2/5/3, B:34, F:Victor F. Lawson.

13. Quine, "History of the College of Physicians and Surgeons of Chicago," 69.

14. Bacon to James, 10 March 1913, 2/5/3, B:30, F:C. S. Bacon.

15. Ibid.

16. Bacon to James, 12 March 1913, 2/5/3, B:30, F:C. S. Bacon.

17. Ibid.

18. Steele to James, 21 April 1915, James to Steele, 7 May 1915, 2/5/6, B:55, F:Steele, DAK February–May 1915.

19. Bacon to James, 15 March 1913, 2/5/3, B:30, F:C. S. Bacon.

20. Bacon to James, 14 May 1913, 2/5/3, B:30, F:C. S. Bacon.

21. Steele to James, n.d. [1 April 1913], James to Steele, 2 April 1913, 2/5/6, B:29, F:D. A. K. Steele.

22. Harry C. Koenig, ed., *A History of the Parishes of the Archdiocese of Chicago,* 2 vols. (Chicago: Archdiocese of Chicago, 1980), 2:1653–56. St. Jarlath Church, founded in 1869, was located at Jackson Boulevard and Hermitage Avenue, a bit north of the College of Medicine. In 1913 the Reverend Thomas F. Cashman was the pastor at St. Jarlath. In 1969 the church was consolidated and its buildings torn down.

23. E. W. Fiegenbaum to Bacon, 15 April 1913, 2/5/3, B:30, F:C. S. Bacon.

24. Bacon to Fiegenbaum, 17 April 1913, 2/5/3, B:30, F:C. S. Bacon.

25. Bacon to James, 17 April 1913, 2/5/3, B:30, F:C. S. Bacon.

26. Edmond Beall to Fiegenbaum, 5 May 1913; James to Arthur W. Stillians, 8 May 1913, 2/5/6, B:28, F:Med School; A. J. Graham to James, 13 May 1913, 2/5/3, B:30, F:C. S. Bacon.

27. *Daily News,* editorials 10, 11, and 13 May 1913; Bacon's letter, 14 May 1913, and clippings in 2/5/3, B:30, F:C. S. Bacon.

28. Bacon to James, 8 April 1913, 2/5/3, B:30, F:C. S. Bacon; 2/5/7, Diary entries, 11 and 17 June 1913; James to A. J. Graham, 18 June 1913, 52/38/20, Archie J. Graham Papers, B:1; *27th Report* (1914), 263; "Medical School to Get Support," *Champaign Daily News,* 13 June 1913, p. 2.

29. James to F. T. Gates, 25 October 1913, 2/5/3, B:45, F:General Education Board.

30. Gates to James, 20 November 1913, Wallace Buttrick to James, 24 January 1914, 2/5/3, B:45, F:General Education Board.

31. [N. P. Colwell], "University of Illinois, College of Medicine. Inspected Friday, Nov. 21, 1913"; Colwell to James, 29 November 1913, 2/5/3, B:50, F:AMA.

32. Steele to James, 15 October 1913, 2/5/6, B:42, F:D. A. K. Steele; Frank B. Earle (secretary of the faculty) to James, 1 July 1913, 2/5/6, B:25. F:DE.

33. Steele to James, 15 October 1913, 2/5/6, B:42, F:D. A. K. Steele. H. B. McGuigan, a professor who joined the faculty of the College of Medicine in 1917, doubted that age was the main factor in Quine's retirement. "I understand he did not envisage the union with the University as favorably as some others." McGuigan to Carl Stephens, 2 March 1942, 26/1/20, Carl Stephens Papers, B:9, F:Medicine.

34. Steele to James, 16 April 1914, 2/5/6, B:42, F:D. A. K. Steele.

35. Adolph Gehrmann, "Presentation of the Bust of Dr. Steele," and Edmund Janes James, "Acceptance of the Bust of Dr. Steele," in "Exercises in Honor of Dr. Steele," *Alumni Quarterly* 8 (July 1914): 187–91.

36. Steele to James, 1 May 1915, 2/5/6, B:55, F:Steele, DAK June–August 1915.

37. Ibid.

38. James to Steele, 3 May 1915, 2/5/6, B:55, F:Steele, DAK June–August 1915.

39. Abbott to James, 26 July 1913, 2/5/3, B:30, F:W. L. Abbott.

40. Montgomery to James, 29 May 1914, 2/5/3, B:50, F:John T. Montgomery.

41. 2/5/7, Diary entries, 4 and 5 August 1913; *27th Report* (1914), 643, 644.

42. *28th Report* (1916), 133; Steele to James, 31 August 1914, James to Steele, 4 September 1914, 2/5/6, B:42, F:D. A. K. Steele.

43. Steele to James, 14 December 1915, 28 January 1916, 23 May 1916, 2/5/3, B:99, F: Steele, D. A. K. 2.

44. James to Steele, 21 October 1915, Steele to James, 25 October 1915, James to Steele, 24 November 1915 (the quotation), 2/5/3, B:99, F:D. A. K. Steele 1; Steele to James, 31 July 1916, 2/5/3, B:99, F:D. A. K. Steele 2.

45. Casey A. Wood to James, 28 August 1915, James to Wood, 31 August 1915, 2/5/3, B:93, F:Med. Coll. Clinic Bldg.

46. Pusey to James, 21 May 1914, 2/5/6, B:39, F:William A. Pusey; 2/5/7, Diary entry, 18 February 1914.

47. 2/5/7, Diary entry, 29 May 1914.

48. 2/5/7, Diary entries, 11 June 1914, 11 July 1914.

49. 2/5/7, Diary entry, 13 July 1914; *28th Report* (1916), 128.

50. Steele to James, 19 June 1915, James to Steele, 21 June 1915, 2/5/6, B:55, F:Steele, DAK, June–August 1915. See also James to Steele, 9 September 1915, 2/5/3, B:99, F:Steele, D. A. K. 1.

51. Steele to James, 23 June 1915, 2/5/6, B:55, F:Steele, DAK June–August 1915.

52. Steele to James, 30 August 1916, 2/5/3, B:99, F:Steele D. A. K. 2.

53. Mall to James, 25 June 1913, Welch to James, 29 June 1913, H. Gideon Wells to James, 30 June 1913, 2/5/3, B:35, F:Med School Reorganization.

54. Bardeen to James, 26 June 1913, 2/5/3, B:35, F:Med School Reorganization.

55. Wells to James, 30 June 1913, 2/5/3, B:35, F:Med School Reorganization.

56. 2/5/7, Diary entries, 28 May 1914, 8 July 1915, and 9 June 1917; James to Ellen M. Henrotin (a trustee), 20 August 1915, 2/5/3, B:64, F:Henrotin, Ellen.

57. James to Eycleshymer, 13 March 1916, Lyon to Eycleshymer, 24 March 1916, 2/5/3, B:83, F:Eycleshymer, A. C.

58. Steele to James, 14 March 1917, 2/5/3, B:135, F:Steele, D. A. K. January–July 1917.

59. 2/5/7, Diary entries, 5 and 30 March 1917; Eycleshymer to James, 27 March 1917, 2/5/3, B:117; F:Eycleshymer, A. C. September 1916–May 1917.

60. James to Eycleshymer, 7 July 1917, Eycleshymer to James, 10 July 1917, James to Members of the Committee, 11 July 1917, 2/5/3, B:117, F:Eycleshymer, A. C. June–August 1917; *29th Report* [1918], 398, 411.

61. Eycleshymer to James, 6 November 1917, James to Eycleshymer, 9 November 1917, 2/5/3, B:154, F:Eycleshymer, A. C. August 1917–November 1917.

62. James to William H. Welch, 24 June 1913, 2/5/3, B:35, F:Med School Reorganization.

63. Mall to James, 25 June 1913, Bardeen to James, 26 June 1913, 2/5/3, B:35, F:Med School Reorganization.

64. Evans to James, 27 July 1913, 2/5/3, B:35, F:Med School Reorganization; *27th Report* (1914), 647.

65. Wells to James, 30 June 1913, Bardeen to James, 26 June, 19 July 1913; Hektoen to James, 24 June 1913, 2/5/3, B:35: F:Med School Reorganization.

66. Opie to James, 31 July 1913; James to Opie, 6 August 1913; James to Opie, 6 August (telegram); Opie to James, 7 August (telegram), 2/5/3, B:35, F:Med School Reorganization.

67. 2/5/7, Diary entry, 9 August 1913.

68. 2/5/7, Diary entry, 18 August 1913.

69. 2/5/7, Diary entries, 25 August, 8 September 1913; James to Davis, 9 September 1913, 2/5/6, B:34, F:D. J. Davis; *27th Report* (1914), 659.

70. In 1922 Rose joined the University of Illinois faculty as professor of physiological chemistry. In 1936 his title was changed to professor of biochemistry. His important study of the role of amino acids in animal growth had practical application in clinical medicine.

71. Chittenden to James, 28 June 1913; Walter Jones to James, 27 June 1913; Mall to James, 25 June 1913; Bardeen to James, 3 July 1913, 2/5/3, B:35, F:Med School Reorganization.

72. *27th Report* (1914), 648. Dreyer's appointment as junior dean, effective on 1 September, became official on 4 October; *27th Report* (1914), 659.

73. *27th Report* (1914), 647, 659.

74. Williamson to James, 16 March 1914, 2/5/5, B:23, F:Medical Curriculum, 1914–15; *28th Report* (1916), 119–21.

75. Most of the letters were sent on 30 April 1914. Copies are in 2/5/5, B:23, F:Medical Curriculum 1914–15.

76. Blumer to James, 7 May 1914, 2/5/5, B:23, F:Medical Curriculum 1914–15. The other responses are in the same folder.

77. James's form letter of invitation and responses are in 2/5/3, B:50, F:Med School Form Letter.

78. "Standards of the Council on Medical Education of the American Medical Association," *JAMA* 63, pt. 1 (22 August 1914): 666–71.

79. James to Colwell, 3 August 1914, 2/5/3, B:50, F:AMA.

80. Colwell to James, 6 August 1914, 2/5/3, B:50, F:AMA.

81. James to Steele, 5 September, 16 October 1914, 2/5/6, B:55, F:Steele, DAK September 1914–January 1915.

82. Steele to James, 25 November 1914, 2/5/6, B:55, F:Steele, DAK September 1914–January 1915.

83. Steele to James, 12 January 1915, 2/5/6, B:55, F:Steele, DAK September 1914–January 1915.

84. Dock to James, 1 February 1915, enclosing "Report on the Examination of Medical School of the University of Illinois, by Dr. E. P. Lyon and Dr. George Dock," 2/5/6, B:52, F:Medical College 1914–15; James to Dock, 2 February 1915, 2/5/6, B:52, F:Medical College, 1914–15.

85. Lyon and Dock, "Report on the Examination of Medical School of the University of Illinois," 1 and 2.

86. Ibid.

87. Lyon to James, 28 January 1915 (quotations on 3 and 4), 2/5/6, B:52, F:Medical College 1914–15.

88. "State Board Statistics for 1913," *JAMA* 62, pt. 2 (23 May 1914): 1639–61.

89. Dreyer to James, 1 March 1915, 2/5/5, B:23, F:Medical Curriculum 1914–15.

90. Carl Beck, "Surgery of To-Day in Germany, Austria and France," *Surgery, Gynecology, and Obstetrics* 14 (March 1912): 294–303 (quotation on 299).

91. Ibid., 294.

92. Steele to James, 25 July 1913, Joseph Beck to Steele, 23 July 1913, 2/5/6, B:29, F:D. A. K. Steele.

93. Steele to James, 24 July 1914, 2/5/6, B:42, F:DAK Steele.

94. Williamson to James, 10 August 1914, 2/5/6, B:43, F:Charles S. Williamson.

95. Fournadjieff to James, 27 October 1913; James to Fournadjieff, 28 October 1913; Fournadjieff to James, 31 October 1913; James to Fournadjieff, 3 November 1913, 2/5/3, B:45, F:D. G. Fournadjieff.

96. Fournadjieff to James, 19 August 1914, 2/5/3, B:45, F:D. G. Fournadjieff.

97. Ibid.

98. James to Fournadjieff, 3 November 1914, 2/5/3, B:45, F:D. G. Fournadjieff.

99. In 1913 the Council of Administration in Urbana approved of a procedure in cases of discipline in the Chicago departments. A committee of five in the College of Medicine was to consider cases and report their recommendations to the council through the dean of men or of women in Urbana. 3/1/1, Council of Administration Minutes, 9 December 1913, Vol. 10, p. 184.

100. 3/1/1, Council of Administration Minutes, 10 March 1914, Vol. 11, p. 57. The men were Victor J. Anderson and Louis S. Fenchel, both of Chicago.

101. 3/1/1, Council of Administration Minutes, 9 June 1914, Vol. 11, p. 144. On Greis, see James to Dreyer, 28 September 1914; Dreyer to James, 29 September 1914, 2/5/6, B:46, F:Dreyer, Geo. P.

102. Dreyer to Clark, 12 June 1914; Clark to Kendrick C. Babcock (secretary of the Council of Administration), 13 June 1914, both in 3/1/1, Council of Administration Minutes, 19 June 1914, Vol. 11, pp. 150, 156.

103. James to Dreyer, 28 September 1914; Dreyer to James, 29 September 1914, 2/5/6, B:46, F:Dreyer, Geo. P. If they exist, Arthurton's letters to James and Dreyer cannot be located in the University of Illinois Archives, Urbana-Champaign.

104. Arthurton to Steele, 29 October 1914, 2/5/6, B:55, F:Steele, DAK September 1914–January 1915.

105. Steele to James, 9 November 1914, 2/5/6, B:55, F:Steele, DAK September 1914–January 1915.

106. James to Steele, 11 November 1914, 2/5/6, B:55, F:Steele, DAK September 1914–January 1915.

107. James to Steele, 18 November 1914; Steele to James, 20 November 1914, 2/5/6, B:55, F:Steele, DAK September 1914–January 1915.

108. "Gladys Owens, Rich California Girl, Says Dr. Arthurton Forced Her to Marry by Threats," *Chicago Defender,* 2 March 1918, p. 1.

Chapter 11. The Continued Quest for Excellence

1. *22nd Report* (1904), 57, 123, 311 (the quotation).

2. Andrew S. Draper to Samuel A. Bullard, 11 April 1904; Steele to Bullard, 28 April 1904, 2/5/5, B:16, F:Hahnemann Medical College.

3. Shears to Draper, 1 June 1904, 2/5/5, B:16, F:Hahnemann Medical College; Draper to Shears, 3 June 1904, 2/4/3, Andrew S. Draper Letterbooks, B:9 Ltrbks.; H. N. Higinbotham to Draper, 3 June 1904, 2/5/3, B:7, F:H. N. Higinbotham in re Hahnemann Medical College; Shears to Bullard, 23 August 1904, 2/5/5, B:16, F:Hahnemann Medical College. Howard R. Chislett [dean of Hahnemann Medical College] to Shears, n.d. [June 1904?]; 2/5/5, B:16, F:Hahnemann Medical College, sending figures on enrollments.

4. *22nd Report* (1904), 302, 310, 334; D. A. K. Steele, Wm. E. Quine, and Wm. Allen Pusey to Samuel A. Bullard, 5 July 1904, 2/5/5, B:16, F:Hahnemann Medical College.

5. George W. Gere to Samuel A. Bullard, 25 June 1904, 2/5/5, B:16, F:Hahnemann Medical College.

6. L. F. Swift to James, 15 November 1904, Edward F. Swift to James, 21 November 1904, 2/5/5, B:16, F:Hahnemann Medical College; H. N. Higinbotham to James, 5, 11 December 1904, 13 February 1905, 2/5/3, B:7, F:H. N. Higinbotham.

7. Bacon to James, 30 December 1904, 2/5/5, B:16, F:Hahnemann Medical College.

8. Higinbotham to James, 3 February 1913, 2/5/3, B:33, F:Harlow N. Higinbotham; Chislett to James, 25 April 1916, 2/5/3, B:78, F:Chislett, Howard R.

9. Chislett to James, 14, 25 April 1916, 2/5/3, B:78, F:Chislett, Howard R.

10. James to Chislett, 18 April, 1, 3 May 1916, 2/5/3, B:78, F:Chislett, Howard R.

11. James to Harris, 22 November 1913; Harris to James, 26 November 1913; James to Harris, 27 April 1914, 2/5/3, B:46, F:A. W. Harris.

12. Ingals to James, 18 April 1914, 2/5/3, B:47, F:I.

13. James to Ingals, 20 April 1914, 2/5/3, B:47, F:I.

14. *27th Report* (1914), 747.

15. Ingals to James, 24 April 1914; James to Ingals, 25 April 1914, 2/5/3, B:47, F:I.

16. Dean J. R. Angell to President Judson, 12 January 1912, and letters from Anton J. Carlson, H. G. Wells, C. Judson Herrick, and Preston Keyes to Dean Angell, 11–18 January 1912, either favoring or opposing union. Presidents' Papers, 1889–1925, B:58, F:5, Special Collections Research Center, University of Chicago Library.

17. Ingals to Harper, 21 October 1899, Presidents' Papers, 1889–1925, B:57, F:12, Special Collections Research Center, University of Chicago Library.

18. Ingals to Harper, 22 February 1901, Presidents' Papers, 1889–1925, B:57, F:14, Special Collections Research Center, University of Chicago Library.

19. Ingals to Harper, 29 September 1903, Ingals to Dear Doctor [Harper], 9 February 1907, Ingals to Harry Pratt Judson, 16 January 1908, Presidents' Papers, 1889–1925, B:57, F:14, Special Collections Research Center, University of Chicago Library; Ingals to Council of Administration of Rush Medical College, 13 December 1906, B:58, F:12, Special Collections Research Center, University of Chicago Library.

20. Ingals to Harper, 18 February 1898, Presidents' Papers, 1889–1925, B:57, F:11, Special Collections Research Center, University of Chicago Library.

21. Ingals to Harper, 3 October 1904, Presidents' Papers, 1889–1925, B:57, F:14, 11, Special Collections Research Center, University of Chicago Library.

22. [Billings] to Harry Pratt Judson, 25 June, 5 July 1907, Presidents' Papers, 1889–1925, B:57, F:14; B:58, F:3, Special Collections Research Center, University of Chicago Library.

23. Steele to James, 14 December 1915, 2/5/3, B:99, F:Steele, D.A.K. 2.

24. 2/5/7, Diary entries, 15 October, 1 November 1913.

25. James to Judson, 22 November 1913, 2/5/3, B:48, F:Harry P. Judson.

26. Judson to James, 28 November 1913, 2/5/3, B:48, F:Harry P. Judson.

27. James to Judson, 1 December 1913, 2/5/3, B:48, F:Harry P. Judson.

28. James to Billings, 1 December 1913 (the quotation), Billings to James, 12 December 1913, 2/5/3, B:93, F:Medical Coll.-Rush Merger.

29. Bevan to James, 16 January 1914; James to Bevan, 19 January 1914; James to Billings, 12 January 1914, 2/5/3, B:93, F:Medical Coll.-Rush Merger.

30. 2/5/7, Diary entries, 6, 7, 8 January, 18 February 1914.

31. Bevan to James, 20 January 1914, James to Judson, 3 February 1914, Judson to James, 5 February 1914, 2/5/3, B:93, F:Medical Coll.-Rush Merger.

32. Bevan to James, 27 January 1914, 7 February 1914, 2/5/3, B:93, F:Medical Coll.-Rush Merger.

33. Bevan to James, 13 January 1914, James to Bevan, 12 February 1914, 14 February 1914, 2/5/3, B:93, F:Medical Coll.-Rush Merger.

34. "Union between Rush Medical College and the University of Illinois," 2 pp., undated, 2/5/3, B:93, F:Medical Coll.-Rush Merger.

35. Bevan to James, 13 February 1914, 2/5/3, B:93, F:Medical Coll.-Rush Merger.

36. 2/5/7, Diary entries, 2 and 8 March 1914; Bevan to James, 26 and 27 February, 2/5/3, B:93, F:Medical Coll.-Rush Merger.

37. Ingals to J. Spencer Dickerson, 2 March 1914, with similar letters to each of the other trustees, Presidents' Papers, 1889–1925, B:58, F:13, Special Collections Research Center, University of Chicago Library.

38. 2/5/7, Diary entry, 17 March 1914.

39. Bevan to James, 7 April 1914, 2/5/3, B:93, F:Medical Coll.-Rush Merger.

40. 2/5/7, Diary entries, 17 and 21 April 1914.

41. *27th Report* (1914), 747.

42. James to Bevan, 23 April 1914; James to Billings, 23 April 1914, 2/5/3, B:93, F:Medical Coll.-Rush Merger.

43. David Kinley et al. to James, 27 April 1914, 2/5/3, B:93, F:Medical Coll.-Rush Merger; 2/5/7, Diary entry, 27 April 1917.

44. Ingals to James, 27 April 1914, 2/5/3, B:93, F:Medical Coll.-Rush Merger.

45. Ingals to James, 29 April 1914, 2/5/3, B:93, F:Medical Coll.-Rush Merger.

46. Bevan to James, 30 April 1914, 2/5/3, B:93, F:Medical Coll.-Rush Merger.

47. Ibid.

48. "Memorandum, in re Rush Medical College," 1 p., undated, 2/5/3, B:93, F:Medical Coll.-Rush Merger.

49. Bevan to James, 30 April 1914, 2/5/3, B:93, F:Medical Coll.–Rush Merger.

50. Bevan to James, 15 May 1914, 2/5/3, B:93, F:Medical Coll.-Rush Merger; James to John T. Montgomery, 15 May 1914, 2/5/3, B:50, F:John T. Montgomery.

51. James to Montgomery, 15 May 1914, 2/5/3, B:50, F:John T. Montgomery.

52. 2/5/7, Diary entry, 29 May 1914; Hektoen to James, 14 July 1914; James to Hektoen, 16 July 1914, 2/5/3, B:46, F:Ludvig Hektoen.

53. James is either wrong, as the vote in the official record of the previous board meeting shows, or he refers to a previous vote.

54. James to Trevett, 23 April 1914, 2/5/3, B:55, F:John R. Trevett.

55. James to Montgomery, 27 April 1914; Montgomery to Trevett, 28 April 1914, 2/5/3, B:50, F:John T. Montgomery.

56. Trevett to James, 28 April 1914, 2/5/3, B:55, F:John R. Trevett; Montgomery to James, 30 April 1914; James to Montgomery, 1 May 1914, 2/5/3, B:50, F:John T. Montgomery.

57. James to Montgomery, 27 April 1914, 2/5/3, B:50, F:John T. Montgomery.

58. Montgomery to James, 28 April 1914, 2/5/3, B:50, F:John T. Montgomery.

59. James to Montgomery, 29 April 1914, 2/5/3, B:50, F:John T. Montgomery.

60. Montgomery to James, 29 May 1914, 2/5/3, B:50, F:John T. Montgomery.

61. 2/5/7, Diary entry, 13 October 1914.

62. Sperry, *A Group of Distinguished Physicians and Surgeons of Chicago,* 189–94; Loyal Davis, *Fellowship of Surgeons: A History of the American College of Surgeons* ([Chicago]: Charles C. Thomas, 1960; American College of Surgeons, 1973, 1981), passim. Franklin H. Martin, *The Joy of Living: An Autobiography,* 2 vols. (Garden City, N.Y.: Doubleday, Doran, 1933). The first, highly readable volume deals with the years covered in the present book.

63. Ochsner to James, 9 February 1915; Martin to James, 9 February, 2 March (list of the original committee members), 3 April 1915, 2/5/6, B:52, F:Medical Cooperation.

64. James to Judson, 5 March 1915; Judson to James, 6 March 1915, 2/5/3, B:65, F:Judson, Harry Pratt.

65. Billings to David A. Robertson (Judson's secretary), 24 March 1915, informing him of his letter to Martin, Presidents' Papers, 1889–1925, B:58, F:3, Special Collections Research Center, University of Chicago Library.

66. Martin to James, 28 May 1915, 2/5/6, B:52, F:Medical Cooperation.

67. *28th Report* (1916), 236–38 (includes the text of the resolutions).

68. *Ibid.,* 237–40; James to Steele, 5 May 1915, 2/5/6, B:55, F:Steele, DAK. February–May 1915.

69. 2/5/7, Diary entry, 23 May 1915.

70. Judson to James, 11 August 1915, 2/5/3, B:65, F:Judson, Harry Pratt.

71. Ochsner to James, 20 September 1915, along with "A Form of Agreement" and "Suggested By-Laws for the Universities Graduate School of Medicine of Chicago," 2/5/6, B:93, F:Medical Cooperation.

72. James to Ochsner, 21 September 1915; James to Martin, 16 December 1915, 2/5/6, B:93, F:Medical Cooperation.

73. "Plan of Agreement for Reorganization of the Medical Colleges of Chicago under Consideration by the Chicago University, the Loyola University, the Northwestern University, the University of Illinois and the Graduate School of Medicine of Chicago: Pre-

sented to Mr. Henry S. Pritchett of the Carnegie Foundation," n.d., 14 pp., 2/5/3, B:93, F: Medical Cooperation. The document bears no author's name and no date, and there is no evidence that it was presented to Pritchett. On 17 February 1915 Pritchett had met with the Universities Committee on Medical Education in Chicago. The document may have been prepared to give to Pritchett at that time.

74. "Plan of Agreement for Reorganization of the Medical Colleges of Chicago under Consideration by the Chicago University, the Loyola University, the Northwestern University, the University of Illinois and the Graduate School of Medicine of Chicago," 2/5/3, B:93, F:Medical Cooperation.

75. James to Martin, 20 December 1915, 2/5/3, B:93, F:Medical Cooperation.

76. 2/5/7, Diary entry, 27 November 1915.

77. Billings to James, 4 December 1915, 2/5/3, B:93, F:Medical Coll.-Rush Merger.

78. 2/5/7, Diary entry, 4 December 1915.

79. James to Glessner, 7 December 1915, Glessner to James, 9 December 1915, 2/5/3, B:93, F:Medical Coll.-Rush Merger; 2/5/7, Diary entry, 17 December 1915.

80. James to Billings, 22 December 1915, 2/5/3, B:93, F:Medical Coll.-Rush Merger.

81. Billings to James, 22 December 1915, 2/5/3, B:93, F:Medical Coll.-Rush Merger.

82. James to Billings, 6 January 1916 (cover letter); James to Billings, 5 January 1916 (initial draft of his response to Billings's questions); James to Billings, 6 January 1916 (response to the questions Billings raised); Billings to James, 7 January 1916, 2/5/3, B:93, F:Medical Coll.-Rush Merger; 2/5/7, Diary entry, 6 January 1916.

83. 2/5/7, Diary entry, 17 January 1916. There is no record of his talk with Pritchett in *The Papers of Henry Smith Pritchett* in the Manuscripts Division of the Library of Congress, Washington, D.C.

84. 2/5/7, Diary entries, 6 and 7 February, 4 March, 24 April 1916.

85. Cornelius W. Vermeulen, *For the Greatest Good to the Largest Number: A History of the Medical Center, the University of Chicago, 1927–1977* (Chicago: Vice President for Public Affairs, University of Chicago, 1977), 5–8.

86. James to Hon. William B. McKinley, 5 September 1916, 2/5/3, B:126, F:McKinley.

87. 2/5/7, Diary entry, 21 February 1917.

88. 2/5/7, Diary entries, 8 and 9 March 1917.

89. *University of Illinois Circular* 1 (March 1915): 5, copy in 2/5/6, B:52, F:Medical College.

90. For the source of enrollment data for the years 1912–13 to 1915–16, see chapter 6, note 15 above. For the data for 1916–17 and 1917–18 see Edmund J. James, "Biennial Report of the University of Illinois," in *Thirty-second Biennial Report of the Superintendent of Public Instruction of the State of Illinois, 1916–1918* (Springfield, 1919), 309. For the data for 1918–20 see David Kinley, "Biennial Report of the University of Illinois," in *Thirty-third Biennial Report of the Superintendent of Public Instruction of the State of Illinois, 1918–1920* (Springfield, 1920), 469, 473. For the number of graduates see the *27th Report* (1914), 239–40; *28th Report* (1916), 74, 82, 303, 308; *29th Report* ([1918]), 362, 815, 824; *30th Report* ([1920]), 425, 431; *Alumni Record,* 192, 200, 207, 213, 221, 224, 226, 229.

91. See the note, "Medical Research Club," part of a report on the Library, attached to George P. Dreyer to E. J. James, 31 July 1916, 2/5/3, B:81, F:Dreyer, Geo. P.

92. Eycleshymer to James, 23 December 1915, 2/5/3, F:83, F:Eycleshymer, A. C.

93. See "Graduate Work in Medicine: The Graduate Summer Quarter," and "Report on Graduate Work in Medical Sciences," undated documents, perhaps written by Dean A. C. Eycleshymer, in 2/5/3, B:117, F:Ecycleshymer, A. C. September 16–May 17.

94. [Council on Medical Education], "State Board Statistics for 1913," *JAMA* 62, pt. 2 (23 May 1914): 1648–49.

95. [Council on Medical Education], "State Board Statistics for 1914," *JAMA* 64, pt. 2 (24 April 1915): 1410.

96. [Council on Medical Education], "State Board Statistics for 1915," *JAMA* 66 (8 April 1916): 1104.

97. [Council on Medical Education], "State Board Statistics for 1916," *JAMA* 68, pt. 2 (14 April 1917): 1110–11; *29th Report* ([1918]), 299.

98. "College of Medicine," *Alumni Quarterly and Fortnightly Notes* 1 (15 July 1916): 446.

99. [Council on Medical Education], "State Board Statistics for 1917," *JAMA* 70, pt. 2 (13 April 1918): 1078–79.

100. Ibid., 1082.

101. *Alumni Record,* 168–76.

Chapter 12. A Clinical Building and a Hospital

1. 2/5/7, Diary entries, 21 June, 10 July 1913; 22 January, 18 and 21 April 1914; 3 July 1915; 12 and 20 January 1916; 6 November 1917.

2. Steele to James, 6 October 1913, 2/5/6, B:42, F:D. A. K. Steele; James to Steele, 7 May 1915, 2/5/6, B:55, F:Steele, DAK February–May 1915.

3. Several folders related to the legislative campaign in 2/5/3, B:66, provide ample evidence on this point.

4. James, To the Members of the General Assembly, 29 May 1915 (a printed letter), 2/5/5, B:21, F:Legislature 1915; James to Arthur Roe (a legislator), 29 May 1915, 2/5/3, B:69, F:Ri–Ro; Steele to James, 3 June 1915, 2/5/6, B:55, F:Steele, DAK June–August 1915.

5. *28th Report* (1916), 225, 233–35, 773–74; *29th Report* ([1918]), 262.

6. *28th Report* (1916), 778; Steele to James, 23 August 1915, 2/5/6, B:55, F:Steele, DAK June–August 1915.

7. *29th Report* ([1918]), 100, 176.

8. Ibid., 232, 409–11.

9. Steele to James, 26 July 1915; James to Steele, 27 July 1915, 2/5/6, B:55, F:Steele, DAK June–August 1915.

10. Special committee telegram to James, 18 September 1915, 2/5/3, B:93, F:Med Coll Clinic Bldg; 2/5/7, Diary entry, 7 September 1915.

11. Steele to James, 4, 15, and 24 May 1915, James to Steele, 18 May 1915, 2/5/6, B:55, F: Steele, DAK February–May 1915; 2/5/7, Diary entries, 26 March and 14 May 1916.

12. Spalding, "The Beginning of the Loyola University Medical School and an Account of the School during the First Ten Years," 18–21; Council, 231–32.

13. W. L. Abbott, "How the University of Illinois Acquired Its College of Medicine," 8 June 1939, p. 11, 2/9/1, Arthur C. Willard General Correspondence, B:37, F:Medicine, College of March-August.

14. "Palatial Park for Champions," *Chicago Daily Tribune,* 24 December 1908, p. 6; "League's Action Checks Murphy," *Chicago Daily Tribune,* 15 February 1912, p. 6; "Baseball Owners Plan Two Moves to Oust Murphy," *Chicago Daily Tribune,* 13 February 1914, p. 15; "Murphy Meets C. P. Taft Today," *Chicago Daily Tribune,* 16 November 1914, p. 16; "Murphy and Taft in Conference," *Chicago Daily Tribune,* 17 November 1914, p. 11; "Even

Million Now Value of Chicago Cubs," *Chicago Daily Tribune,* 7 January 1916, p. 13; Art Ahrens, "Chicago Cubs: Sic Transit Gloria Mundi," in *Encyclopedia of Major League Baseball Team Histories,* ed. Peter C. Bjarkman, 143–47 (Westport, CT: Meckler, 1991); Donald Dewey and Nicholas Acocella, *The Biographical History of Baseball* (Chicago: Triumph Books, 2002), 297–98, 449.

15. "Palatial Park for Champions," *Chicago Daily Tribune,* 24 December 1908; "Comiskey Buys New Grounds for White Sox," *Chicago Daily Tribune,* 29 December 1908; "But It's a False Joy That Is Garnered from That Sort of Victory: Baseball Owners Plan Two Moves to Oust Murphy," *Chicago Daily Tribune,* 13 February 1914; "Ogden Armour Et Al. Cited by Murphy in Suit against Cubs," *Chicago Daily Tribune,* 19 January 1918; "Former Owner Cubs Seeks to Prevent North Side Games," *Chicago Daily Tribune,* 10 February 1920; "Taft's Share of Old 'Cubs' Park Sold to Murphy," *Chicago Daily Tribune,* 16 July 1920; "C. W. Murphy, Cubs' Owner in 1906–1914, Dies," *Chicago Daily Tribune,* 17 October 1931; Jerome Holtzman and George Vass, *The Chicago Cubs Encyclopedia* (Philadelphia: Temple University Press, 1997), 322–23, 324–25. According to the *Chicago Daily Tribune,* 20 July 1916, p. 16, Taft and Murphy purchased the property from the Equitable Trust Company; each acquired an undivided half interest. The site, 550 by 620 feet, was under lease to the Chicago National League baseball club. The lease had eighty more years to run, and the rental was $12,000 a year. Another account says that the Equitable Trust Company leased the property to the Chicago League Ball Club for seventeen years, from 1 February 1905. By a special warranty deed dated 15 December 1908 for a consideration of $150,000 the property was conveyed to Anna Sinton Taft (wife of Charles P. Taft of Cincinnati) and Charles W. Murphy, share and share alike, subject to lease dated 1 February 1905 for a total rental of $155,050 in four payments of $1,966.10 or $7,864.40 annually up to 31 January 1912 and four payments of $2,500 each the first of February, May, August, and November, or $10,000 a year, until 31 January 1922, together with all taxes and assessments and water tax. Edmund J. James to Odgen Armour, 31 March 1916, 2/5/3, B:74, F:Armour, J. Ogden.

16. "Gives $200,000 to Disease War; James A. Patten Founds Chair of Experimental Pathology at Northwestern," *Chicago Daily Tribune,* 8 November 1910; "Patten's Northwestern Gift Told in Formal Statement; University Trustees Hear of $200,000 Fund Which Will Be Utilized for Advancement of Medical Research," *Chicago Daily Tribune,* 23 November 1910; "Noted Surgeons Meet; Well-Known Society in Session at Medical School," *Daily Northwestern,* 11 November 1910; "Big Gift by Mr. Patten; Evanstonian Adds $50,000 to Donation to Medical School," *Daily Northwestern,* 23 March 1911; Northwestern University Board of Trustees, Minutes, 22 November 1910, p. 92, and 23 March 1911, p. 157; James to Patten, 9 November 1910, 31 March 1911, 2/5/3, B:23, F:James A. Patten. I am indebted to Mr. Kevin B. Leonard, associate archivist, Northwestern University, for all of the references in this note except for the two James letters.

17. James to Patten, 27 April 1914, 2/5/3, B:52, F:Pa–Pe.

18. 2/5/7, Diary entries, 11, 12, and 13 January 1916.

19. James to Armour, 24 January 1916, Armour to James, 10 February 1916, James to Armour, 31 March, 1 April, 17 April 1916, 2/5/3, B:74, F:Armour, J. Ogden.

20. Armour to James, 27 April 1916, 2/5/3, B:74, F:Armour, J. Ogden.

21. 2/5/7, Diary entry, 13 May 1916.

22. James to Patten, 19 and 23 May 1916, 2/5/3, B:96, F:James A. Patten.

23. Patten to James, 25 May 1916, 2/5/3, B:96, F:James A. Patten.

24. *29th Report* ([1918]), 6, 69–70.

25. James to Armour, 26 July 1916; Armour to James, 8 August 1916, 2/5/3, B:74, F: Armour, J. Ogden.

26. 2/5/7, Diary entry, 20 November 1916; University of Illinois, *Transactions of the Board of Trustees, 1916–1918,* 104; "Taft's Share of Old 'Cubs' Park Sold to Murphy," *Chicago Daily Tribune,* 20 July 1916, p. 16.

27. "State Medical School Plans New Buildings," *Chicago Daily Tribune,* 14 June 1916.

28. *29th Report* ([1918]), 199, 232, 240–41; James to Henrotin, 10 March 1917, Henrotin to James, Sunday [n.d., before 19 March 1917], 2/5/3, B:121, F:Henrotin, Ellen M.

29. William T. Hutchinson, *Lowden of Illinois: The Life of Frank O. Lowden,* 2 vols. (Chicago: University of Chicago Press, 1957), 1:307.

30. State of Illinois, *Report of the Department of Public Welfare, 1919–1920* (Springfield, 1921), 7, 15–16 (also in State of Illinois, *Third Administrative Report of the Directors of Departments under the Civil Administration Code, July 1, 1919 to June 30, 1920* [Springfield, 1921], 283, 291–92); Charles H. Thorne, "The Research and Educational Hospitals of the State of Illinois: Part Two, From the Standpoint of the Department of Public Welfare," *Modern Hospital* 15 (December, 1920): 450–52.

31. State of Illinois, *Report of the Department of Public Welfare, 1917–1918* (Springfield, 1918), 226–27 (also in State of Illinois, *First Administrative Report of the Directors of Departments under the Civil Administration Code, July 1, 1917 to June 30, 1918* [Springfield, 1918], 226–27).

32. 2/5/7, Diary entry, 1 August 1917; *29th Report* ([1918]), 511–12.

33. *Chicago Herald,* 11 August 1917; unidentified newspaper clipping, 16 September [1917], in 2/5/5, B:17, F:Hospitals Chicago 1917–19.

34. Magnuson to James, 11 August 1917, 2/5/5, B:17, F:Hospitals Chicago 1917–19.

35. *Chicago Herald,* 11 August 1917, clipping in 2/5/5, B:17, F:Hospitals Chicago 1917–19.

36. Abbott to James, 4 September 1917, 2/5/5, B:17, F:Hospitals Chicago 1917–19.

37. Abbott to James, 17 September 1917, Eycleshymer to James, 14 September 1917, 2/5/5, B:17, F:Hospitals Chicago 1917–19.

38. James to Brackett, 19 September 1917; Eycleshymer to James, 14 September 1917, 2/5/5, B:17, F:Hospitals Chicago 1917–19.

39. James to Shanahan, 27 September 1917; James to Oglesby, 27 September 1917, 2/5/5, B:17, F:Hospitals Chicago 1917–19.

40. King to James, 15 November 1917; James to King, 11 December 1917; King to James, 15 December 1917, 2/5/5, B:17, F:Hospitals Chicago 1917–19.

41. 2/5/7, Diary entry, 4 October 1917. James was probably inaccurate. The block in question was bounded by Polk, Wolcott (later Lincoln), Taylor, and Wood streets.

42. *29th Report* ([1918]), 544–45, 617–18.

43. 2/5/7, Diary entries, 14 and 23 December 1917.

44. Abbott, "How the University Acquired Its College of Medicine," 11; James to Abbott, 8 October 1917, 2/5/3, B:142, F:Abbott, W. L.; Holtzman and Vass, *The Chicago Cubs Encyclopedia,* 327.

45. Abbott to James, 12 December 1917, 2/5/3, B:142, F:Abbott, W. L; Holtzman and Vass, *The Chicago Cubs Encyclopedia,* 327. See also *Chicago Daily News,* 28 December 1916, clipping in 2/5/3, B:109, F:Browne, Wm. H. January–April 1917.

46. James to Abbott, 17 December 1917, 2/5/3, B:142, F:Abbott, W. L.

47. James to Abbott, 14 December 1917, 2/5/3, B:142, F:Abbott, W. L.

48. Abbott to James, 4 January 1918, 2/5/3, B:142, F:Abbott, W. L.

49. 2/5/7, Diary entry, 8 January 1918.

50. Abbott to James, 2 March 1918, James to Abbott, 4 March 1918, 2/5/3, B:142, F:Abbott, W. L.

51. 2/5/7, Diary entry, 7 February 1918.

52. *29th Report* ([1918]), 667. The blueprints of White's plan are in 2/5/5, B:17, F:Hospitals Chicago 1917–19. White envisioned a facility that would provide 250 beds at a cost of $1,107 per bed, for a total cost of $276,750 or $276,800.

53. 2/5/7, Diary entries, 21, 22, and 28 April 1918; James to Dunham, 27 April 1918, 2/5/5, B:17, F:Hospitals Chicago 1917–19.

54. *28th Report* (1916), 126–27. See also Bonner, *Medicine in Chicago*, 147–74.

55. C. G. Graves to D. A. K. Steele, 24 June 1913, 2/5/6, B:29, F:D. A. K. Steele.

56. Council, 300.

57. Ibid., 316–17.

58. "Medical Schools of the United States," *JAMA* 47, pt. 1 (25 August 1906): 615. For a list of hospitals and infirmaries in Chicago, see Illinois State Board of Health, *Bulletin* 8 (August 1912): 662–63.

59. *29th Report* ([1918]), 729.

60. 2/5/7, Diary entries, 20 March, 4, 20, 22, and 30 April, 4 May 1918; Davison to James, 27 April 1918, 2/5/5, B:17, F:Hospitals Chicago 1917; Hyman L. Meites, ed., *History of the Jews of Chicago* (Chicago: Chicago Jewish Historical Society and Wellington Publishing, 1990 [originally published 1924]), 630–33; Ruth M. Rothstein, "Hospitals," in *The Sentinel's History of Chicago Jewry, 1911–1986* (Chicago: Sentinel Publishing, [1986]), 244–46.

61. 2/5/7, Diary entries, 4 and 20 April 1918.

62. James to Abbott, 25 April 1918, 2/5/3, B:142, F:Abbottt, W. L. The letter is marked, "Not sent."

63. 2/5/7, Diary entry, 4 May 1918.

64. Arthur Meeker, *Chicago, with Love: A Polite and Personal History* (New York: Knopf, 1955), 94–98 (quotations on 97–98).

65. 2/5/7, Diary entry, 14 May 1918.

66. James to Dunham, 28 June 1918, Dunham to James, 5 July 1918, 2/5/5, B:17, F:Hospitals Chicago 1917–19.

67. 2/5/7, Diary entry, 5 August 1918.

68. *Journal of the House of Representatives of the Fifty-first General Assembly of the State of Illinois* (Springfield, 1919), 189, 657, 689, 704, 729, 1103; *29th Report* ([1918]), 395–96, 440–41; Albert C. Eycleshymer, "The Research and Educational Hospitals of the State of Illinois: Part One, From the Standpoint of the University," *Modern Hospital* 15 (December 1920): 447–49.

69. *30th Report* ([1920]), 318–19.

70. Ibid., 487–90.

71. The new buildings, which became the home of the University of Illinois College of Medicine, were erected on the site of the former West Side Grounds. In an effort to ascertain who bought the property from Charles W. Murphy, I pursued the matter in the office of the Cook County Recorder of Deeds. After obtaining the property index number of the West Side Grounds, I searched the records of the deeds for the site from the 1850s to the 1950s. I found nothing that indicated the sale of the entire site and did

not find the name of either Charles W. Murphy or Anna Siton Taft. I did find evidence of the sale of many small plots over the years (there were small plots in an area south of the ballpark and north of Taylor Street). In the 1940s and 1950s Newton C. Farr, a Chicago realtor acting as agent for the board of trustees, purchased parcels of property in the area of the former West Side Grounds for the Medical Center District. These parcels may have been in the area south of the ballpark and north of Taylor Street. Property Insight, a Chicago firm that searches title records for a fee, offered to see if they could solve the matter, but they could not promise a successful outcome. I pursued the matter no further.

72. State of Illinois, *Fourth Annual Report of the Department of Public Welfare, 1920–1921* (Springfield, 1922), 23–29; Edgar Martin, "The Research and Educational Hospitals of the State of Illinois: Part Three, From the Standpoint of the Architects," *Modern Hospital* 15 (December 1920): 452–58; "New Research and Educational Hospitals—State Institution Statistics," *Blue Book of the State of Illinois, 1925–1926,* 448–51; David J. Davis and William F. Peterson, "The Research and Educational Hospital and the Research Laboratory and Library of the University of Illinois and the State Department of Public Welfare," in *Methods and Problems of Medical Education,* Tenth Series (Division of Medical Education: Rockefeller Foundation, 1928), 253–307.

73. *30th Report* ([1920]), 416, 709–10, 715.

74. "Health's Temple," *Chicago Daily Tribune,* 7 December 1920, p. 7; "New Research and Educational Hospitals," *Blue Book of the State of Illinois, 1925–1926,* 448, 451.

INDEX

Abbott, William L., 123, 134, 157, 171, 174, 179, 187–88, 189, 235, 236, 237, 238, 240, 241
Abel, John J., 162
Adkins, Charles, 129
Adler, Abraham K., 240
affiliation of P&S and the University. *See* College of Physicians and Surgeons of Chicago (P&S)
African-Americans at P&S, 94
Agnew, William H., 245
Alexander III, Czar, 42
Allen, Frances M., 90, 91
allopathy. *See* medicine, regular
Alpha Omega Alpha, 112–13
alternative medicine, 10–16
Altgeld, John P., 77, 246
Alumni Association of the College of Medicine, 34, 168, 171, 172
Alumni Record, 34
American Baptist Education Society, 26
American College of Medicine and Surgery. *See* Chicago College of Medicine and Surgery(Valparaiso)
American College of Surgeons, 68, 73, 215
American Dermatological Association, 70
American Gynecological Association, 84
American Institute of Homeopathy, 14
American Medical Association (AMA), 14, 68, 70, 85, 119, 134, 140, 157, 179, 181, 182–83
American Medical Institute, 11
American Medical Missionary College, 20
American Medical Women's National Association, 93
American Practice of Medicine, 11
American School of Osteopathy, 15
American Surgical Association, 68, 85
American Text-Book of Gynecology, Medical and Surgical, for Practitioners and Students, 66
Andrews, Edmund, 65
Angear, John James M., 45

Angell, James, 3
Anthony, George A., 172
apprentice system, 7–8
Archives of Dermatology and Syphilology, 70
Arey, Leslie B., 63
Armour, J. Ogden, 231, 232–33, 238, 240, 241
Armstrong, James E., 78
Arthur, Chester A., 42
Art Institute of Chicago, 42
Arthurton, Robert N., 94, 201–02
Ashcraft, Edwin M., 159–60, 168
Association of American Medical Colleges, 135, 141
Association of American Universities, 4

Babcock, Elmer E., 59
Babcock, K. C., 212
Babcock, Robert H., 59
Bacon, Charles S., 60, 86, 127, 128, 134, 168, 169, 170–71, 180, 181, 182, 183, 189, 192, 193, 204, 239
bacteriology, 2, 17, 31, 59, 60, 62, 64, 66, 162, 247
ballpark. *See* West Side Grounds
Banting, Frederick G., 245
Bardeen, Charles, R., 162, 166, 190
Barrett, Channing W., 199
basic medical sciences, 8
Bass, Charles C., 191
Battle Creek Sanitarium, 20
Beall, Edmond, 184
Beck, Carl, 72–75, 102, 198–99
Beck, Emil G., 73, 74
Beck-Jianu operation, 74
Beck, Joseph C., 73, 74, 199
Beech, Wooster, 11
Beedy, Lora L., 88, 89, 90, 91
Belfield, William T., 25.
Benedict, A. L., 104
Bennett College of Eclectic Medicine and Surgery, 20–21
Bennett, Edward H., 236

WINTON U. SOLBERG is Distinguished Historian and Professor
Emeritus, University of Illinois, Urbana-Champaign. His many
publications include *The Federal Convention and the Formation
of the Union of the American States; Redeem the Time: The
Puritan Sabbath in Early America; Cotton Mather: The Christian
Philosopher;* and two volumes of the early history of the University
of Illinois. He has taught at Harvard, Yale, and West Point and
at the Johns Hopkins Center in Bologna, Italy. He has been a
Fulbright Professor at Moscow State University (U.S.S.R.) and at
Calcutta University in India.

The University of Illinois Press
is a founding member of the
Association of American University Presses.

Composed in 10.5/13 Adobe Minion Pro
by BookComp, Inc.
Manufactured by Thomson-Shore, Inc.

University of Illinois Press
1325 South Oak Street
Champaign, IL 61820-6903
www.press.uillinois.edu